THE NEUROBIOLOGY OF COGNITION AND BEHAVIOR

THE NEUROBIOLOGY OF COGNITION AND BEHAVIOR

JOHN HART, JR., MD
Jane and Bud Smith Distinguished Chair
Center for BrainHealth
Professor of Behavioral and Brain Sciences
University of Texas at Dallas
Professor of Neurology and Neurotherapeutics
University of Texas Southwestern Medical Center

OXFORD
UNIVERSITY PRESS

OXFORD
UNIVERSITY PRESS

Oxford University Press is a department of the University of Oxford. It furthers the University's objective of excellence in research, scholarship, and education by publishing worldwide.

Oxford New York
Auckland Cape Town Dar es Salaam Hong Kong Karachi
Kuala Lumpur Madrid Melbourne Mexico City Nairobi
New Delhi Shanghai Taipei Toronto

With offices in
Argentina Austria Brazil Chile Czech Republic France Greece
Guatemala Hungary Italy Japan Poland Portugal Singapore
South Korea Switzerland Thailand Turkey Ukraine Vietnam

Oxford is a registered trademark of Oxford University Press in the UK and certain other countries.

Published in the United States of America by
Oxford University Press
198 Madison Avenue, New York, NY 10016

Library of Congress Cataloging-in-Publication Data
Hart, John, Jr., 1957– , author.
The Neurobiology of cognition and behavior / John Hart, Jr.
p. ; cm.
ISBN 978-0-19-021903-1 (alk. paper)
I. Title.
[DNLM: 1. Cognition—physiology. 2. Behavior—physiology. 3. Brain—physiopathology.
4. Brain Mapping. 5. Mental Processes—physiology. WL 337]
QP360.5
612.8′233—dc23
2014043541

1 3 5 7 9 8 6 4 2
Printed in the United States of America
on acid-free paper

This book is dedicated to Laura, Jack, and Charlie,
Jack and Julie,
David, and
All the Mikes

DIGITAL MEDIA ACCOMPANYING THE BOOK

Individual purchasers of this book are entitled to free personal access to accompanying digital media in the online edition. Please refer to the access token card for instructions on token redemption and access.

These online ancillary materials, where available, are noted with iconography throughout the book.

Video

The corresponding media can be found on Oxford Medicine Online at: www.oxfordmedicine.com/neurobiologyofcognitionandbehavior

If you are interested in access to the complete online edition, please consult with your librarian.

CONTENTS

PREFACE

This book could not have been completed without the continued discussions with colleagues in the fields of cognitive/behavioral neurology and cognitive neuroscience and the need to produce an integration of the findings of the multiple investigations into cognition. A consensus emerged that the basic framework of cognition and behavior is taking the numerous findings from functional imaging localizations of cognition and combining them with confirmatory lesion studies to form a basic architecture of cognition. This framework provided a basis to build further upon for activated regions associated with a cognitive operation but did not result in a decrement of performance when lesioned and more complex network models associated with a cognitive operation.

This desire for confirming the localizations identified with functional activation studies for cognition and behavior by assessing whether a lesion in that region would reliably disrupt those cognitive operations. This would provide a basic framework on which to build other aspects of cognition, such as brain regions not associated with a loss of function when being lesioned or more complex network models. These ideas extended from numerous discussions with leading colleagues in the field for whom I and others have the utmost respect, including but not limited to Mark D'Esposito, Branch Coslett, Anjan Chatterjee, Vic Henderson, Elliot Ross, Dan Kaufer, Kirk Daffner, Dave Arciniegas, Bruce Crosson, Munro Cullum, and Ken Heilman.

As the field of exploring brain–behavior relationships has exploded with a wealth of information, the need for a basic volume to organize this information was evident. In addition, the proliferation of neuroscience programs, cognitive neuroscience courses and programs, and individuals training in cognitive neurology and neuropsychiatry has led to a large and growing audience for this material. This book adopts the approach of using cognitive neuroscience principles to define dissociable, fine-grained cognitive units and associating these units with brain regions encoding for these units or aspects of the units from both functional imaging and lesion studies.

These cognitive–brain relationships are integrated into accounting for the symptoms in clinical neuropsychiatric syndromes, with the added feature of presenting patient videos, when relevant and available, demonstrating the clinical findings.

This textbook is intended to provide a framework of the basic architecture of cognition in the brain upon which network and other models can be incorporated. This basic set of principles is useful for students studying the interaction of cognitive science and neuroanatomy as well as relevant to the experienced neuroscientist researcher or clinician.

ACKNOWLEDGMENTS

This book could not have been completed without the help of several individuals. I thank Sharon O'Meara for her invaluable assistance on book preparation and keeping everyone on schedule. I am truly grateful to the students in my lab who inspired and edited for clarity each chapter in the book—Sheng Chiang, Jeremy Strain, Neena Rao, Bambi DeLaRosa, and Justin Eroh. I thank Dr. Gail Tillman for proofing the first and last chapters and Athula Pudhiyidath for her help in preparing the manuscript.

Throughout the years, there have been invaluable influences on me that have led to this book: Guy McKhann, who took a chance on me, supported and guided me, has been an incredible role model and academic godfather; Alfonso Caramazza, who took in an 18-year-old South Baltimore kid and taught him how to think; Rita Berndt, who taught me the most invaluable lessons that I use every day—how to design experiments, perform studies, and do them right; Dick Johnson and Jack Griffin for their continued support and confidence; Justin McArthur for his invaluable advice and guidance, care, and compassion; and Dave Zee and Bob Fisher—I could not have asked for a greater set of teachers. I thank Lauren Moo for having faith in me by choosing me to teach her, my first real teaching assignment; Scott Slotnick for his brilliance and the advanced intermediate lindy hop; Ola Selnes for teaching me clinical evaluations, neuropsychology, and always showing his kindness; and Barry Gordon for his support and guidance throughout the years. My thanks to Vic Henderson for choosing me to join him and our enjoyable times in the "Rock" and to Tim Kimbrell and Tom Freeman for teaching me neuropsychiatry.

I am indebted to John Santruck for setting me on this path of writing a textbook. I thank Mandy Maguire, Raksha Mudar, Dan Krawczyk, Bart Rypma, and Francesca Filbey, who have been the most terrific colleagues in Dallas; Mike Motes for challenging and thoughtful discussions and his strong chin; Lance, Don, and Doug for putting up with my golfing, complaining about this book, and their friendship; Michael, Harry, Rich, and Tanner, Tuscano for the greatest gift of lifelong friendship and always keeping me grounded; Kyle Womack for teaching me molecular dementia; Tom Campbell and Leo Estevez for entertaining and counseling my ideas and theories; and Nyaz Didehbani, Tina Bass, and Heather Conover for taking care of everything while I wrote this book. I also thank Elliot Frohman and Munro Cullum for their friendship, partnership, and "the love"; Sandi Chapman for choosing me as a partner and giving me the gift of allowing me to help her in building her center; Bruce Gnade and Bert Moore for being the best bosses, an extremely tough and thankless job, and teaching me how to be a better one; Mike Kraut, my twin brother from a different mother, who is and always will be my creative partner, and first cognitive neuroradiologist; and my family—Laura, Jack, and Charlie, Jack, Julie, substitute dad and big brother—the Mikes, Honora who never went by that name but was one of the most honorable people I know, and Dave—for putting up with me and their support over all of these years.

THE NEUROBIOLOGY OF COGNITION AND BEHAVIOR

1

Cognition, Behavior, Brain, and Networks

Humans have long been fascinated about our most unique qualities—how we think and behave. The brain's organization and dynamic state changes allow for the nimble changes in our thoughts and behavior in response to the world. For this to occur at the speed at which we think requires some degree of regularity of brain regions and pathways for the structure necessary to function successfully in everyday life. This regularity is also consistent with how similar we are in many regards as humans in our thinking and behaviors.

As part of our search for understanding the basis of cognition and behavior, there has been a recent proliferation of functional neuroimaging studies (e.g., positron emission tomography (PET) and functional magnetic resonance imaging (fMRI)) investigating the localizations of cognitive operations and behaviors in the human brain. By functional neuroimaging studies, we are referring to individuals (normal or impaired) lying in an imaging instrument and performing a cognitive/behavioral task so that one can image what regions of the brain are more activated while the task is being performed. Prior to these developments, understanding of the relationship between cognition, behavior, and brain anatomy came from correlations between patients with specific anatomic lesions and the subsequent cognitive and behavioral deficits generated by such lesions. Today, these anatomic correlates would typically be obtained from autopsy or computed tomography (CT) or MRI scans. These correlations, which date back to the late 1800s with the works of Paul Broca, Carl Wernicke, Joseph Dejerine, Pierre Marie, and colleagues, provided our basic understanding of which brain regions are responsible for specific cognitive tasks or operations.

The approach of correlating a lesion in the brain with a co-occurring behavioral deficit has existed throughout the years due to the detailed work of investigators who not only provided comprehensive descriptions of the brain-lesioned patients' cognitive deficits and behavioral abnormalities but also performed the most accurate anatomical localizations of their lesions with the best techniques available at that time. These behavioral descriptions included detailed observations of patients' performance, administration of neurological tests, and assessment of behavioral and cognitive status with testing that could be performed by healthy normal individuals or with tests that had been normed in comparable control populations. Prior to the advent of functional brain scanning, successful brain–behavior localization required that patients be assessed soon after developing a deficit, typically from a stroke. This was followed by testing the patients potentially several more times until death to assess for changes in performance that may indicate a new deficit from a new lesion or to determine if the deficit represented a progressive decline associated with a degenerative disease or an expanding lesion such as a tumor.

Determining the anatomical extent of patients' lesions prior to the development of CT and MRI scanning required careful follow-up by the investigator, who monitored patients' behavior until their death, obtained autopsies, and performed careful dissection of their brains. After obtaining these anatomic localizations, the investigator correlated the behavioral and cognitive deficits with the lesion location. The resultant conclusions were that the damaged brain region was responsible for the functions that patients could no longer perform or the atypical behavior they displayed.

As noted previously, the tasks that can no longer be performed by the patient, and any aberrant behavior identified, defined the extent of the behavioral deficit that presumably is the result of the lesion. The characterization of this cognitive deficit phenotype of the patient was determined by the sophistication and extent of testing administered to the patient. As the field of cognitive neuroscience has advanced, not only has the precision of these behavioral observations improved but also there has been a clearer delineation of the types of cognitive operations that underlie the performance of the cognitive tasks being used to test patients. One reason for this refinement in cognitive descriptions is the ongoing parcellation of increasingly finer distinctions in defining cognition operations. In addition, advancements in the field of cognitive science have produced other useful advances inducing investigators to derive models of cognition consisting of components or units allowing for testable hypotheses and predictions. This has led to a better understanding of the tests that are administered to patients to assess cognition and behavior with the improved characterization of units or components that are needed to perform a cognitive task and how these units are coupled together to perform these tasks.

As we proceed forward, these cognitive units are being continually refined to best approximate the roles we are identifying for anatomic structures. This has led not only to better specified characterizations of the behavioral performance and phenotypes of patients who develop impairments but also to a better understanding of normal cognition. The closer the delineation of cognitive units to approximate neural functions that are being attributed to neuronal firing and transmission in the brain, the closer cognitive neuroscience approaches a better understanding of cognition and behavior.

In parallel to the advancements in defining aspects of cognition, sophistication of anatomic specification has evolved greatly throughout the years. Anatomic specification from the 1800s to the present has always included evaluation of autopsy specimens of patients after death. Whereas there have been considerable changes in the staining techniques of brain specimens that have resulted in changes in the microscopic specification of lesions, there have been few changes in the macroscopic examination of the size and location of lesions that have changed the anatomic specification throughout the years. Thus, the major advance in the ability to make brain–behavior correlations was not in changes in autopsy techniques but, rather, in the advent of modern neuroimaging.

CT is based on mathematics developed in the early 1900s by Johann Radon, but the first practical CT scanners were not developed and manufactured until the early 1970s (Figure 1.1). It was at that point that the technological advances in computers, radiological equipment, and software had advanced

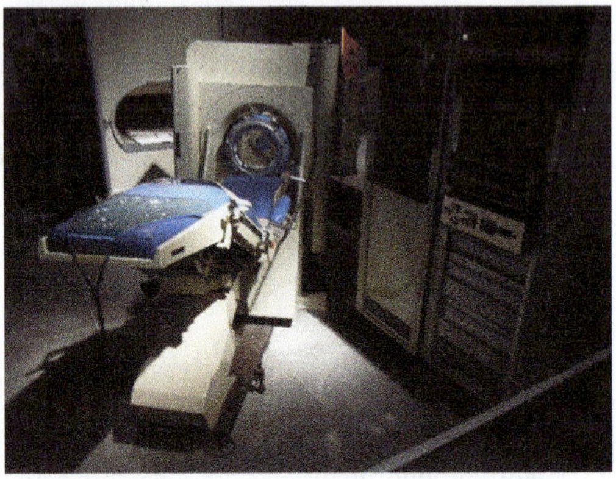

FIGURE 1.1: Photograph of one of the original EMI CT scanners.

so that computer processing of the x-ray images could be reconstructed to form tomographic slices of the brain without excessive radiation exposure to the patient. For CT scans, elements of x-ray images are obtained as the x-ray machine spins around a single axis of rotation for 360 degrees. In the middle of this circle is the patient's head. The series of x-rays is reconstructed using computer processing, and an image is generated that represents a slice of brain (a tomograph). The first patient CT scan of the brain was performed in 1971 and announced in 1972. This represented the first time that images of the brain could be acquired without requiring cutting the head open as performed at an autopsy.

The first company to produce commercial CT scanners for widespread use in hospitals was EMI, which also produced the recordings of The Beatles. For years, it was rumored that it took the profits generated from The Beatles record sales for EMI to have the revenue to launch the production of CT scans, although this rumor has subsequently been questioned.

CT scans offered the first view of the human brain while the patient was still alive. However, the resolution of the CT image did not easily allow for specific gyral and sulcal localization of lesions. The path that led to advancing beyond CT scanning started with Herman Carr's 1952 Ph.D. thesis describing the development of a magnetic resonance (MR) image. Since that point, the ability to acquire and refine MR images (Figure 1.2 shows an MR scanner) has led to a revolution in the ability to image in detail the human brain in living people. MRI uses a combination of magnetic fields and radio frequency (RF) pulses to align and then perturb the alignments of protons within the body

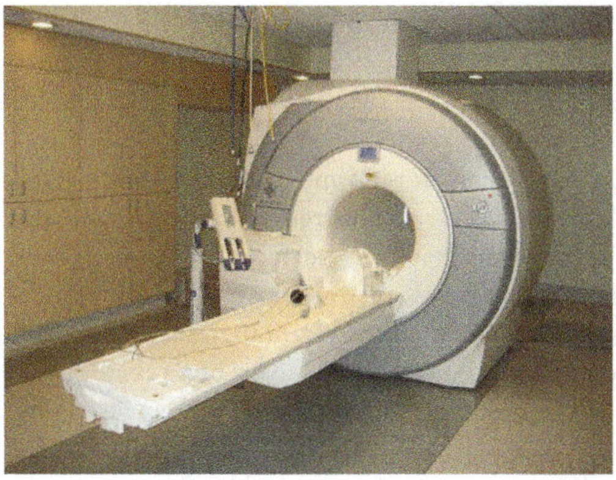

FIGURE 1.2: Photograph of an MRI scanner.

part to be imaged. Upon recovering from their perturbations, the protons give off RF signals (like those received in a radio) that are detected by the MRI instrument. The magnetic fields are calibrated to have slightly different values at different locations within the bore of the MR instrument; thus, the protons at each location spin at slightly different frequencies. It is the small differences in these frequencies that allow the MR system to determine from where in the body the signals originated and thus to create an image. In general, MRI operates by exciting and receiving signals from protons in water molecules because they are the most ubiquitous and thus will emit the strongest signal, but in principle (and occasionally in practice), MRI can be used to detect signals from any nuclei with odd numbers of nucleons (protons and neutrons). Thus, although most MR images depend on hydrogen protons, MR imaging is based on detection of protons in sodium (23 nucleons) and helium-3 (3 nucleons instead of the usual 4). Currently, however, most clinical and research MR imaging is based on the signals from excited water protons.

The first widespread usage of MRIs in the 1980s was a major advance in markedly improving the spatial resolution obtained from imaging studies, providing the basis for the more precise anatomical localizations that we have today. This anatomic specificity combined with detailed cognitive assessments of what a patient cannot perform has led to the current advances in lesion-based brain–behavior correlations and more sophisticated models of cognitive localization (e.g., from disconnection models to network approaches).

The focus of the account of the neurobiology of cognition and behavior presented in this book is based on information derived from localization of functions, which is in turn based on the convergence of studies demonstrating on a consistent basis that a brain region is essential to performing a cognitive operation. This can be shown to some degree by functional neuroimaging studies, but it is best to be confirmed by lesion studies. The reasoning for this approach is that functional activation studies (e.g., PET and fMRI performed while a subject is performing a task) demonstrate brain regions that are *involved* in performing a cognitive task as well as those that are *essential* to performing the task. Lesion–deficit models demonstrate within those activated regions the ones that are essential to performing the task. Requiring the lesion correlation provides brain–behavior localizations that are the most consistent because the regions are essential to performing the task. This may lead to an underestimate of regions associated with cognitive operations, but it provides a basic neural architecture of cognition and behavior on which to build.

Thus, the consistent brain–behavior correlations referred to in this book can extend from multiple activation studies but with confirmation using lesion studies, unless otherwise specified. These findings are listed within each chapter in a summary table labeling the cognitive unit and anatomic region for that cognitive domain. We discuss further the use of other applications of MRI imaging sequences such as fMRI, functional connectivity MRI, and diffusion tensor imaging as they apply in the support of these localizations, the differing aspects of models of brain–behavior correlations, or the mapping of specific cognitive domains.

The following sections describe the logic and organization of this neurobiological approach to cognition and behavior, the cognitive units that are used, the processing schemata in which these units function when they are connected together in accomplishing a cognitive task, the anatomic units and the processing schemata they use, and the resultant cognitive anatomic units that are the basis of this book.

LOGIC OF LESION–DEFICIT CORRELATIONS

The logic of the lesion–deficit associations is that one can link a specific behavioral/cognitive deficit with a brain lesion, with the resultant conclusion being that the brain region identified is essential to performing that cognitive operation. Although this approach has been used for more than a century, it is best applied for cognition and behavior in the classic work of Norman Geschwind (Geschwind, 1965) (Figure 1.3).

The lesion–deficit approach thus assumes that when a part of the brain is removed, the cognitive operations that the patient is no longer able to perform were subsumed by that removed brain region. This type of logic presupposes some assumptions, with the following key assumption addressed first: There are no compensatory strategies or recovery that occur after a lesion. This is clearly not the case for many lesions that occur acutely in the brain because the deficit seen immediately after a lesion can be more severe than the one seen when retesting the patient several months later. This is likely due to brain structures reorganizing to take over the functions that were previously performed by the damaged region, other regions or pathways in the brain that could also perform the function starting to perform the function, and/or brain regions that were injured but not destroyed by the acute lesion recovering and being functional after inflammation and ischemia (a reduction in blood supply to tissues usually due to a restriction in flow in the blood vessels) are no longer present. Attempts have been made to overcome this problem of time affecting the primary characteristics of the lesion. There are some circumstances that allow for assessment of cognitive status following the "hyperacute" state of a lesion that potentially would provide for a clear brain–behavior association without the opportunity for recovery or compensation (Hillis, 2005; Lesser et al., 2011). However, there are not enough of these instances to cover all cognitive operations.

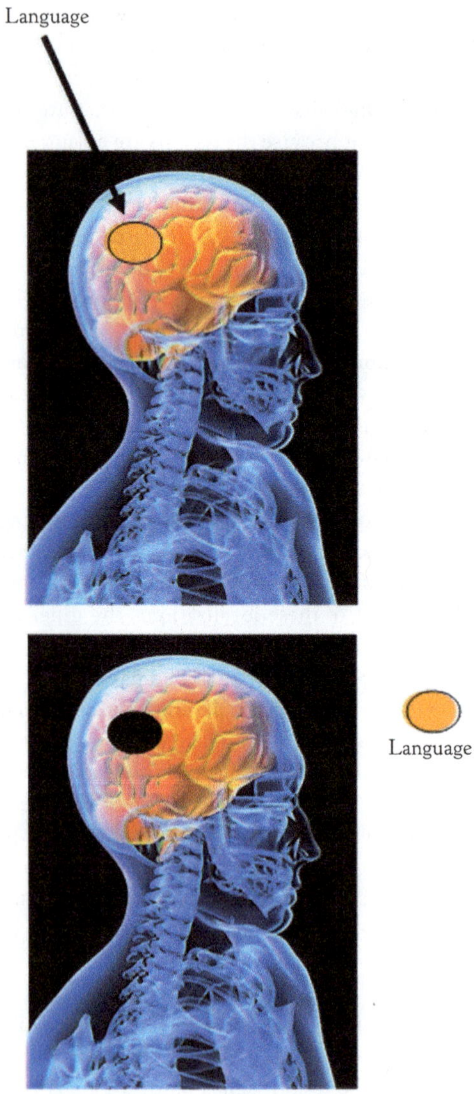

FIGURE 1.3: A schematic of the assumptions of the lesion–deficit model using language as the example. The lesion–deficit approach suggests that when a lesion of the language system occurs, if you test what the patient cannot do with this area of the brain lesioned, then you can infer what that brain region did.

Irrespective of the recovery issue, there are some clear conclusions that can be drawn from lesion studies, based on the following logic. Given that recovery/compensation does occur following many brain lesions and that the mechanism by which this occurs is not the same for each lesion or individual, *we take it as compelling evidence when relatively consistent behavioral/cognitive deficits exist months to years after lesions occur in the same general region across a number of individuals.* An alternative account that appears unlikely but possible, which would challenge this logic to some degree, is that after a specific lesion, a relatively consistent pattern of recovery occurs and produces a consistent impairment across individuals, but this recovered function bears no relationship to the cognitive function originally performed by the lesioned region. One can conceive that this could occur from a brain region that was part of a network and the network reorganizes across individuals in a consistent manner. However, the most likely explanation for a consistent deficit that occurs across multiple individuals is that the lesioned brain region encodes for a common cognitive construct that is localized in the same region across individuals.

Thus, the optimal circumstance to verify this localization of a cognitive operation is see if multiple observations or studies of different individuals with the same lesion report the same deficit in these people. The more reported studies and/or the more individuals with a consistent brain–behavior association, the stronger the evidence for the association. Only brain–behavior correlations found in multiple individuals/studies are included in this book, unless otherwise specified.

It is imperative to have clear definitions and an organizational framework to proceed to delineate a group of brain–behavior correlations. The following provides the framework used for this book to establish these brain–behavior correlations with working definitions for cognitive and anatomic constructs.

BEHAVIORAL/ COGNITIVE UNITS

A key factor in any approach to describing how complex functions such as behavior and cognition are organized in the brain is how well one can define and characterize the units that are being used. Anatomically, these units have been described in great detail throughout the years down to the cellular and molecular level, as brain specification has developed to account not only for cognition and behavior but also for all brain functions. On the other hand, whereas descriptions of the anatomy of the brain have changed little in the recent past, the units describing cognition and behavior have continued to evolve throughout the years, as stated previously.

Traditionally, the delineation of cognitive deficits occurs after a patient has been administered cognitive or behavioral tasks to perform. The first level of definition we use in our approach to the neurobiology of cognition and behavior is thus the *task* level:

> *Task*: A test of cognition or behavior that is administered to a subject to assess the ability of the individual to use their cognitive functions to adequately produce a correct outcome to the request of the task. A task typically engages multiple cognitive units or functions, but it can consist conceivably of just one unit.

Tasks have evolved throughout the years as investigators have continued to dissect human behavior increasingly further in order to advance their understanding of thinking and behavior. As these tasks have advanced, so has the ability of investigators to further divide aspects of a task into component parts that can be defined and that can be isolated as separate components of cognition that are separable from other isolatable components. These are referred to operationally as *cognitive units* and defined as follows:

> *Cognitive unit*: A component of cognition (representation, function, processing, etc.) that can be reproducibly delineated in terms of its role or operation in cognition and can be demonstrated as functionally distinct from other cognitive units. An example of a cognitive unit is "inhibition," "selection," or "accessing a lexicon (store of words)."

The existence of cognitive units—in essence some divisions of cognition other than one homogeneous, amorphous cognitive system—is accepted in most models of cognition, except for extreme versions of parallel distributed processing (PDP) models. In some pure PDP models of cognition, all units of cognition have an equal role in contributing to all thought, without distinctions for representations, processing, or even differing domains of cognition. There is not overwhelming empirical support for a pure PDP organization to the brain because there is clearly not an absence of units or divisions in cognition or other functions in the brain.

A clear set of divisions of the functions that the brain performs is that there are *domains* of cognition that are clearly dissociable from each other, categorized by general distinctions such as language, memory, attention, visuospatial, and higher-order cognition associated with sensory domains. These are definable by the presence of a number of cognitive units engaged in performing cognitive tasks of the same general target function. These large classifications of cognitive units performing similar, related target functions have been shown to be dissociable and are referred to as domains (language, memory, etc.). These domains are featured in most of the chapters in this book to describe the cognitive units that have been delineated within those domains.

It is important to note that not all cognitive units are specific to one domain. Some cognitive units are referred to as *domain general* as opposed to *domain specific*. Domain-general cognitive units subsume functions/operations/representations that can engage in tasks in several different cognitive domains. An example of a domain-general function is "selection," a cognitive control function that is engaged in choosing from among multiple alternative choices. Such a cognitive unit can be engaged in language tasks, memory tasks, and reasoning tasks, for example.

The distinction that cognitive units are domain specific or domain general brings with it several implications. If a domain-specific unit is lesioned, then one would hypothesize that the only tasks that would be disrupted would be those within the specific domain that the unit serves and that performance of tasks in other cognitive domains would not be affected. Lesions in domain-general units would likely result in impaired performance to some degree in tasks from several cognitive domains.

Specifying the operation that a cognitive unit performs and the domain(s) to which it corresponds allows for creating informed models of the units needed to perform a task, assigning the types of roles that units subsume in the task, and hypothesizing more clearly what deficits would exist after a lesion occurs. Because performing a cognitive task of any degree of complexity can require more than one of these defined cognitive units, units need to be linked together effectively for efficiency of performance and for speed of processing. How these units are linked together is referred to as *processing schemata* or *processing streams*. These processing streams allow for modeling how units are connected, the directions in which information is streamed, and the feedback that may occur between units. They also allow for attributing an impairment in performance to dysfunction in a specific cognitive processing stream.

> *Cognitive processing streams*: Manner in which cognitive units are linked to, interact with, and transfer information among one another.

The most basic type of processing stream is referred to as *serial processing* (Figure 1.4). In this processing schema, each cognitive unit does its processing sequentially, with a unit beginning processing only when the results are received from the temporally preceding unit, only after that stage has totally completed its processing. Thus, a key aspect of serial processing schemata is that units send information only in a unidirectional manner. This type of serial processing does exist in the human brain, but for only some cognitive tasks. Techniques that reveal aspects of timing, such as event-related potentials, have been used in conjunction with lesion studies to demonstrate the existence of independent cognitive units arranged serially in terms

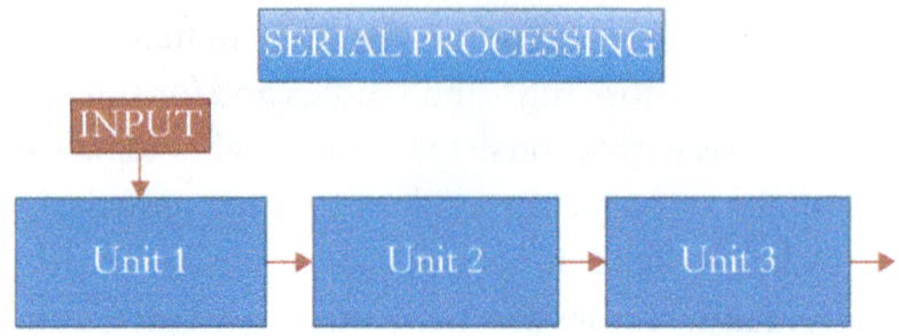

FIGURE 1.4: Input comes into the cognitive system, and processing of that input begins at Unit 1. The other units are inactive until the processing at Unit 1 is completed. When Unit 1 processing is completed, the output of that is sent in its entirety to Unit 2. Unit 2 processing then begins with Units 1 and 3 now inactive. Once Unit 2 is complete, it sends its output to Unit 3, which then begins its processing while Units 1 and 2 are inactive, and so on if there are further units.

of information transfer as well as a specific temporal ordering of the processing of these units.

A cognitive task that requires multiple cognitive units and proceeds by serial processing is an optimal one to use in assessing patients. The logic of how they would be used and interpreted is as follows: While investigating the cognitive deficits associated with a lesion, a patient is given a task that, for example, consists of three cognitive units that are arranged in serial processing. If the patient performs the task well, this leads to the conclusion that the functions of all three cognitive units are intact. Subsequently, another task can be administered that consists of four cognitive components arranged in serial processing, with the first three components being the same as those of the last task but with one new component added to the end. If the subject cannot perform this new task, then by comparing performance on these two tasks, one can assume by a subtraction type of logic that the lesion is located in a region that supports this additional fourth cognitive unit. For this conclusion to be valid, the remaining unaffected components must not have reorganized or adapted, an alternate pathway of the brain is not available to accomplish the task, and the impaired component has not recovered after being lesioned. Tasks that employ cognitive units arranged in a serial processing schema allow for the most straightforward interpretation when a deficit in performance is present.

Several other types of processing schemata have been purported to occur in the human brain, with two key examples being parallel and cascade processing. In *parallel processing*, multiple cognitive units perform different cognitive operations

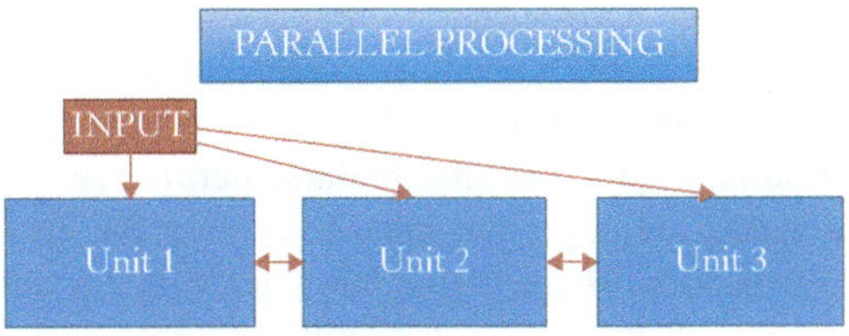

FIGURE 1.5: Input comes into the cognitive system, and processing of that input begins at all units. All units work simultaneously on their processing of the input. Each unit can communicate with the partial processing of the other units throughout. Once a satisfactory final product is reached, an output is forwarded and processing in all units stops.

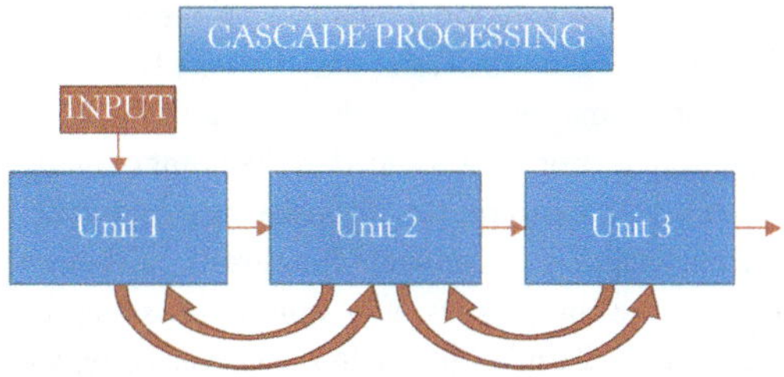

FIGURE 1.6: Input comes into the cognitive system, and processing of that input begins at Unit 1. The other stages downstream can receive partial information from previous units to inform their processing (partial information can feed backward to inform previous units' processing also) from other units. Processing then proceeds down each unit until completed processing at Unit 3 is sent as output.

simultaneously (Figure 1.5). In a parallel schema, each of the units can pass partial or complete information of the processing it has performed to any of the other units in the stream so that those units might take that partial information to complete their processing. When one of the cognitive units in a parallel processing stream is lesioned, a variety of deficits may occur due to the complex interactive and collaborative relationships that the cognitive units have with one another.

Another major type of processing stream between cognitive units is referred to as *cascade processing* (Figure 1.6). This is a hybrid schema between serial processing and parallel processing streams. In cascade processing, each cognitive unit processes input separately but passes along partial output in a feeding-information-forward-to-other-units (referred henceforth as feed-forward). These receiving units can use this information to further their processing of partial information gained from earlier processing units. In addition, units downstream in the processing stream can feed information backward to earlier processing units in a feed-backward manner to complete their processing. Again, drawing conclusions from lesions in units in these types of processing streams can be difficult without careful specification of the operations of each unit and the interrelationships with other units in the processing stream.

There can be other processing schemata for cognitive units that can be the result of combining different combinations of the schemata previously described, possibly including additional factors such as monitoring units and different speeds of connections. Given that these more complex processing stream models do not necessarily have adequate brain–behavior specifications at present, we continue with the present level of complexity of the three presented processing stream models (serial, parallel, and cascade) as described unless otherwise specified.

ANATOMIC SPECIFICATION

The anatomy of the human brain has not changed like the evolving specification that has occurred in the area of describing cognitive units. As noted previously, the improvements in anatomical specification have been mostly in the technical aspects of superior neuroimaging of the brain while a person is alive. Neuroimaging techniques have improved with MRI and, with increasing Tesla strength, continue to offer better anatomic resolution with the most current imaging tools. With these changes, the specification of the anatomic localization continues to improve, and the resolution of the size of the anatomic units has allowed for finer distinction of smaller dissociable units. The following delineates the definitions and organizational structure used for anatomic specification for cognition and behavior in this book:

> *Anatomic units*: An anatomic region that can be defined on neuroimaging or autopsy with reproducibility across investigators in terms of the localization and extent of the region.

The size of the anatomic units that can be correlated with cognitive units will continue to get smaller as the resolution of neuroimaging improves. Currently, the resolution appears to consist of circumscribed regions of adjacent populations of neurons, with resolution dependent on the strength of the MRI scanner in Teslas and the slice thickness of the brain images acquired during scanning. MRI resolution has not yet advanced to the point of being able to isolate anatomic units consisting of networks of transynaptically connected neurons, although in the future these types of anatomic units may be detectable and undoubtedly informative. Here, we consider the anatomic resolution from neuroimaging to be at the several-millimeter level, which captures a population of neighboring neurons.

Anatomic specification with MRI allows for localization of lesions to specific gyri and sulci or to other areas of interest in an individual's brain anatomy. This ability to specify anatomical localizations in individual subjects allows for the potential collection of multiple cases of patients with lesions in a specific location. These data can then be analyzed among large numbers of subjects to find converging evidence that a lesion in a specific region is correlated with specific neurobehavioral findings. However, certain factors need to be addressed to optimize the ability to make the most accurate localizations. To arrive at cognition–brain correlations, one can (1) map a cognitive deficit of an individual to a lesion identified in that individual's brain, (2) collect deficit–lesion mapping of many individuals with that deficit (or that lesion), and (3) assess across all individuals for consistent association between deficit and lesion.

There are key assumptions and caveats that must be considered in the process of anatomic specification of brain regions, which are detailed as follows. To critically assess this fitting of brains into a template, one must also assess the assumptions made and limitations of placing varying-sized brains into a common brain template. For example, it is important to understand how the varying sizes and gyral variability in individuals are accounted for in "warping" brains to a common template. A typical approach of placing multiple brains into a common template is to globally shrink or expand brains to fit an overall cortical outline. A currently available technique that may best account for mapping misalignment is to designate "anchors," anatomical landmarks (the temporal pole, ventricular system, etc.) to which all brains are mapped to minimize distortions that may lead to false localizations and conclusions.

Anatomic specifications used to derive brain behavior correlations have to contend with several other issues. One is that all brains are not structurally the same in terms of the interrelationship between brain regions. Although there is a conventional acceptance that brain structures (gyri, sulci, etc.) are all present, are in the same place, and have the same shape across individuals, this is an oversimplification. The variability inherent naturally in a normal individual's brain organization is best illustrated by viewing intraoperative photos of individuals who are about to undergo surgical resection for medial temporal sclerosis (Figure 1.7). It can be seen from viewing actual brains that there exists some variability in the shape and length of the Sylvian fissures alone across these individuals. In addition, this type of variability can exist for each gyrus in terms of its presence, length, and relative location compared to other gyri. As can also be detected from the photos, although gyri appear in schematics to always be oriented so that the cortical surface faces outward toward the skull, this is not always the case. It can be seen that gyri sometimes fold inward from the skull surface, at times reemerging later to a surface orientation. Because the templates to which brains are coregistered for studies of localization all use a standard orientation of each gyrus with the cortex facing toward the skull, it is unclear how these regions are mapped into templates for analysis. One should consider this imprecise template mapping if distinct localization of a specific area is an important issue in a study.

The issue of variable brain shapes and sizes in individuals requires further discussion because of the possible negative consequences this factor may have if improper registration of brains occurs when analyzing multiple individuals in a group study. Because many group brain studies require the brains to be globally shrunk or enlarged to match a standardized brain size, there can be some key regions—particularly the Sylvian fissure, which separates the frontal lobe from the temporal lobe—where a small of misalignment can lead to a marked difference in location. For example, a lesion that was in the superior aspect of the temporal lobe could be moved to the inferior aspect of the frontal lobe in a brain warping process.

Another anatomic question that arises is whether a region associated with a specific function is anchored to a specific *distance from* an anatomical marker or the location is *relative to the length* of the gyrus (e.g., always located in the middle of the gyrus irrespective of the gyrus length). For

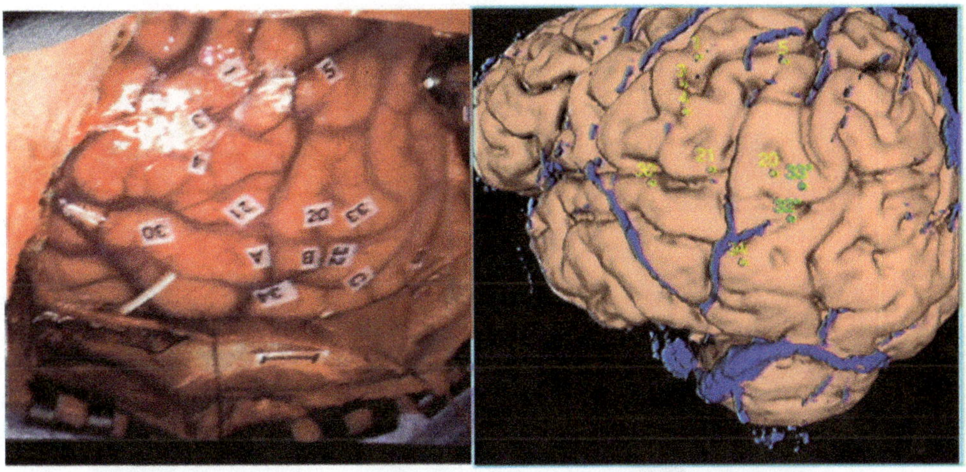

FIGURE 1.7: The photo on the left is an example of cortical mapping intraoperatively. The numbers represent regions where cortical electrical stimulation was performed to identify the function of those regions. The cortical veins are shown in blue, and the gyri can be visualized. The figure on the right is a 3-D reconstruction of the same brain from imaging that shows the cortical gyral pattern with an overlay of blood vessels in blue. What is to be gleaned from these two sets of figures is that in an individual, one can see that the gyral pattern does not always resemble the templates used.

Source: http://www.biomedcentral.com.

instance, if one found that a function was localized in one individual at a region 2 cm from the tip of the posterior termination of the Sylvian fissure in the superior temporal gyrus, which also happened to be in the middle of that gyrus in terms of the gyrus' length, then in other individuals with different-sized brains, would the region always be 2 cm from the posterior tip of their Sylvian fissure (Figure 1.8) or always be in the middle of the superior temporal gyrus, irrespective of the length of that gyrus?

For many cases of behavioral–anatomic localization, it is unknown whether areas specified to be associated with an assigned function are fixed to a certain distance from a certain brain marker or shift in location based on the size of the brain or specific gyrus with which it is associated (e.g., the auditory cortex; Wessinger et al., 2001) (Figure 1.9). Thus, when group analyses of behavior–brain correlations are performed, it is important to know how the brains were normalized to one another. Were the brains and lesions fit to a common brain template, were the locations of the areas of interest first mapped to the individual's structural scan to best localize the lesion, or were the lesions and brains together warped to a common template? Being aware of how these issues were addressed best allows for critical assessment of the findings of a study as to how the anatomic localizations were derived.

Another factor that will continue to evolve in neuroimaging is the improving resolution of anatomic specification to correlate with cognition and behavior. In anticipation of the need to relate present findings to future findings as anatomic

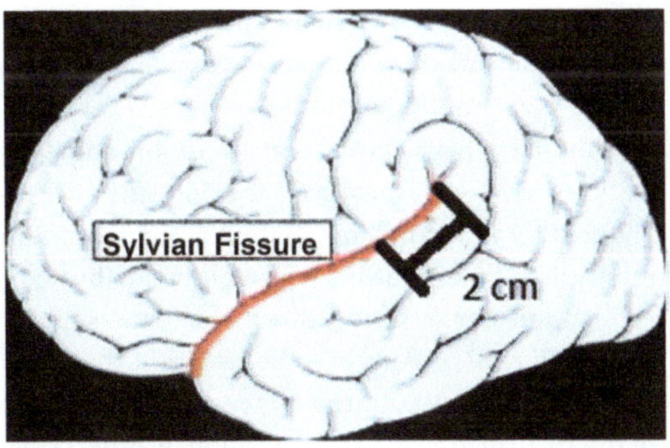

FIGURE 1.8: At the end of the red line denoting the Sylvian fissure, one can see the forked split into two sulci, which is reported in approximately 40% of individuals. Triradiate ends have been reported but are uncommon. Single termination is reported in the majority of individuals. However, other studies report the split ending in the majority of cases. The angle of the ending, although typically tilting superiorly, can also end in a neutral or inferior deflection. The length of the anterior ascending ramus varies from 10 to 30 mm, and that of the anterior horizontal varies from 10 to 25 mm. The Sylvian fissures are typically longer in the left than the right hemisphere.

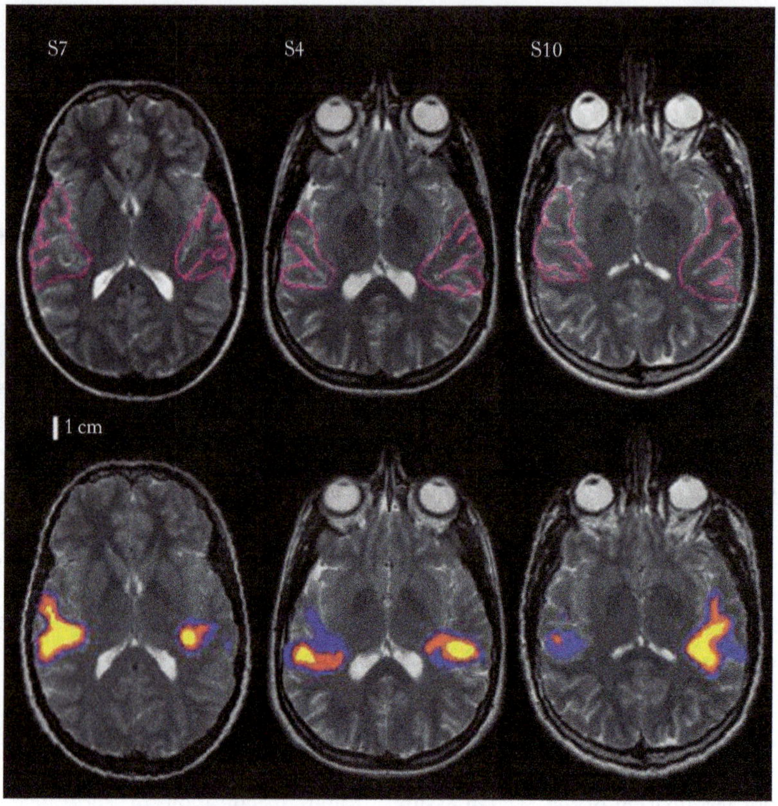

FIGURE 1.9: This figure shows the variability across individuals of a basic representation—primary auditory cortex. Oblique-axial slices approximately parallel to the supratemporal plane showing anatomical images (top) and regions of activation (bottom) produced by auditory stimulation in three representative subjects. Thresholded Z maps are co-registered and overlaid on coplanar anatomical images from each individual subject. Because the border of Heschl's region is not well defined in the anterolateral direction, its outline is continued to the edge of the slice (Wessinger et al., 2001).

resolution changes, uniform methods and standardization of anatomic specification exist and have been adopted for reporting localizations. The most commonly used technique is to report location by hemisphere and gyrus of location (e.g., right superior temporal gyrus). Another specification, based on cytoarchitectonic patterns of neurons in the layers of the cortical gray matter of a region, was described by Brodmann and is referred to as Brodmann areas (see Figure 1.10 for both gyral and Brodmann designations). Neuroanatomy is reviewed in more detail in Chapter 2, which discusses these distinctions on how to specify anatomic localizations.

Anatomic regions communicate with each other to effectively transmit neural signals supporting cognitive operations. As such, it is essential to optimally delineate the manner that these anatomic regions interrelate. The following provides a framework for how these regions interact for successful neural processing.

Anatomic processing schema: The way that neuronal firing patterns (spatially and/or temporally) in a brain region are linked to other anatomic regions to transfer information between regions.

The neurons in the regions associated with cognitive operations and processing fire via action potentials in the same manner as do neurons in other brain systems. The neurons within anatomic regions engaged in cognition will send signals via action potentials to neighboring neurons within the circumscribed region that is engaged in the cognitive operation. This allows for populations of neighboring neurons to fire in an organized manner to perform cognitive operations. These units of contiguous neurons fire in a variety of patterns that are still being explored.

There are patterns of neuronal firing localized to a specific region that are correlated with an outcome (motor movement, cognitive operation, etc.) and are considered to be performing the function of

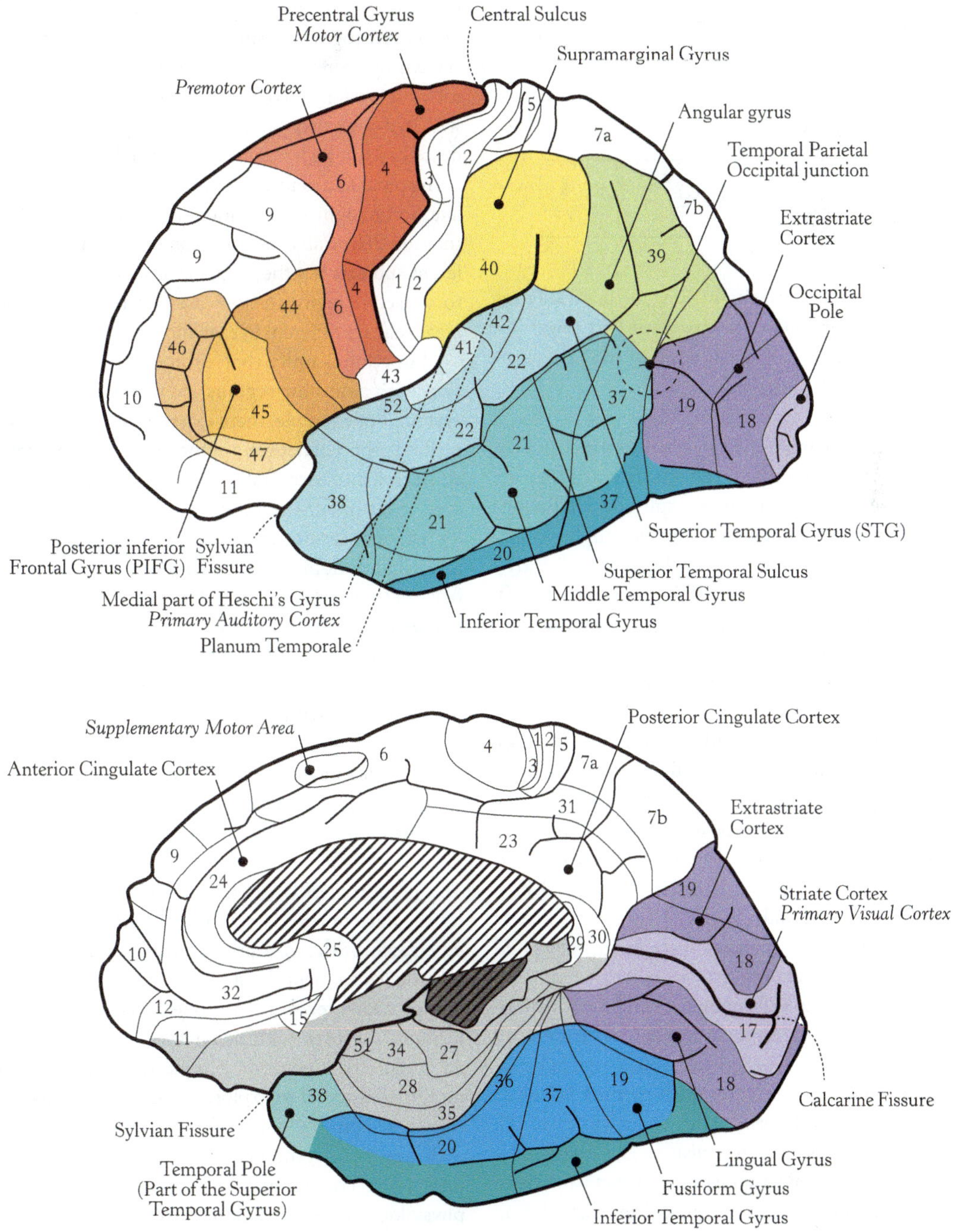

FIGURE 1.10: Brodmann areas denoted on lateral and medial surfaces of the brain, along with gyral names.

that region. There are also neuronal firing patterns between regions that communicate the output of one region to another. This provides the manner by which anatomic units communicate in a processing stream.

One of the methods through which anatomic units communicate in a processing stream with each other is via neurons sending signals through single action potentials. Another key method by which groups of neurons send signals to other brain regions is through synchronized neural firing in a rhythmic pattern, referred to as neural oscillations. Through synaptic connections, the rhythm of firing of neurons in a region can become synchronized, with their aggregate action potentials creating rhythmic signals. This

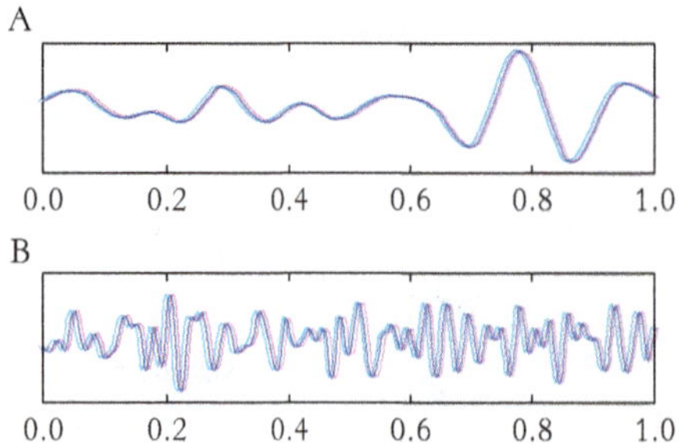

FIGURE 1.11: Examples of EEG rhythms. The top image (A) is of an EEG theta wave (4- to 7-Hz range). The bottom image (B) is an EEG beta wave (16- to 31-Hz range).

synchronized firing results in synchronized oscillating inputs to other cortical regions to which they are connected, resulting in large-amplitude oscillations of the local field potentials (an electrophysiological signal from the current flowing from all nearby dendritic synaptic activity within a volume of brain tissue) that are routinely measured outside the scalp with electroencephalography (EEG).

EEG oscillatory activity in several specific frequency bands has been well-described, and their rhythms have been detected from scalp recordings. The most commonly known frequency band is alpha (8–13 Hz), which is usually assessed by recording EEG from the occipital lobe while a subject is awake with eyes closed. Other commonly described frequency bands are delta (1–4 Hz), theta (4–8 Hz), beta (13–30 Hz), and gamma (30–70 Hz) (Figure 1.11). All these frequencies have been associated with multiple cognitive processes, with the most common being alpha frequency changes with attention (Klimesch, 2012), theta and beta with memory (Buszaki, 2006; Slotnick et al., 2002), sensory perceptual binding of features with gamma (Gray et al., 1992), and inhibition with theta (Brier et al., 2010), for example. Sleep is clearly characterized by increasing slow wave signals such as theta and delta and decreasing beta and alpha. These oscillating rhythms have proven to be informative in accounting for some neural mechanisms that support communication and operations in cognition and behavior. When relevant, these associated rhythms are noted throughout the book.

COGNITIVE–ANATOMIC CORRELATIONS

As noted previously, advances in experimental cognitive neuroscience allow investigators to design multiple experiments to tease apart units of what are purported cognitive units. However, there remains a "matching" component to identifying a discrete cognitive operation and the brain region that is associated with it, if one exists. Some cognitive operations can be described after a lesion has occurred, but it does not correspond to a detectable, *consistent* anatomic correlate. Some cognitive operations are identifiable in that they are dissociable after a lesion occurs in many different subjects but these operations are not localized to a discrete region, or they are localized to discrete areas that are different in each individual person.

Functional units that exhibit a clear relationship with anatomic regions are those in the motor system. For example, there exists a discrete, circumscribed group of neurons in the motor system that is dedicated and essential to moving the hand. If that area is lesioned, the individual loses hand mobility, whereas lesions in other areas typically do not affect hand mobility. This demonstrates the specificity of that relationship and independence to some degree of that functional anatomic unit from other brain areas. To detect similar—although not always independent—units in the cognitive domain, we define the following construct:

> *Cognitive–anatomic units (CAU)*: A delineated cognitive unit that is consistently associated with an anatomic unit.

This definition of CAUs is an operational definition for the current text. It requires a brain region that is detectable with currently available neuroimaging techniques to meet the anatomic unit criteria. This will of course evolve over time as anatomic specification improves with advances in neuroimaging. Although the definition emphasizes an anatomic unit, it is essential to explore the neurophysiological role that these regions perform in order to provide a clearer understanding of the actual mechanisms underlying cognition. When available, the neurophysiological mechanism for each CAU in this book is described. It is essential to extend beyond the mere mapping of locations and correlations of cognition to the actual patterns of neuronal firing (e.g., EEG power frequencies, neurotransmitter systems, etc.). As the field of understanding cognition evolves, there will also be further refinement of the cognitive units into definitions that more closely reflect neural firing.

With all of the assumptions listed being addressed, this CAU identification approach is one of the optimal methods to discover consistent localizations that minimize variability and to determine whether a specific function associated with the same brain region has occurred across multiple individuals. CAUs are best derived when localizations that correlate with cognition were consistent across individuals, when the studies were obtained for each individual at approximately the same time after the lesion occurred, and when these localizations occurred across multiple studies leading to a convergence of the same findings. The approach of using the single case study to delineate CAUs has evolved to studying groups of patients who share an impairment in a common cognitive unit and assessing whether and where a common lesioned region exists across these patients. Advances in neuroimaging analytical methods have allowed for improved and an increased number of studies using a large number of lesioned subjects to identify CAUs. Voxel-based lesion–symptom mapping (Bates et al., 2003) uses the approach of taking patients with a common symptom, which could be a simple cognitive unit, and then mapping the lesions of each brain into a common space. The space is divided into small cuboid shapes of equal size referred to as voxels. The technique allows for finding a region defined by the voxels where the lesions overlap in these patients who exhibit the cognitive symptom of interest. This identifies the most convergent region across individuals that is associated with the symptom. Although this may result in a smaller region than is the case in each individual patient, it reduces variability due to recovery, anatomic differences by individual, and warping to common space. Thus, the resultant region common across multiple studies will be most consistent with the deficits and the best correlation acceptable.

The types of cognitive operations that CAUs represent are varied and described throughout the remainder of this book. The following are examples of what these CAUs could assume: (1) encoding a representation at some level (e.g., premotor region encoding for how to position the hand or fingers to hold an item); (2) processing information or performing some operation (e.g., gating access of information from one region to another, blocking transfer of information, selecting among multiple choices, and searching); (3) integrating input from multiple representational levels or modalities; (4) detecting a specific category, trait, or feature and other attributes of items as they are delineated (an item is an animal, an item is threatening, etc.); and (5) accessing encodings of individual entities that are represented by spatially or spatially and temporally distributed patterns of neuronal firing that is not located in that specific region (Hart et al., 2007).

This latter point of a region accessing encoding of individual units of information (e.g., the word "dog" and that "ketchup is red") where the individual unit representations do not reside in the CAU is a key organizational mechanism proposed for storing and accessing knowledge in the brain. One way to encode these units of knowledge is via neurons that transmit signals transynaptically to neurons connected to, but not necessarily contiguous to, the neuron initiating the signal. These signals to distant yet synaptically connected neurons allow for incorporating distant regions in encoding for representations. This organization leads to multiple combinations of neurons connected synaptically to encode units of cognitive information, providing the option to store vast amounts of information. When a collection of neurons are used to encode information, then patterns of activation and inactivation in groups of neurons can encode for extremely large numbers of individual entities. This has been referred to as a "coarse coding" model of information storage (Hinton, 1981). In this type of schema, relevant neurons (or groups of neurons) representing a unit of information can be physically different locations. The firing pattern of all of the relevant neurons for a unit of information—that is, the "on" and "off" of all of the neurons taken together at a given time—signifies a specific entity (e.g., pattern A is the word "cup" in Figure 1.12, and see examples in Chapter 4). Neurons can be associated with other neurons in different "on" and "off" patterns that, when firing, signify a different specific entity. This allows for the capacity to encode for large amounts of information, and the multiple neurons and multiple locations involved in encoding a single entity protect against damage causing loss of individual entities/items. Neurons that are not contiguous to each other would not be disrupted by a circumscribed, discrete lesion.

Other plausible theoretical organizations of brain–behavior correlations are mentioned now, although to date, they have not been consistently established. This is particularly true for some cognitive units that do not clearly map onto a focal, discrete neural entity. One example of this type of brain–behavior correlation is where there is a clearly delineated cognitive unit but it is supported neurally by nondiscrete and noncontiguous anatomical areas. Another example of this type of correlation

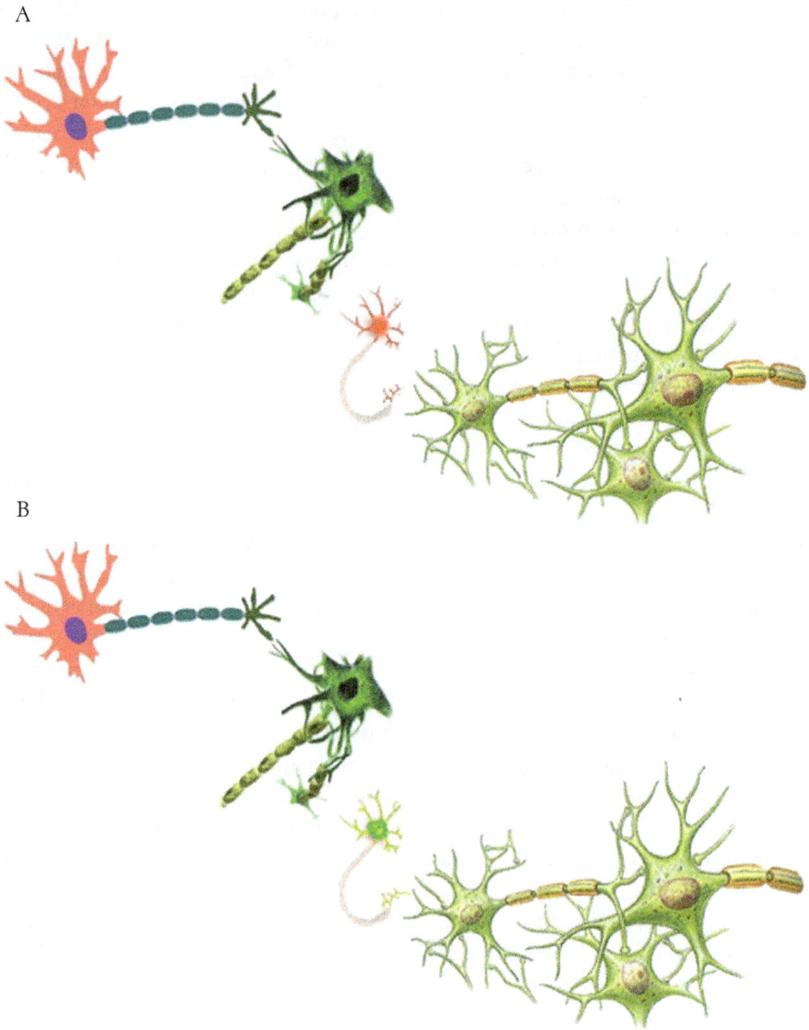

FIGURE 1.12: In this schema, the color of the neurons could signify that the neuron is active (green for on) or inactive (red for off). The neurons in these patterns may or may not be contiguous; each could be in different parts of the brain. Each pattern is referred to as a neural unit. The pattern of all the "on" and "off" neurons in the neural units taken together signifies a specific semantic entity (e.g., pattern A is the word "glass"). In this example, the same neurons firing in a different pattern in that neural unit (e.g., pattern B) would signify another distinct entity (e.g., "cow"). These are same neurons, as it is likely in the brain that each neuron dedicated to encoding semantic entities may be involved in different groupings for each specific semantic entity. In this manner, one can encode an extremely large number of unique entities with many fewer neurons than entities. Also, by being in spatially different locations, this type of coding protects against losing individual entities when there is focal brain damage.

is where there is a clearly delineated cognitive unit supported neurally by nondiscrete and noncontiguous anatomical areas that produce synchronized neuronal firing in a coherent synchronized brain rhythm (alpha, theta, etc.) that leads to supporting a cognitive operation. Although we have described this type of activity that is generated by discrete anatomic foci, we have to be mindful that this could occur from distributed neurons not localized in one region.

The CAUs that are included in this book meet the criteria of being a defined cognitive unit and an isolatable anatomic unit that are associated together. These have been typically arrived at by a convergence of studies that have resulted in a consistent association of cognitive unit with anatomic unit. Functional imaging studies such as fMRI and PET that have been obtained during cognitive task performance contribute to the association. These activation studies that show both regions that are essential to and regions that are involved with performing a cognitive task are interpreted in conjunction with lesion studies to find those regions that are essential to performing the task, that if lesioned will result in a consistent disruption of the cognitive operation, and thus allowing for the establishment of an optimal brain–behavior correlation. The confirmation of both an activation study and lesion studies to arrive at a CAU is both a more conservative and a more definitive way to establish brain–behavior correlations.

CAU PROCESSING STREAMS

A single CAU may be all that is needed in single simple task. An established relationship in which a lesion to the anatomic correlate of a CAU consistently disrupts the cognitive unit associated with it, resulting in impaired performance, allows for the most straightforward predictions from a lesion perspective in describing cognitive outcome.

When the cognitive unit of a CAU is involved with other CAUs in performing a complex cognitive task, this is typically referred to as a type of network. If a CAU functioning in a network with other CAUs is lesioned, then that unit's cognitive function would be "reduced" in participating with the cognitive functions of the other units in the network. Depending on the type of cognitive processing stream involved (serial, parallel, cascade, etc.), one can then predict the type of behavioral dysfunction that will result with this damaged network. In addition, one would be able to assess the type of performance that would be found with a task when that CAU is disconnected to some degree from the other CAUs due to white matter damage.

The concepts described thus far consist of cognitive units, anatomic units, processing schemata, and CAUs. Tasks typically involve multiple CAUs connected in a network whose interactions with each other are delineated by the processing schema. When a lesion affects an anatomic region associated with a particular CAU, dysfunction of the cognitive unit can lead to deficits. The lesioned CAUs that are part of a network will lead to disruption of that network function, which can be complex or more straightforward in terms of overall task performance changes depending on the CAU's characteristics and network connections.

Historically, understanding CAUs in a network relied on several assumptions. First, it was assumed that the CAUs in a network each had the anatomic region being solely responsible for completing all of the cognitive unit's functions. Second, it was assumed that the CAUs were independent of each other. This is the simplest configuration of a network and could allow one to most straightforwardly assess how a lesion to one CAU would result in a change in output and impaired performance. This was particularly true if the task was the product of serial processing and the disrupted CAU was the last one in the processing chain.

Further advances in cognitive neuroscience have helped to better define the characteristics of what we attribute to a cognition–brain correlation, including whether multiple brain regions contribute to a cognitive unit or whether multiple cognitive units are associated with one brain region. There were some clearly defined cognitive units that were not dependent on only one brain region to be fully performed but were involved with two or more brain regions in performing that cognitive operation. Thus, the concept of a definable cognitive unit being supported by, and requiring, multiple brain regions for that operation to be accomplished successfully emerged and led to a more sophisticated consideration of networks of brain regions encoding for a cognitive operation as well as for cognitive tasks.

NETWORK ORGANIZATION

There is a broader definition of networks in cognition and behavior, in which the definition of CAUs used in this book is expanded. What has been previously described for CAUs still holds in these network models, in which each node represents a CAU, but "networks" can also refer to supporting other cognition–brain relationships in which a single *cognitive unit does not correspond to a single anatomic unit but to multiple anatomic units*. Thus, this single cognitive unit can be represented in a distributed manner across several anatomic regions, which in itself represents a network of regions encoding for a single, defined cognitive unit.

A more typical usage of networks is a more global version in which multiple cognitive units supported by multiple brain regions in a variety of different combinations can be linked together in a network, processing information in order to perform a specific cognitive task. These anatomic regions have been given a variety of names, with the best fit in a network organization being that the regions represent "nodes." Basically, networks are composed of two components: the elements of the network and the relationships between them. These elements are typically referred to as nodes and the relationships as links (Stanley et al., 2013). One of the key functions of a node is to engage in performing cognitive processing of some type or in representing cognitive constructs. Another key function to consider is that a node may function simply as a connecting node that links other nodes together. (This can also be a function of some CAUs.) The connections that typically link the multiple, distinctly located nodes in the cortex and subcortical regions are white matter tracts (Figure 1.13). The architecture of how the neurons in a node are connected and may fire in a pattern, and the multiple different patterns in which groups of neurons in a node may fire, account for the types of operations a node may perform. The connectional pattern that groups a node to others defines how that node can function in an interactive way with other nodes to perform a variety of cognitive tasks.

In addition, *some nodes may be engaged in a number of different domains of cognition and behavior (multiple-domain nodes), with the function for each of those domains being subserved by anatomically distinct subpopulations of neurons within the node and/or distinct firing patterns that those neurons assume for each cognitive operation in which they can be engaged.* Thus, if damage occurs to part of a node, then the functions that were subsumed by that part of the node are the functions that would be disrupted. A decrement in performance would be expected in the different domains and cognitive tasks that the

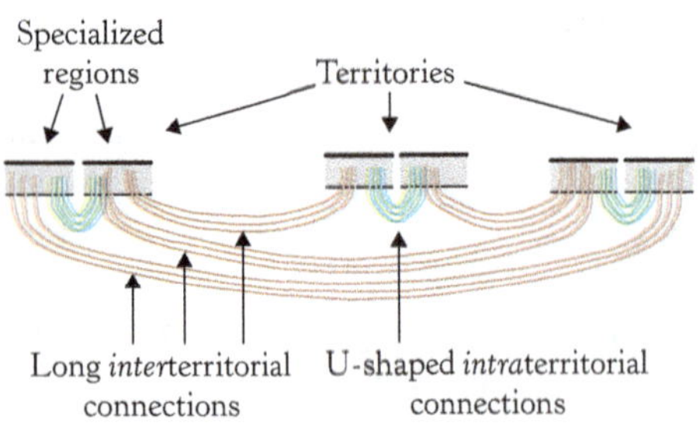

FIGURE 1.13: A view of specialized cortical regions and their connections. Different subpopulations of neurons in specialized regions are designated as gray rectangles. These regions are connected to neighboring regions by white matter U-shaped fibers (green). Connections to distant cortical regions are via longer white matter interterritorial tracts (red).

Source: Catani and ffytche (2005).

damaged part of the node was engaged in when it was supposed to be active.

When a region of neurons in a whole node or part of a node are engaged in performing multiple, different cognitive operations, several factors are essential in determining the role of an anatomic region at a particular time. Some, but not all, of the factors that are important include (1) other neurons, or more likely groups of neurons, at other locations that are associated with performing the cognitive operation to be performed; (2) the pattern of firing of those neurons in the node engaged in each operation; and (3) the time at which the neurons fire when involved with one set of regions performing one cognitive operation vis-à-vis when they fire with another set of neurons performing a different cognitive operation. For example, when neurons in a region fire in a certain pattern or rhythm (e.g., beta rhythm) and are connected to two other brain regions, the cognitive unit that they support may function to select from among multiple target word choices the best word. However, these same neurons may play a role in another cognitive operation. In that operation, they may fire only after receiving a signal from a distant brain region, their output is a different pattern or rhythm (e.g., theta rhythm), and the function in that operation is to inhibit a response. This attribute is referred to as dual functioning of neuron groups in multiple cognitive operations. A lesion in a brain region in which these neurons are located would possibly lead to disruption of two entirely unrelated cognitive operations. In addition, this same type of multiple patterns of neuronal firing for multiple cognitive operations can occur in a node, not necessarily from the same neurons but from different subpopulations of neurons in that node for each cognitive operation. Taking into account all of these multiple roles of neurons in a node further complicates the ability to isolate brain regions associated with a specific operation.

The most common cognition–behavioral correlation encompassed in networks, which is also relevant in a modified version in CAUs, is that some cognitive operations may require multiple nodes for that operation to be successfully performed. Each of the nodes can assume a variety of roles individually so that the aggregate product is the cognitive unit being performed normally. Most of the nodes have been assumed to perform partial processing in these networks and to participate in the interactive processing between the nodes to complete the cognitive operation. It is imperative as network models are proposed that the particular role within cognitive operations that the nodes play (partial processing, hierarchical, connecting, etc.) be specified as detailed as possible if networks are to be useful to account for dysfunctional cognition or to allow for useful predictions.

With all of these factors considered, there are multiple combinations of neural regions to support cognitive functions. The previous combinations are delineated to demonstrate the possible complexity that can belie networks and that the role each node plays in the network need to be defined as best possible. This complexity also leads to the limited number of CAUs that can be presently described.

Lesions to one of the nodes in the network can lead to partial impairment of the performance of that cognitive operation and a partial deficit in the execution of the cognitive task of which the particular cognitive operation was a part. The following discussion describes in general principles conclusions about networks that can be derived from lesions.

Damage to a Network

Clinical manifestations of lesions in the different nodes of a network are determined by three core factors: which node is interfered with, which subpopulation of neurons within that node or its connecting axons are destroyed, and what cognitive functions that node might perform on its own or might contribute to with other nodes. A cortical lesion affecting a node may thus be expected to have a major impact not only because the lesion disrupts the unique set of cognitive operations in which that node is involved to varying degrees but also because it affects the widespread connections throughout the particular distributed network for which that cortical area serves as connecting nodes. Disrupting a single node in a network can then lead to a host of complex deficits.

Models of Nodal Damage in a Network

Networks can consist of nodes that are characteristic of a CAU where lesioning a node consistently disrupts one key cognitive function (Figure 1.14). In Catani et al.'s (2012) model, this type of network is referred to as a holistic network. In addition, another type of "pure" network is parallel distributed encoding of cognitive units in nodes, which is represented in Figures 1.14E and 1.14F. In this model, each node is contributing only an incomplete aspect of a cognitive operation; the summed contribution of all the nodes in the network is required to completely perform the specific operation. A lesion of a node then affects only part of the performance of the operation in which the network is engaged and can result in a general type of degradation of that operation's performance.

It is also very important to consider that a lesion to a node in this type of network may result in remote effects in other tasks that this node is partially engaged with. This type of "remote deficit" that occurs from a brain region that on the surface appears to have no relationship to regions typically performing a task is referred to as *diaschisis* (Nomura et al., 2010). These types of network models can provide a clear account of why a lesion located far away in the brain from where one would associate with a specific cognitive operation can still affect that cognitive operation. It is due to the fact that a node that is damaged may function in multiple networks, particularly those networks that require multiple nodes to perform a cognitive operation.

The other type of model to consider for nodes in a network is the associationist network, in which each node performs one cognitive function, needs no assistance to perform it, and also functions as a connector node. Thus, a lesion to that node not only will lead to a loss of function that the affected node subsumes (black circle in the diagram in Figure 1.14) but also will secondarily affect to some degree those nodes to which it is connected because communication no longer passes through the connection provided by that node.

Having delineated these three network prototypes, which are only a subset of possible network organizations, the picture of predicting the effects of a lesion on a network node becomes more complex. The level of complexity increases even higher when a network has nodes in it that are a mix of the three types of nodes described in these prototypes. For example, there can be a network in which some nodes function as holistic-type nodes (similar to the CAU units described), some are distributed types, and some are connector types.

Focal pure cortical lesions are rare and usually are the result of a small stroke due to a blockage in a small cortical artery or a brain neoplasm (tumor or metastasis) that spare long white matter fibers. Many lesions involve both cortical and subcortical structures as well as short and long white fiber tracts, which typically can result in widespread dysfunction, especially because disruption in the white matter connections in the network can be as detrimental as lesions to nodes, as detailed next.

White Matter Damage in a Network

In a network framework, one must consider areas other than nodes that can be damaged by a brain lesion and result in cognitive dysfunction. One of the key sets of structures to consider is the bidirectional white matter tracts that function to connect

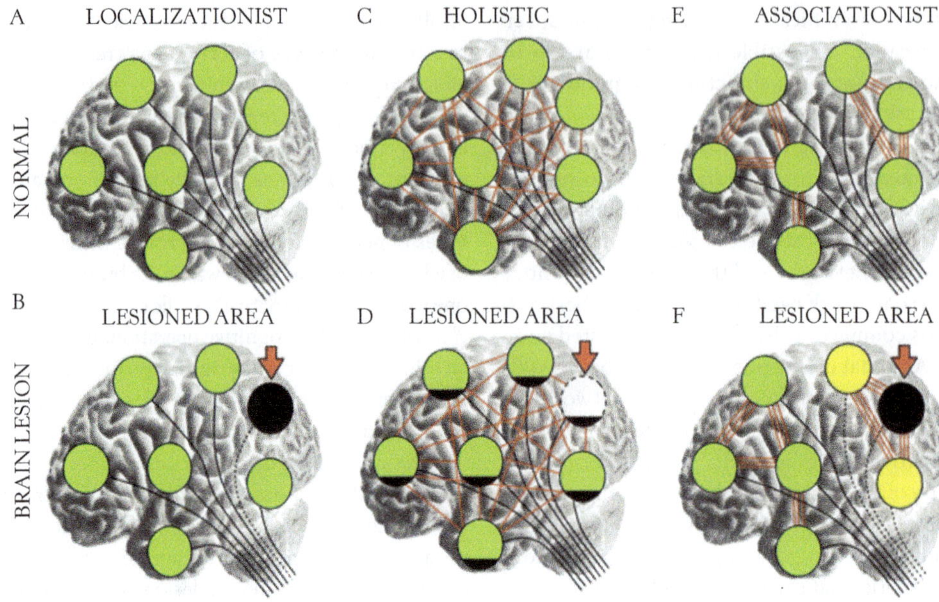

FIGURE 1.14: Theories of brain function and consequences of a discrete cortical lesion. (A and B) Localizationist models give little importance to interregional connections because each function is carried out by discrete independent regions, whose damage (black) results in a complete loss of a specific function leaving the others intact. Hence, localization of symptoms corresponds to localization of functions. (C and D) Holistic models consider all regions as mutually interconnected through a network of homogeneously distributed association fibers. Cognitive functions are the result of the simultaneous activity of all regions acting as a whole through the association pathways. In case of damage to one area (white), the network allows the redistribution of the lost function to the undamaged brain regions. It follows that for holistic approaches, function cannot be localized with clinical–anatomical correlative methods because the symptoms result from the loss of a "quantity" of cerebral cortex rather than a localized area. (E and F) Associationist models consider the brain organized in parallel distributed networks around cortical epicenters. Primary sensory and motor functions are localized (Hatsopoulos, 2010; Penfield & Boldrey, 1937; Plow et al., 2010), but higher cognitive functions are distributed within large-scale networks. Discrete lesions cause loss of specialized functions, whereas complex cognitive functions cannot be localized within single areas. A cortical lesion causes functional loss of the damaged area (black) and partial dysfunction of other interconnected regions (yellow).

Source: Catani et al. (2012).

the nodes in a network. There are a variety of white matter connections between nodes in a network. To illustrate these principles, Catani and ffytche (2005) proposed a framework for two specialized cortical regions that would represent types of nodes (see Figure 1.13). In Figure 1.13, territories are simplified as being composed of two specialized areas or subregions. It is unclear whether different specialized subregions are always anatomically distinct within a node, overlap, or are scattered patches of neurons. Irrespective, the predominant intraterritorial connections between nodes and parts of nodes are likely to be U-shaped association fibers. Tractography evidence suggests that more distant territories are connected by multiple parallel long association fiber pathways. It has been difficult to determine clearly the impact that disruptions to the subcortical U-fibers, which are short-range connections between nodal regions, have on network processing. This will improve with better specification of the type of functions that nodes subserve and specification of the role of subregions of neurons within nodes.

White matter long tract lesions disrupting connections between distant cortical regions can be dysfunctional due to a failure or excess of transfer of outputs from one area to another. The impact of disruption to these connections can be delineated in terms of performance disruption because these can lead to nodal disconnection. Tasks that require continuous, two-way communication and cooperation between nodes (e.g., synchronous bidirectional coordination) can be greatly disrupted by a white matter lesion—even if the gray matter nodes are intact—due to the disconnection of the flow of information between nodes. Of interest, although there may be a profound disruption of performance when the white matter tract separating two nodes is lesioned, it applies only to tasks requiring both connected nodes. If one of these nodes is involved in other networks supporting other tasks in which the white matter connections are not damaged, then performance for that task network will be perfectly intact (this represents a form of diaschisis; Nomura et al., 2010; Price et al., 2001).

Thus far, mostly loss of function with white matter lesions of networks has been discussed; however, this is not the only finding that can occur with network white matter lesions. Lesions can also result in phenomena known as white matter hyperconnectivity and cortical hyperfunction, in which there is an overactivity of the output of a network. These dysfunctions can include positive symptoms, such as face hallucinations related to the hyperexcitibility and spontaneous activation of face-specialized cortex (ffytche et al., 1998).

Overall, one can see that the network approach to cognition can be quite powerful. Networks, and all of the varieties of nodes and connections that can be linked together in them, can account for performance of an unlimited number of cognitive tasks. These networks also allow for accounting for individual variability in both cognitive functions and anatomic organization across individuals. However, as can be seen by the descriptions, there can be numerous modes of performance that can occur from lesioning a network model.

ROLE OF FUNCTIONAL IMAGING STUDIES

Many of the studies discussed with regard to both determining CAUs and delineating networks have been performed based on the findings of functional imaging studies. At this point, it is appropriate to frame the role these studies play in this text. For our approach to establishing that an anatomic region is essential to the cognitive operation, we are requiring a corroborating lesion study. However, there are those who would rely only on fMRI activation studies. The proliferation of functional neuroimaging gave rise to activation studies, which are studies in which a cognitive task is performed while the subject is in an MRI scanner. Given the role of these studies in localizing cognitive functions, the logic behind how these studies are performed, what they measure, and how their findings can be incorporated into helping establish consistent brain–behavior correlations is explained next.

For typical structural MRI of the brain, the RF signals received in the MRI collector are used to construct corresponding brain regions to specific signals. For fMRI, a patient performs a task in the MR scanner while RF signals are being collected. The RF target for the fMRI technique is blood, and thus a marker of blood oxygenation level-dependent (BOLD) response is the target of the RF signal collection. BOLD is a marker of neuronal metabolism based on the principle that neurons that are becoming more active require nutrients from blood rapidly to support their energy requirements. As part of this hemodynamic energy response, active neurons will extract oxygen quickly from the blood. This leaves in the region of the active neurons more oxyhemoglobin compared to deoxyhemoglobin, with each of these displaying different magnetic properties. This variation in magnetic signal can be detected using MRI to obtain what is referred to as the BOLD signal for each voxel. When one compares the BOLD signal during task performance within a voxel to the BOLD signal in that same voxel during a baseline or compared to that of another task or a baseline, one can determine regions that are more "active" during the targeted task performance and refer to these as task-related signal change. As experimental design has improved, the comparisons (one task to another task, a task to a baseline, etc.) have enabled investigators to focus on isolating regions associated with specific cognitive operations.

These BOLD signals are indirect measures of neuronal activity, not absolute measures of neuronal activation. In addition, these indirect measures are relative in that they reflect an increase in activity compared to some baseline or comparison task. Although these are limitations that have been addressed with a variety of statistical approaches, it is important to keep in mind when interpreting results from these activation studies that the signal changes detected with fMRI are typically derived from comparing increased signals on one condition to those of another condition.

It bears repeating that these functional imaging studies identify brain regions associated with performing a cognitive task that are both involved with and essential to performing that task. Subtraction logic in the lesion–deficit model attempts to isolate those brain regions essential to performing the cognitive operation under study. This is because only those functions that cannot be performed are associated with the brain area identified as being damaged. Thus, there exists a complementary relationship between activation and lesion–deficit studies, where the lesion–deficit results can be used to determine which of the findings in an activation study are, if damaged, will result in a consistent decrement in the cognitive operation. As a consequence, these complementary techniques can provide a great deal of insight into CAUs. They may also provide useful insights into how CAUs function in processing streams.

LIMITATIONS

With the variety of nodes and connections that can be constructed to form a network model of task performance, there is little that networks cannot account for in the realm of cognition and behavior. Unfortunately, that also means that these models can be limited in their predictions. When a behavior is observed, a variety of lesions and various other adaptations within a network can conceivably account for the behavior. When the nodes, connections, and roles of these components of a network are thoroughly specified predictions can be more easily made based on a predetermined set of network parameters.

Most in the field of cognitive neuroscience agree that network processing may underlie a variety of cognitive tasks and behaviors. Assigning the roles of the components of these networks is the next major innovation that network models need in order to fill in the missing gaps in networks, making them more useful in practical application. This specification of networks and network components will be a huge thrust in cognitive neuroscience in the future, which will expand the applicability of network models.

Currently, the network models that have been most effective in accounting for task performance and in providing a more clear understanding of the neurobiology of cognition have been those in which the nodes are represented by CAUs, where the processing stream is more in line with serial processing, and the network processing model resembles the holistic network described previously and in Figure 1.14. Even in this setting—interpreting these models of multiple cognitive operations—there are certain conditions that lead to effectively delineating that a specific lesion has disrupted a given CAU: serial processing of cognitive operations, independence of CAUs, a lesion affecting only a single component of the network, and no reorganization/recovery of function.

Another key component to consider in determining whether a lesion is affecting a particular cognitive operation is ensuring that the task chosen for the patients to perform is a true reflection of their abilities. The lack of pre-lesion a priori testing in lesion patients limits the tasks to be assessed to only those tasks and stimuli that are of limited complexity and can be performed by the average individual. As a consequence, only cognitive operations that are common and believed to be ubiquitous are reported as consistent lesion–deficit correlations.

Although the previous limitations apply to the network organization of combining multiple nodes together with connections, there are also limitations that arise from the definition of the nodes that constitute a network. We have delimited that there are several types of nodes in terms of the cognitive functions in which they are engaged and the anatomic organization of the node. Each node needs to have clear delineation of these components if there is to be any useful account of what that node does normally and what may occur if it were lesioned. The nodes that allow for the best accounting of cognitive and behavioral performance are those that meet the criteria outlined for CAUs. The majority of what are described in this book, unless otherwise specified, are CAUs. However, it is acknowledged that a limitation is that CAUs are not the only way in which cognition and anatomy are organized. The aim of the anatomical specification field is to better account for these cognitive operations and their supporting anatomic structures in a manner that specifies the neural roles of the anatomic region other than "if it is lesioned, the cognitive operation is disrupted." This refined specification can occur at both the cognitive descriptive level and the anatomic specification level. Not all anatomical correlates of cognition are circumscribed delimited cortical regions that are within the spatial resolution of the currently available anatomical measurement tools. Thus, throughout the book, when a cognitive unit is accounted for by multiple anatomic regions that when lesioned result in a consistent deficit, these are also described as brain–behavior correlations and noted in the text along with the CAUs. One method to find deficits that might occur after lesioning specific nodes in a network is to assess performance after applying a temporary, safe technique such as repetitive transcranial magnetic stimulation to a node.

SUMMARY

Cognition and behavior are the most complex functions that the human brain performs. As a result, models that account for cognitive operations range from more straightforward brain–behavior correlations to rather complex ones. Determining what brain regions are associated consistently with cognition and behavior requires a series of conditions being met and a number of variables minimized. The variables best minimized for making the optimal brain–behavior correlations include, but are not limited to, the following: (1) no compensatory or recovery strategies that occur after a lesion happens, (2) independence, (3) serial processing, (4) the same gyral pattern and size of brain for all participants in a study, (5) a discrete brain region subserving an entire cognitive process (e.g., CAU), and (6) the entire anatomic region is responsible for just the one cognitive function that the region supports. These are just optimal, not required conditions. A range of conditions exist where CAUs are identified, it just requires that all conditions and assumptions are carefully considered.

The definable CAU was developed where there was a delineated cognitive unit associated with an isolatable, circumscribed anatomic region. These have been developed via a "matching process" involved with the unit of cognitive operation and the anatomical region isolated by structural imaging or autopsy. It is acknowledged that the delineation of cognitive units continues to evolve, and the scales of size and anatomic resolution are not uniform for the anatomic units. Therefore, there is a great deal of heterogeneity in the CAUs in terms of scope of cognitive function performed and anatomic substrate.

Given the approximately 120 years of study, the findings reported here are ones that have been shown to be consistently present across multiple studies. In many cases, these cognitive anatomic correlations were confirmed by both activation studies (fMRI and PET) and lesion studies. There are others that are not included due to inconsistent reports from studies on the correlation, an insufficient number of reports to date to support a consistent association, and/or differing accounts of the findings.

Network models consisting of nodes (CAUs and other cognitive–brain correlation units) and connections (white matter pathways, nodes, etc.) can be constructed to link together cognitive anatomic units to account for task performance. There are localizationist network models consisting predominantly of CAUs; holistic networks that are more consistent with nodes that each contribute to a cognitive operation (distributed processing); and associationist networks in which nodes account for all of a cognitive operation like CAUs but also function as connectors to other nodes so that lesions affect both a cognitive operation and the link to the cognitive operation of other nodes.

Accordingly, the aforementioned accounts of processing models may all exist and also may exist as a combination of aspects of each model in one network. Thus, the entire cognitive system in the brain is not conducive to a simplistic one-processing-model account. It is acknowledged that the brain–behavior relationships as a whole exist as a hybrid of multiple models of cognitive processing and neural encodings in brain regions associated with cognition—from a discrete circumscribed brain region with a specific function to a spatially and temporally distributed network of neurons.

The importance of these CAU findings and the reasons to study them are twofold. First, this basic set of behavioral–anatomic correlations is the foundation on which to build more complex maps of cognition–brain relationships. Second, these correlations are reliable to the point that they are essentially the basis of the field of behavioral and cognitive neurology and are consistently used to diagnose and localize lesions in the brain based on behavioral testing. Thus, the true test of these findings has been the reliability of these localizations to make clinical localizations and lead to successful medical decision-making.

REFERENCES

Bates, E., Wilson, S., Saygin, A., Dick, F., Sereno, M., Knight, R., et al. (2003). Voxel-based lesion-symptom mapping. *Nature Neuroscience, 6*(5), 448–450.

Brier, M., Ferree, T., Maguire, M., Moore, P., Spence, J., Tillman, G., et al. (2010). Frontal theta and alpha power and coherence changes are modulated by semantic complexity in Go/NoGo tasks. *International Journal of Psychophysiology, 78*(3), 215–224.

Buszaki, G. (2006). *Rhythms of the brain.* Oxford, England: Oxford University Press.

Catani, M., Dell'Acqua, F., Bizzi, A., Forkel, S., Williams, S., Simmons, A., et al. (2012). Beyond cortical localization in clinico-anatomical correlation. *Cortex, 48,* 1262–1287.

Catani, M., & ffytche, D. (2005). The rises and falls of disconnection syndromes. *Brain, 128*, 2224–2239.

ffytche, D., Howard, R., Brammer, M., David, A., Woodruff, P., & Williams, S. (1998). The anatomy of conscious vision: An fMRI study of visual hallucinations. *Nature Neuroscience, 1*(8), 738–742.

Geschwind, N. (1965). Disconnexion syndromes in animals and man. *Brain, 88*, 237–294, 585–644.

Gray, C., Engel, A., König, P., & Singer, W. (1992). Synchronization of oscillatory neuronal responses in cat striate cortex: Temporal properties. *Visual Neuroscience, 8*(4), 337–347.

Hart, J., Jr., Anand, R., Zoccoli, S., Maguire, M., Gamino, J., Tillman, G., et al. (2007). Neural substrates of semantic memory. *Journal of the International Neuropsychological Society, 13*(5), 865–880.

Hatsopoulos, N. (2010). Columnar organization in the motor cortex. *Cortex, 46*(2), 270–271.

Hillis, A. (2005). Brain/language relationships identified with diffusion and perfusion MRI: Clinical applications in neurology and neurosurgery. *Annals of the New York Academy of Sciences, 1064*, 149–161.

Hinton, G. E. (1981). Implementing semantic networks in parallel hardware. In G. E. Hinton & J. A. Anderson (Eds.), *Parallel models of associative memory*. Hillsdale, NJ: Erlbaum.

Klimesch, W. (2012). α-Band oscillations, attention, and controlled access to stored information. *Trends in Cognitive Science, 16*(12), 606–617.

Lesser, R., Crone, N., & Webber, W. (2011). Using subdural electrodes to assess the safety of resections. *Epilepsy & Behavior, 20*(2), 223–229.

Nomura, E., Gratton, C., Visser, R., Kayser, A., Perez, F., & D'Esposito, M. (2010). Double dissociation of two cognitive control networks in patients with focal brain lesions. *Proceedings of the National Academy of Sciences of the USA, 107*, 12017–12022.

Penfield, W., & Boldrey, E. (1937). Somatic motor and sensory representation in the cerebral cortex of man as studied by electrical stimulation. *Brain, 60*, 389–443.

Plow, E., Arora, P., Pline, M., Binenstock, M., & Carey, J. (2010). Within-limb somatotopy in primary motor cortex—revealed using fMRI. *Cortex, 46*(3), 310–321.

Price, C., Warburton, E., Moore, C., Frackowiak, R., & Friston, K. (2001). Dynamic diaschisis: Anatomically remote and context-sensitive human brain lesions. *Journal of Cognitive Neuroscience, 13*, 419–429.

Slotnick, S., Moo, L., Kraut, M., Lesser, R., & Hart, J. (2002). Thalamic modulation of cortical rhythms during semantic memory recall in humans. *Proceedings of the National Academy of Sciences of the USA, 99*(9), 6440–6443.

Stanley, M., Moussa, M., Paolini, B., Lyday, R., Burdette, J., & Laurienti, P. (2013). Defining nodes in complex brain networks. *Frontiers in Computational Neuroscience, 7*, 169.

Wessinger, C., Van Meter, J., Tian, B., Van Lare, J., Pekar, J., & Rauschecker, J. (2001). Hierarchical organization of the human auditory cortex revealed by functional magnetic resonance imaging. *Journal of Cognitive Neuroscience, 13*(1), 1–7.

2

Basic Neuroanatomy Review

The following is a review of the neuroanatomy that is considered to be the most relevant to cognition. Neuroanatomy is not easily learned by reading a text because it is a three-dimensional (3-D) set of relationships. This text assumes some background in neuroanatomy and is not a substitute as an initial comprehensive presentation of neuroanatomy. If one is unfamiliar with neuroanatomy, there will be a reasonable amount of memorization required or at least use of this chapter as a reference to locate regions when anatomic references are made in later chapters.

Although knowledge of the locations of anatomic regions is essential to understanding neuroanatomy, understanding the connections between regions and how regions interact with each other provides the optimal grasp of neuroanatomy. This 3-D grasp of how regions are related in space to each other and interconnect will allow for the optimal understanding of how cognitive–anatomic units (CAUs) connect and interrelate to perform a task. Having a 3-D model in hand while going through this chapter may greatly aid in both grasping the localization of regions and understanding their connections.

The key neuroanatomic structures that are most commonly associated with cognitive processing and behavior are the cerebral cortex, white matter, and subcortical nuclei. One approach of a 3-D conceptualization of the brain is to start with the most deep and midline structures and build layers on top of them. That starting point is the subcortical nuclei. Overlaying these structures are the white matter connections, and then the most external layer is the cortices of the frontal, parietal, temporal, and occipital lobes. If you keep this layering model in mind, it provides both a structural organization on how to envision the neuroanatomic regions and a clearer understanding of how regions are connected and communicate with each other. The layers chosen anatomically also segregate three general functional divisions (cortex—cognitive processing and representation, white matter—connections, and subcortical nuclei—relay and control circuits). We will revisit and elaborate on this layering of brain regions as a guide to organizing and learning neuroanatomy.

Before describing these anatomic structures, some basic principles describing directions and orientation of brain structures are established. Many of the anatomic figures used in this text are from radiological images, and thus brain orientation and directionality are explained as applied in that framework.

Figure 2.1 demonstrates the lateral view of the human brain with the directional terms used to orient one in relative terms to a particular brain region. Regions located more at the front of the brain are referred to as anterior (or rostral) in location (direction of forehead), with the back of the brain referred to as the posterior (or caudal) direction. The top of the brain is referred to as the superior (or dorsal) direction (toward the crown of the head), with the bottom of the brain being the inferior (or ventral) direction. Regions that are more toward the midline of the brain are referred to as more medial, and those toward the outside (nearest cortex) of the brain are said to be more lateral.

Most of the images of the brain presented in this book are from magnetic resonance imaging (MRI) or computed tomography (CT) scans. The presentation of the MRI images varies depending on the orientation in which the brain is "sliced" when the image was acquired or "re-sliced" to assess structures from a different perspective. The typical view in which most MRI/CT images are acquired and presented is the axial view, in which the images are oriented through the brain from anterior to posterior that is parallel to the ground if a person is standing upright (Figure 2.2).

Sagittal images are vertically oriented from superior to inferior with the plane of the slices

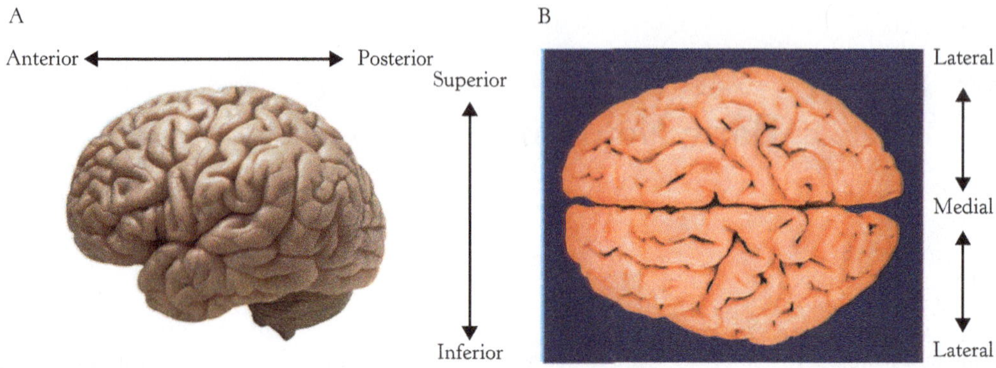

FIGURE 2.1: Labels for directional orientation used in referring to brain structures. Anterior (rostral) refers to being more toward the front (forehead) aspect of the brain, with posterior (caudal) toward the back of the brain and head. Superior (dorsal) refers to the topward direction of the brain (crown of the head) and inferior (ventral) toward the bottom of the brain. When referring to more midline brain structures, the term medial is used. The term lateral is used to refer to the outside aspects of the brain, toward cortical areas.

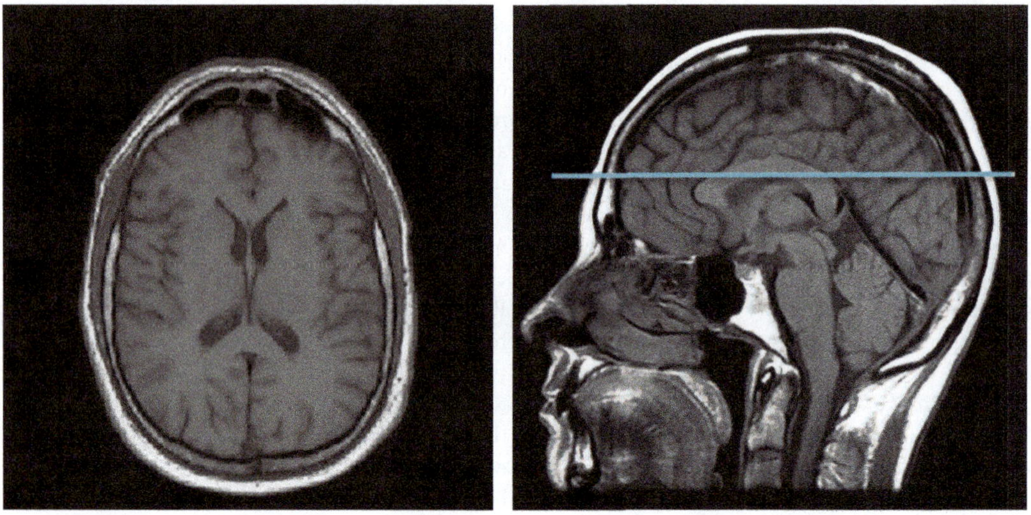

FIGURE 2.2: The left image shows the axial view of the brain. The right image shows a side view of the brain; the blue line designates the plane through the brain that the axial slice is oriented.

dividing the brain into right and left halves (Figure 2.3). Another common orientation is referred to as the coronal plane, which is oriented vertically from superior to inferior but compared to the sagittal is oriented to slice the brain from front to back (Figure 2.4).

There is one additional point to consider when viewing MRI images in this text and elsewhere. If the MRI images are in "radiological" convention, then the right side of the images is actually depicting the left side of the brain. Standard or conventional orientation has the left side of the brain represented on the left side of the image. When a figure is in radiological orientation, it is noted in the figure legend. If there is no notation, then the image is in conventional orientation.

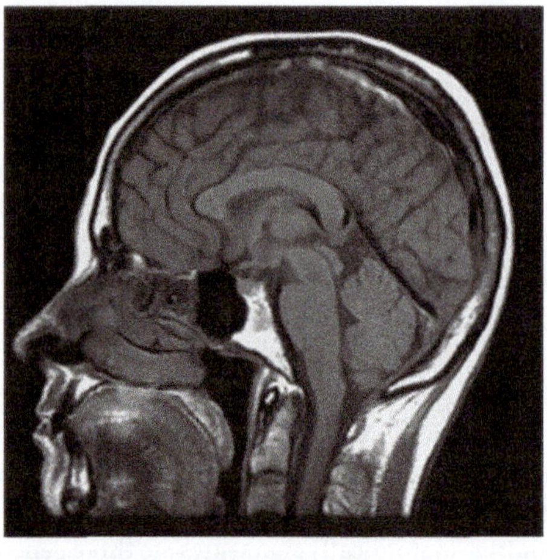

FIGURE 2.3: This orientation is the sagittal axis view of the brain.

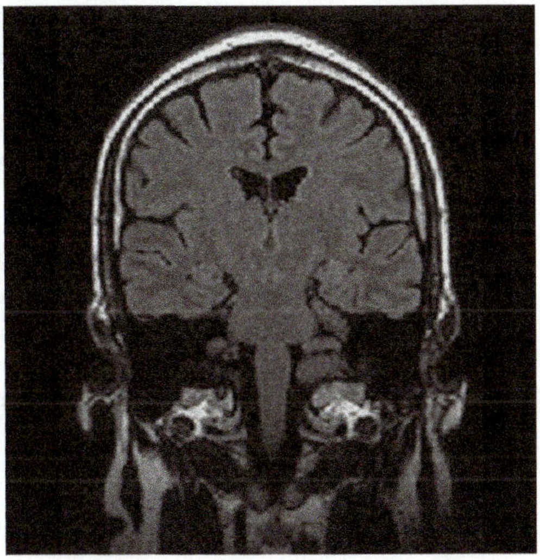

FIGURE 2.4: Coronal orientation view of the brain.

BRAIN LOBES

The basic organization used in this text for cognition is cortex, white matter, and subcortical structures. The organization of the cortex is discussed first, beginning with a description of the general organization of the brain into two halves, or hemispheres, split down the middle of the brain from the anterior to posterior aspects, dividing it into two relatively equal halves—the right and left hemispheres. Each hemisphere is divided into four lobes: the frontal, parietal, temporal, and occipital lobes (Figure 2.5). Each of these lobes consists of gyri, which are outfoldings of cerebral cortex consisting of gray matter and its adjacent, underlying white matter. When two gyri meet, the contour that forms between them is referred to as a sulcus (Figure 2.6). Each lobe and its gyral/sulcal organization are discussed in the following sections.

Frontal Lobe

The frontal lobes (one in the right hemisphere and the other in the left) are in the most anterior aspect of the brain, the largest brain lobes, and typically support higher-order cognitive functions controlling numerous cognitive control operations. The frontal lobe is bordered on the posterior aspect by the central sulcus, which separates it from the parietal lobe, and inferiorly by the Sylvian fissure, which is its border separating it from the temporal lobe (see Figure 2.5).

In the posterior aspect of the frontal lobe, there are two prominent vertically oriented gyri, one in front of the other—the motor cortex, referred to as the precentral gyrus because it is just in front of the central sulcus, and the premotor cortex, which lies just anterior to the precentral gyrus (Figure 2.7).

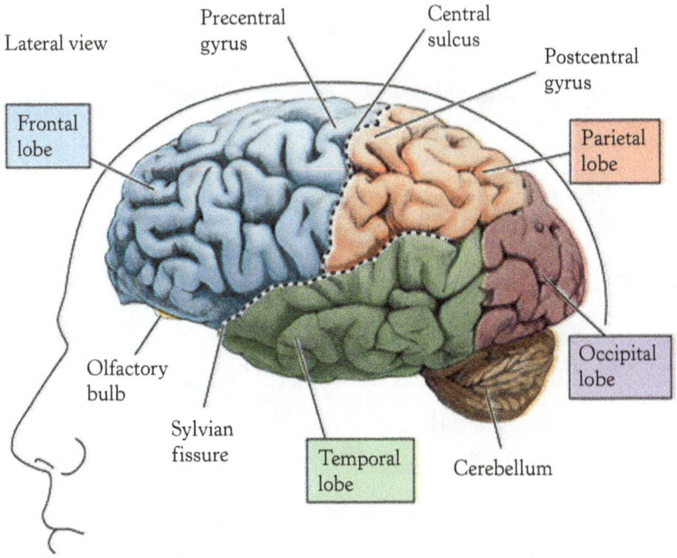

FIGURE 2.5: Lateral view of the brain separated into lobes. The frontal lobe is separated from the parietal lobe by the north–south-oriented central sulcus. The central sulcus extends from the superior aspect of the brain inferiorly to the Sylvian fissure. The horizontally oriented Sylvian fissure separates the temporal lobe from both the frontal and parietal lobes. The parietal lobe is separated from the occipital lobe by the horizontally oriented parieto-occipital sulcus.

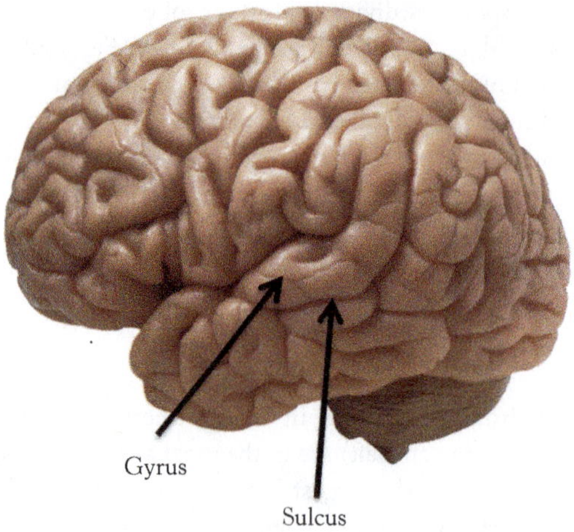

FIGURE 2.6: A gyrus, depicted in the photo of a brain, is the rounded, elevated convolutions on the surfaces of the cerebral hemispheres of the brain. A sulcus is the crevice between two gyri.

The motor cortex encodes the motor functions for the opposite side of the body and is organized by body region, referred to as the homunculus (Figure 2.8). The homunculus demonstrates what part of the body is represented for its motor control by a specific region of the motor cortex. In general, the face and mouth region is located at the most inferior aspect of the gyrus, the hand in the middle, and the leg at the most superior aspect. The largest part of the motor cortex is dedicated to the part of the body that requires the most motor control. Thus, the largest regions of the motor cortex are dedicated to the tongue, face, and hand, as would be expected considering the degree of complexity required to control the motor aspects of these regions. From a spatial perspective, starting at the most inferior aspect of the motor gyrus, the order of representation extending up superiorly is the tongue, face, hand, arm, hip, leg, and foot.

The premotor cortex, anterior to the motor cortex, aids in planning and preparation of motor movements. It follows the same general orientation as the motor cortex, and the functions of planning for motor movement for each body region align in the same general location where that body region is located in the motor cortex.

Anterior to the premotor gyrus are three horizontally oriented gyri that extend up to the most anterior aspects of the frontal lobe—the superior, middle, and inferior frontal gyri (Figure 2.9). A key

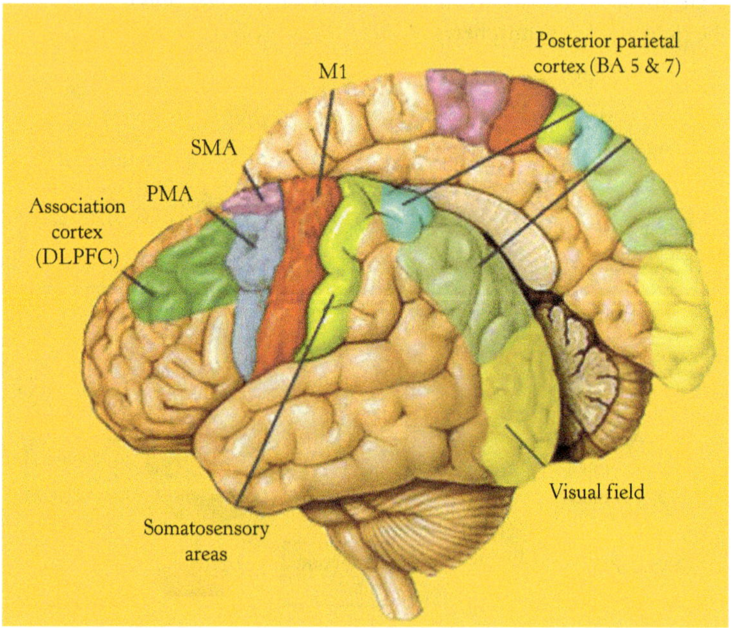

FIGURE 2.7: The red gyrus labeled M1 (to designate primary motor cortex) is the precentral gyrus that encodes for primary motor system control. The light blue gyrus labeled PMA is the premotor gyrus. The purple region at the top of the premotor gyrus is the supplementary motor area (SMA). The green area designates the dorsolateral prefrontal cortex (DLPFC).

Source: http://brainmaps.com.

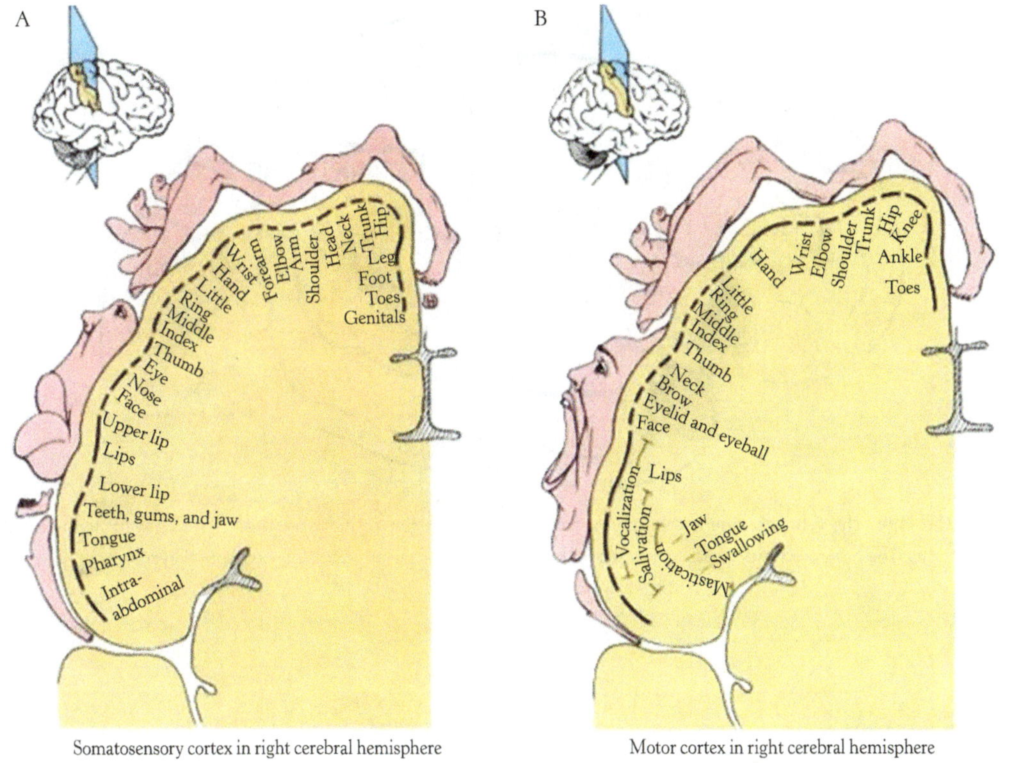

FIGURE 2.8: The homunculus organization to the motor cortex. At the most inferior aspect of the gyrus are the representations of the tongue and face region. Proceeding superiorly up the motor cortex, the hand, arm, hip, leg, and foot are represented in that order.

Source: http://harmonicresolution.com.

region in cognition is the most posterior aspect of the inferior frontal gyrus in the left hemisphere, referred to as Broca's area (Figure 2.10). This is the region described by Paul Broca in the 1890s as being associated with speech production, and it represents one of the first instances of a brain–behavior correlation.

Another region of the frontal lobe that is involved in cognitive operations is the dorsolateral prefrontal cortex (DLPFC). The DLPFC is not strictly defined anatomically by gyral/sulcal borders but, rather, has been delineated based on the functional activities associated with the region. Although there is not a clear definition for the boundaries of the DLPFC, it is generally postulated to include the middle frontal gyrus, including the lateral part of Brodmann area (BA) 9 and BA 46 (see the introduction to the Brodmann system later in this chapter; Figure 2.11). Other investigators have defined the borders of the DLPFC to include regions of BA 8, 9, and 10 (Cieslik et al., 2013). The DLPFC has been associated with a variety of cognitive control and other operations, including working memory, decision-making, planning, abstract reasoning, and inhibition.

The medial aspect of the frontal lobe consists of a prominent gyrus on its most inferior aspect—the cingulate gyrus (Figure 2.12). This gyrus lies directly on top of the largest white matter tract connecting the two hemispheres—the corpus callosum. The white matter fibers of the corpus callosum carry tracts that communicate between the cortices of the two hemispheres for mediating cognitive processes that require cross-hemispheric coordination. In addition, there are two superior medial cortical regions that are engaged directly or indirectly with cognitive functions—the supplementary motor area (SMA) and the pre-supplementary motor area (pre-SMA). The SMA lies just in front of the primary motor cortex and is engaged in the control of movement. The pre-SMA lies anterior to the SMA and is involved with planning of motor acts as well as several cognitive operations to be addressed later in this text.

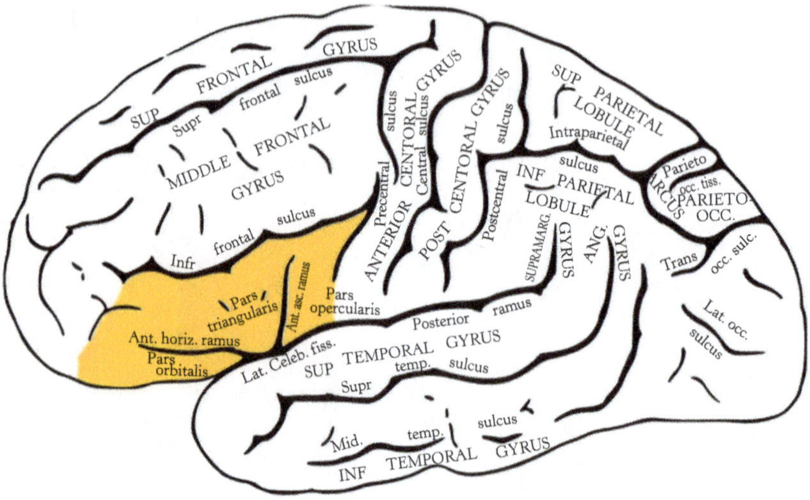

FIGURE 2.9: The yellow region is the inferior frontal gyrus. The horizontally oriented gyrus above it is the middle frontal gyrus. The horizontally oriented gyrus above the middle frontal gyrus is the superior frontal gyrus.

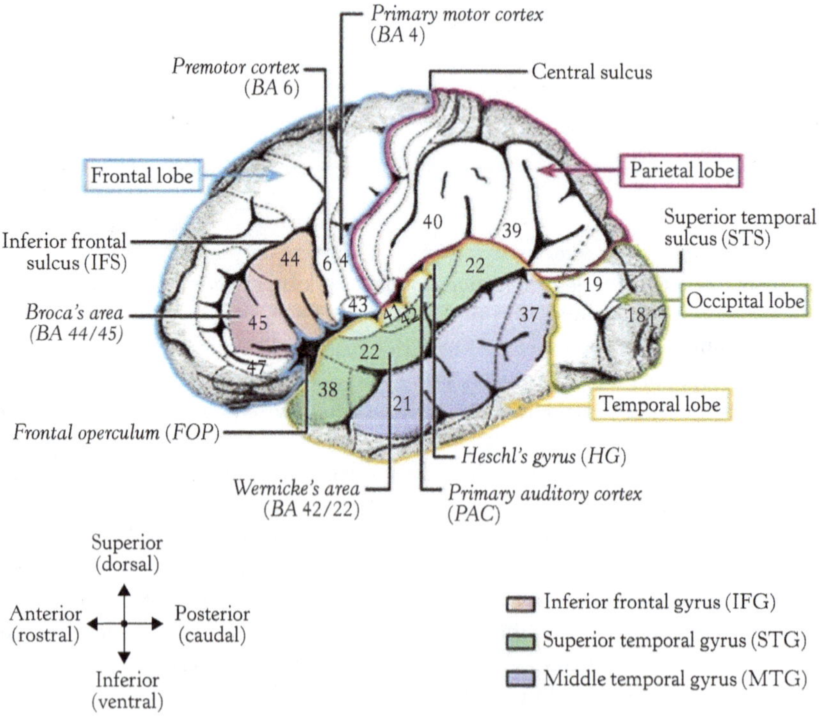

FIGURE 2.10: The purple region located at the posterior aspect of the left inferior frontal gyrus is termed Broca's area. It is in this region where the inferior frontal gyrus undulates upwards and downwards. The area marked 44, Brodmann's area 44, which is the posterior "curve" to the inferior frontal gyrus, is called the pars opercularis. Brodmann area 45, at the bottom of the next to the last curve of the inferior frontal gyrus, is called the pars triangularis. These two regions together constitute the majority of Broca's area.

Source: https://www.quora.com.

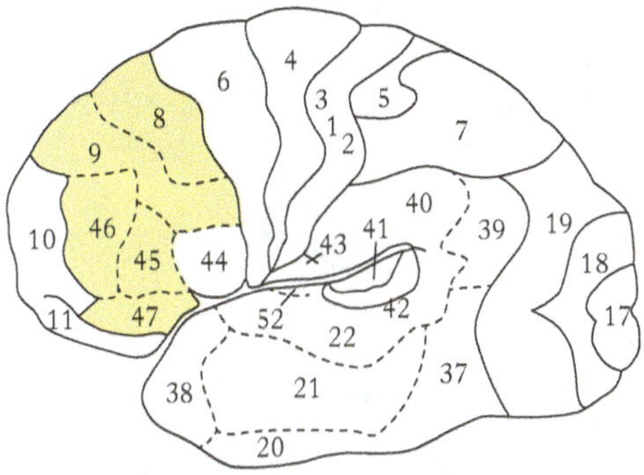

FIGURE 2.11: Regions that have been purported to be the DLPFC. It is a generally held belief that BA 9 and 46 constitute the DLPFC, but some have suggested that BA 8, 9, and 10 better represent the DLPFC.

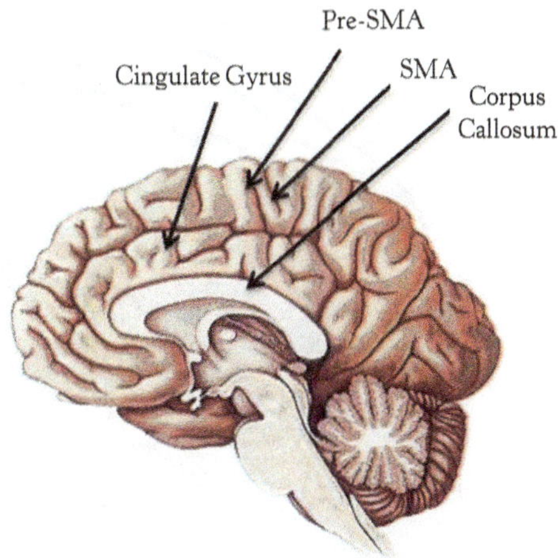

FIGURE 2.12: Medial aspects of the frontal lobe. The corpus callosum is the dominant white matter tract connecting the two hemispheres. Just superior to the corpus callosum is the horizontally oriented cingulate gyrus. The supplementary motor area (SMA) is a superior region just anterior to the motor cortex and is engaged in movement control. Anterior to the SMA is the pre-SMA, which is involved in planning motor acts and cognition.

The inferior aspects of the frontal lobes consist of four gyri—anterior, lateral, posterior, and medial orbitofrontal gyri (Figure 2.13). As a group, these gyri are also referred to as the ventromedial frontal lobe and play a key role in decision-making that is discussed in further detail later. Posterior to the orbitofrontal cortices lies the insular cortex, a region that when viewed from a lateral perspective lies underneath (medial to) the temporal and frontal lobes. The insular cortex has been imputed to be engaged in a variety of functions, most notably language- and speech-related functions as well as body awareness.

Parietal Lobe

The parietal lobe is delineated by three borders. It is separated from the frontal lobe on its anterior aspect by the central sulcus. Its inferior border dividing the parietal from the temporal lobe is the Sylvian fissure. The posterior border separating the parietal from the occipital lobe is the parieto-occipital sulcus (Figure 2.14).

The gyral pattern of the parietal lobe consists of the postcentral gyrus, which is at the anterior aspect of the parietal lobe and is oriented vertically. This region is also referred to as the primary somatosensory cortex because it encodes the sensory representations for touch for the opposite side of the body. Posterior to the somatosensory cortex is a region described collectively as the posterior parietal cortex. This general region is subdivided into the superior parietal lobule and the inferior parietal lobule, which are separated by the intraparietal sulcus. The inferior parietal lobule consists of two gyri of great significance in cognition—the supramarginal and

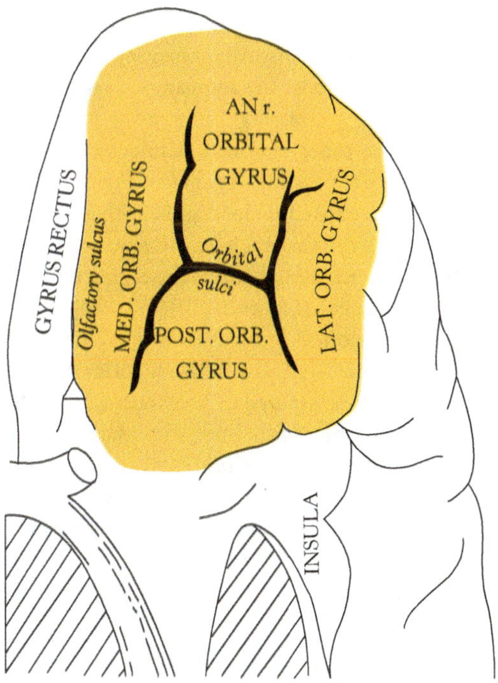

FIGURE 2.13: The inferior frontal lobe has four gyri: the anterior, posterior, medial, and lateral orbitofrontal gyri. Posterior to the orbitofrontal gyri is the insula. If the Sylvian fissure is separated, the insula can be seen underlying the superior temporal and inferior frontal gyri.

Source: http://www.wikipedia.org.

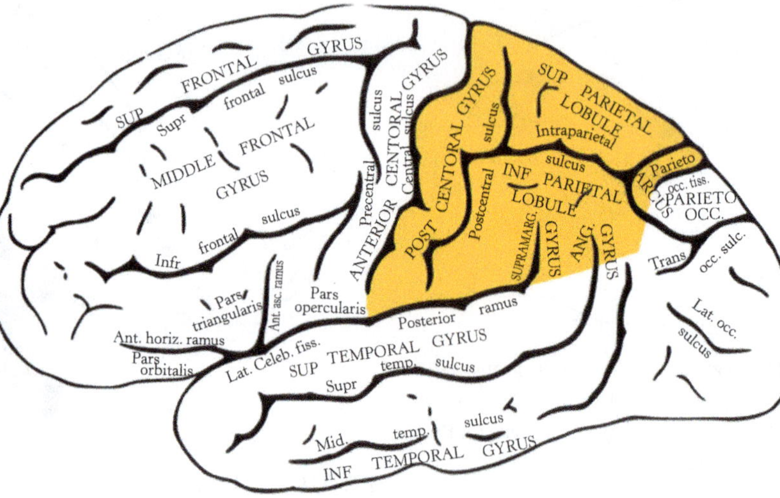

FIGURE 2.14: Gyri of the parietal lobe. The post-central gyrus is a vertically oriented region that encodes for somatosensory (touch) representations for the opposite side of the body. The inferior parietal lobule consists of the supramarginal gyrus, which wraps around the end of the Sylvian fissure, and the angular gyrus, which beings at the end of the superior temporal sulcus and extends up superiorly. The superior parietal lobule is situated above the intraparietal sulcus and is posteriorly bounded by the parieto-occipital sulcus.

Source: http://www.ruf.rice.edu/~lngbrain/cglidden/parietal.html.

angular gyri. The supramarginal gyrus wraps around the end of the Sylvian fissure connecting the temporal to the parietal lobe. The angular gyrus is situated posterior to the supramarginal gyrus as it starts at the end of the superior temporal sulcus extending superiorly into the parietal region (see Figure 2.14).

Another key structure for cognition that is medially located in the parietal lobe and is just superior to the parieto-occipital sulcus is the region referred to as the precuneus (Figure 2.15B). This region borders superiorly on the cuneus area of the occipital lobe and is considered part of the superior parietal lobule. It has been imputed to contribute to episodic and working memory functions, but it has received recent interest in studies of functional connectivity networks in the brain. It is one of the least well cognitively mapped areas in the cortex, mostly attributable to its deep location leaving it rarely damaged by either trauma or stroke.

Occipital Lobe

The occipital is the smallest lobe and is primarily responsible for visual processing. Although the gyral organization to the occipital lobe is covered here, it is typically and most effectively described using Brodmann area distinctions that are explained further later in this chapter.

The most posterior aspect of the occipital lobe is the primary visual cortex, also referred to as the striate cortex due to the striations in the cortices. This region encodes for the low-level (color, orientation, etc.) visual characteristics received directly from the optic radiations that transmit information derived originally from the peripheral visual system. Another name applied to the wedge-shaped region that encompasses the primary visual cortex (BA 17) is the cuneus, which is the region that extends from the parieto-occipital sulcus superiorly to the calcarine sulcus inferiorly (see Figure 2.15B).

The visual information processed in the primary visual cortex extends out to the visual association cortices neighboring the striate cortices, which are named the lateral occipital gyri. Information then proceeds inferiorly to the base of the occipital lobe. The gyri located in this region include the lingual gyrus, which is medial and anterior to lateral occipital gyri. The fusiform gyrus is lateral to the lingual gyrus, and the occipitotemporal gyrus is lateral to the fusiform gyrus (see Figure 2.15A). The fusiform gyrus extends anteriorly to become part of the temporal lobe. At its most anterior aspect, the fusiform gyrus lies between the inferior temporal (laterally) and the parahippocampal (medially) gyri.

These regions (lingual, fusiform, and occipitotemporal gyri) perform higher-order visual

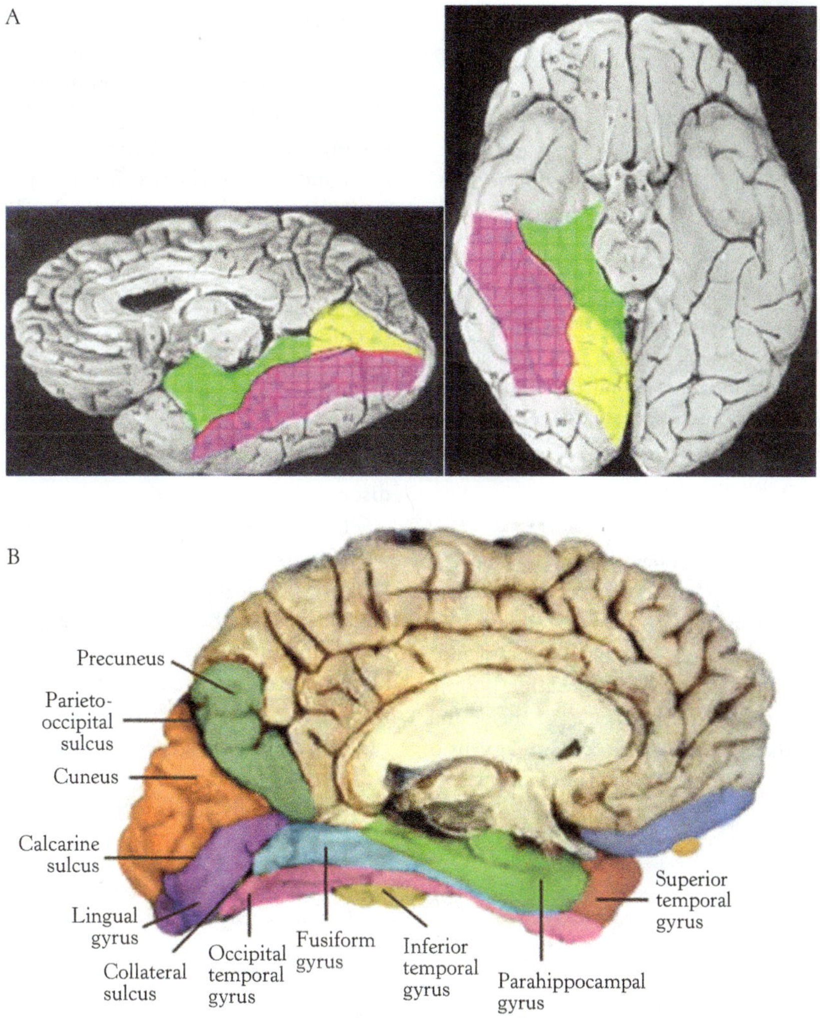

FIGURE 2.15: (A) Gyri of the medial and inferior occipital lobe. The yellow region is the lingual gyrus, the purple region is the fusiform gyrus, and the green region is the parahippocampal gyrus (part of the temporal lobe). (B) Medial view of the occipital lobe. The cuneus is colored orange and located at the posterior aspect of the occipital lobe and includes the primary visual cortex. Anterior to the cuneus at the most medial aspect is the lingual gyrus, with the fusiform gyrus immediately lateral and the occipito-temporal gyrus the most lateral.

processing from the previous analyses performed in the early visual cortices and have been referred to as the "what" system. The "what" system is the region where visual information is integrated to form whole object representations and where the visual memories for these objects are stored. There are further subdivisions of these regions that will be specified throughout the text.

The other method by which the visual system is segregated and described as opposed to gyri is via Brodmann areas. The BA numbers cross gyral boundaries but best describe the functional role each region plays in visual processing. Primary visual cortex is referred to as BA 17, with the regions proceeding more anteriorly being areas BA 18 and BA 19 (see Figure 2.26). As the BA numbers increase, the regions designated by them perform more complex visual processing.

Temporal Lobe

The temporal lobes from the lateral view have three horizontally oriented gyri—the superior, middle, and inferior temporal gyri (Figure 2.16). These regions, particularly in the left hemisphere, have been associated with language-related cognitive operations, with several key areas being associated

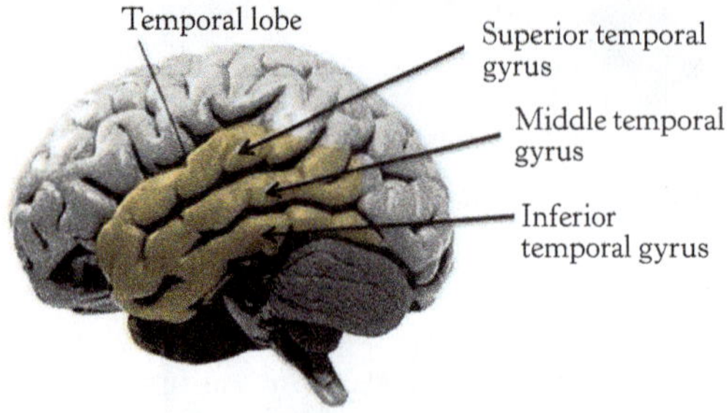

FIGURE 2.16: Lateral view of the temporal lobe. The horizontally oriented superior gyrus is the superior temporal gyrus, with the gyrus just inferior to it being the middle temporal gyrus and the most inferior gyrus being the inferior temporal gyrus.

Source: Cable News Network.

with specific cognitive operations. The superior temporal region is where the primary auditory cortex resides. This region encodes sounds that are delivered in raw form from the peripheral auditory system and processes the information in units that are organized by the frequency of the sound. It is referred to as the transverse temporal gyrus of Heschl and is located in the superior aspect of the superior temporal gyrus and tucked into the Sylvian fissure (BA 42). Another part of the superior temporal gyrus, the posterior and superior aspect, forms a region referred to as the planum temporale, which also plays a role in language-related auditory processing and is larger on the left than right side in most individuals (Figure 2.17). The surrounding cortices, referred to as secondary auditory association cortices, are where these basic frequencies are integrated into meaningful sounds.

Also localized at the most posterior aspect of the superior temporal gyrus is Wernicke's area. This region, described by Wernicke in the 1800s, has been associated with language comprehension and converting sounds to meaning (see Figure 2.10). More details of its role in cognitive operations are discussed in later chapters.

The basal surface of the temporal lobes consists of the hippocampus at its most medial aspect with the amygdala just anterior to it but still on the most medial aspect of the temporal lobe. The next gyrus lateral and inferior to the hippocampus is the parahippocampal gyrus, which extends from the temporal pole posteriorly back to the posterior aspect of the corpus callosum (Figure 2.18). The anterior aspect of the parahippocampal gyrus has a protrusion that projects medially and is called the uncus. Lateral to

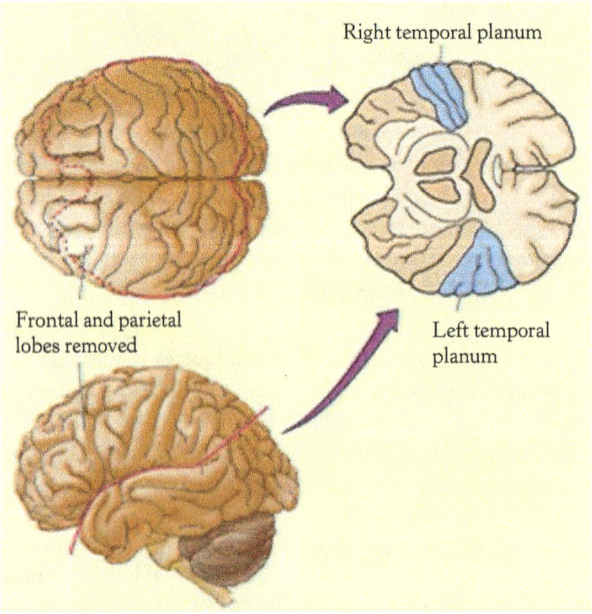

FIGURE 2.17: Location of the planum temporale. The brain drawings show the location and relative size of the planum temporale region of the superior aspect of the superior temporal gyri that has been implicated in language processing. The left planum temporale is typically larger than the right side.

Source: http://brainmind.com.

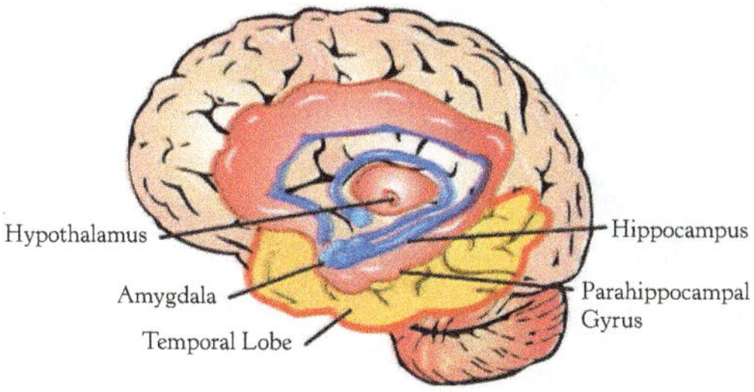

FIGURE 2.18: Caricature of the relative locations of the parahippocampal and hippocampal gyri. The parahippocampal gyrus lies adjacent to (inferior and lateral to) the hippocampus. The hippocampus lies in the medial aspect of the temporal lobe.

Source: http://medchrome.com.

the parahippocampal gyrus is the inferior temporal gyrus, with the border between these two gyri forming the junction of lateral and basal temporal lobe.

The hippocampus is divided into three parts—head, body, and tail. The head is referred to as the pes hippocampus. The body of the hippocampus extends medially, narrowing into the tail that disappears as a ventricular structure (Figure 2.18). The hippocampus, the parahippocampal gyrus, and other related structures form the hippocampal formation. These regions are essential to episodic memory functions and are disrupted in patients with amnesia and Alzheimer's disease.

These medial temporal lobe structures are discussed and described in more detail in Chapter 6.

Another key structure located in the temporal lobe that has a substantial impact on cognition and behavior is the amygdala. This almond-shaped structure, located immediately anterior to the pes hippocampus in the medial temporal lobe, is involved in memory and emotional responses such as arousal and fear.

SUBCORTICAL NUCLEI

The basal ganglia and thalamus are gray matter nuclei located deep in the brain and are supportive of numerous cognitive and behavioral operations. The following discussion does not detail all of the regions of these subcortical areas but, rather, highlights those that are most central to cognition and behavior.

Basal Ganglia

The basal ganglia consists of the striatum (caudate and putamen), globus pallidus (internal and external), substantia nigra, subthalamic nucleus, nucleus accumbens, and the ventral tegmental area (Figure 2.19). The caudate nucleus has a head and tail component, with the tail extending through the frontal gyrus and curving into the temporal lobe terminating next to the amygdala. The next most medial nucleus of the basal ganglia group is the globus pallidus. The globus pallidus is separated into two segments—an internal and an external segment. The putamen is the most lateral of the basal ganglia nuclei, lateral to the external segment of the globus pallidus. These three sets of nuclei have been shown to be engaged in cognitive control functions, procedural memory, and action selection.

Inferiorly (situated near the brain stem) and midline in location is another set of basal ganglia nuclei—the substantia nigra. The substantia nigra is located in the brain stem, midbrain region, and neighboring the cerebral peduncles, with its major function to provide dopamine via its projections to the basal ganglia (see Figure 2.19). This is the brain area that shows significant loss of dopamine neurons in patients with Parkinson's disease, resulting in motor dysfunction due to this lack of dopamine. Another deep basal ganglia nucleus is the subthalamic nucleus, which is located more inferior to the striatum and globus pallidus, inferior to the thalamus, and superior to the substantia nigra. It functions in mediating movements via its inputs to other basal ganglia structures. If unilaterally damaged, the patient develops a movement disorder termed hemiballismus. Degenerative changes in the subthalamic nucleus are associated with progressive supranuclear palsy, a progressive movement and cognitive disorder.

The substantia nigra's role is to provide dopamine input to the basal ganglia structures. The caudate and putamen receive input from the cortices, with outputs to other basal ganglia structures only. The role of the globus pallidus is to provide inhibitory motor control. The subthalamic nucleus projects to the globus pallidus while receiving input mainly from the cerebral cortex. With this rich set of interactions with other cortical and subcortical structures related to motor movements, it is important to note that these structures are also engaged in a vast array of cognitive operations and behaviors, including but not limited to cognitive control/executive functions, processing speed, coordination of cognitive and motor operations, procedural memory, motivation, and emotion processing.

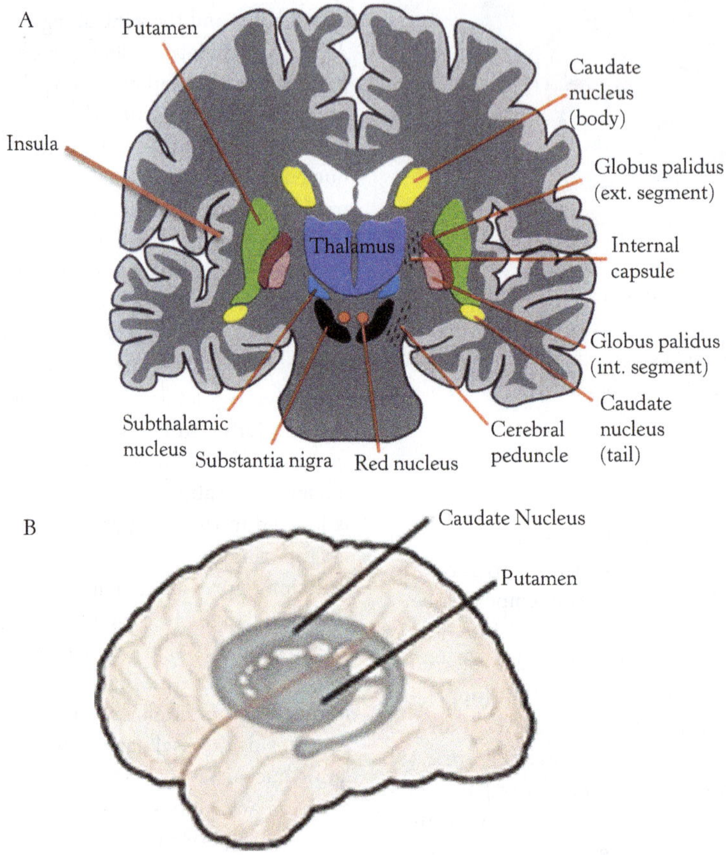

FIGURE 2.19: (A) Basal ganglia structures. The heads of the caudate nuclei are located next to ventricles and extend around in a curved manner to terminate at the amygdala. The middle set of nuclei are at the most medial aspect the internal segment of the globus pallidus, with the external segment of the globus pallidus being just lateral to that, and the most lateral of the group being the putamen. The subthalamic nucleus lies just inferior to the thalamus, and the substantia nigra is located in the midbrain. (Note that the thalamus, red nucleus, and cerebral peduncle are not part of the basal ganglia.) (B) Caricature of the caudate nucleus. The caudate consists of the head, body, and tail. The head starts at the superior and anterior aspect of the caudate, with the body encompassing the extent of the curved aspect of the caudate and the tail terminating at the amygdala.

Thalamus

The thalamus, known as the brain's relay station, is a set of nuclei located centrally in the brain between the cerebral cortex and midbrain. The thalamus maintains an extensive set of connections between its numerous nuclei and the cerebral cortices, providing a rich set of bidirectional circuits. One set of major functions of the thalamus is to relay sensory and/or motor signals to cortical structures. Other functions subsumed by the thalamus and its cortical connections are to relay synchronizing rhythms from the brain stem to mediate sleep/wake states, level of alertness, and aspects of cognition.

Some of the major nuclei of the thalamus act purely as relays of sensory perceptual information to their cortical end target region. For example, the lateral geniculate nucleus acts as a relay nucleus between the retina to the primary visual cortex. The medial geniculate nucleus functions as an auditory relay between midbrain structures and primary auditory cortex. Ventral posterior nucleus is a relay to somatosensory cortex.

Several of the nuclei of the thalamus play essential roles in behavior and cognition (Figures 2.20 and 2.21). The dorsomedial nucleus is associated with episodic memory via its connections to medial temporal lobe and frontal lobe structures. The pulvinar nucleus has widespread connections to visual, posterior parietal, cingulate, and prefrontal cortices and is associated with a variety of

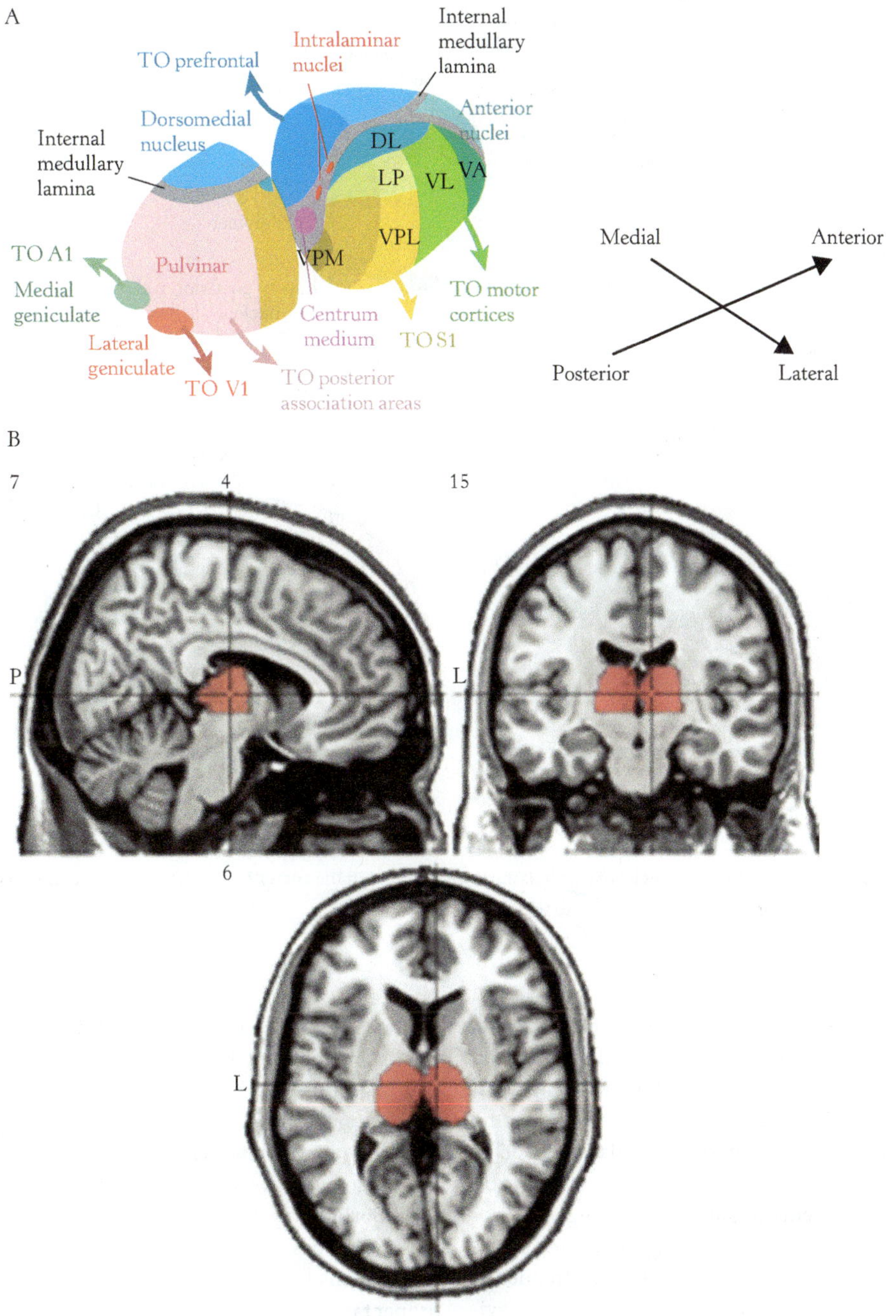

FIGURE 2.20: (A) Depiction of thalamic nuclei and their destination outputs. With regard to cognition and behavior, the most relevant nuclei are the dorsomedial (blue; connecting to prefrontal and medial temporal areas), pulvinar (pink; connecting to posterior association cortices and cingulate and prefrontal cortices), anterior (green; connecting to mammillary bodies and cingulate), and dorsal lateral nuclei (aqua; connecting to visual and parietal cortices). (B) MR images in sagittal, coronal, and axial orientation depicting in red the location of the thalamus.

cognitive functions, including attention, memory, and higher-order visual processing. The anterior nuclei play a key role in learning and memory due to their connections with the mammillary bodies and cingulate gyrus. The dorsal lateral nucleus receives input from visual cortex and has output to parietal cortices that are engaged in emotion and behavioral functions.

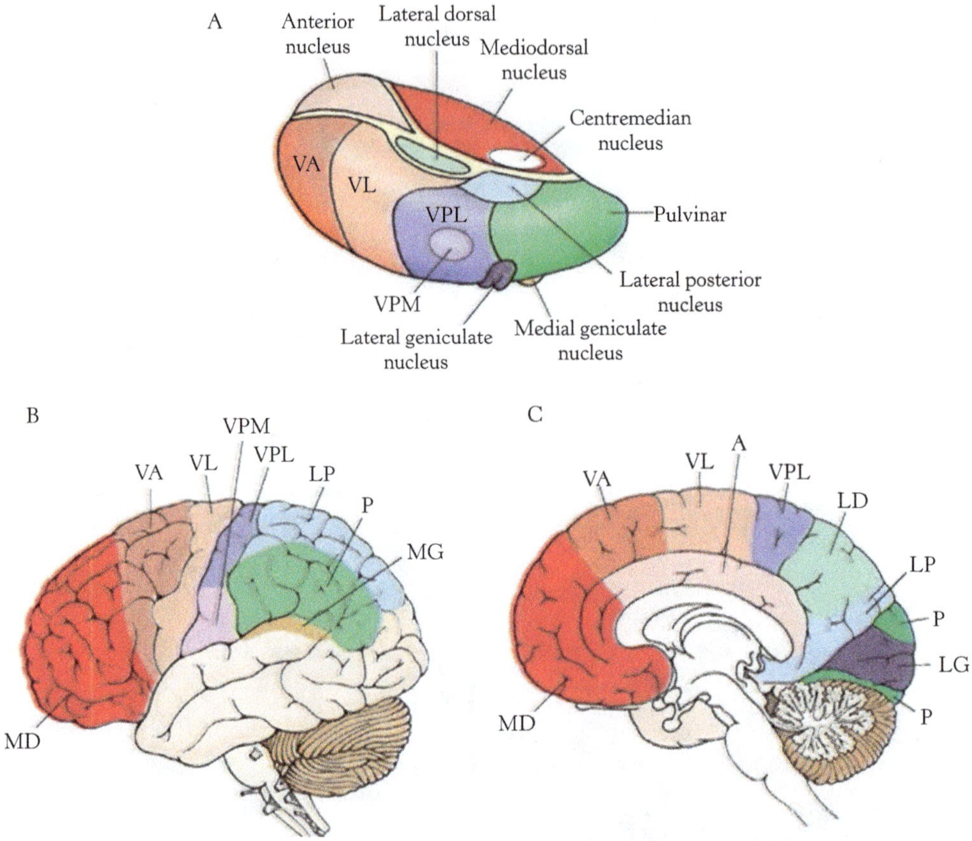

FIGURE 2.21: Depiction of the nuclei of the thalamus and the areas in the cortex to which they project. The color of the nucleus matches the color of the cortical region to which it connects.

Source: http://where-what-how-why.com.

Overall, thalamic involvement in cognition, other than its role as a relay station of information derived from the senses, is evolving with improved experimental designs and advanced neuroimaging techniques. The area where the thalamus appears to have a continually evolving role in cognition and behavior is in mediating and modulating synchronized electrical oscillations (e.g., electroencephalography (EEG) power spectra and time frequency oscillations; Başar et al., 2013). It is becoming evident from a variety of electrophysiological (e.g., EEG and magnetoencephalography) and from a different aspect neuroimaging studies (e.g., functional connectivity MRI; Buckner et al., 2013) that synchronized firing of groups of neurons in a rhythmic pattern communicates signals between cortical regions for cognitive operations and may in fact be a method of encoding object representations (e.g., integrated object concept; Hart et al., 2007, 2013; see also Griessenberger et al., 2012).

WHITE MATTER

White matter tract integrity is essential to effective cognition and behavior. Whereas gray matter has demonstrated notable adaptability and plasticity after injury, white matter does not demonstrate significant reorganization and plasticity. Even if neighboring gray matter cortices develop adaptive, plastic changes, if there are inadequate white matter connections to connect the adapted regions to the proper targets, then functions such as cognition and behavior do not recover.

In addition to the increasingly evident importance of the white matter's role in cognition, it is clear that there are specializations as to the types of white matter tracts present in the brain. Currently, three major different types of white matter tracts can be specified: (1) projection tracts that extend vertically between cortical regions and lower brain/spinal cord centers (e.g., spinocerebellar tracts), (2) commissural tracts crossing from one cerebral

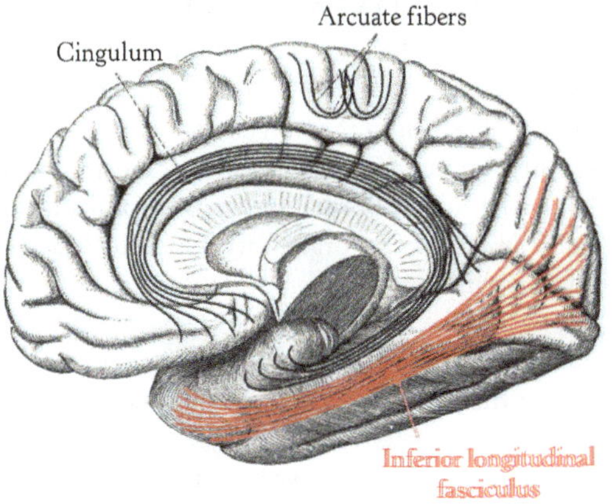

FIGURE 2.22: Diagram of the inferior longitudinal fasciculus (red)—the white matter tract connecting the visual system to the temporal lobe.

Source: http://www.wikipedia.org.

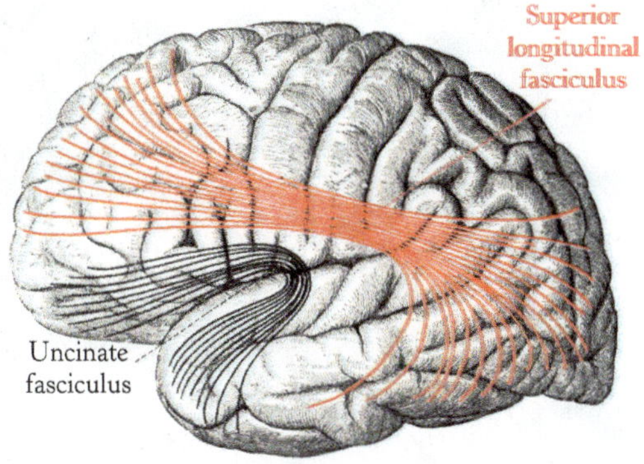

FIGURE 2.23: Diagram of the superior longitudinal fasciculus (red)—the white matter tract connecting the occipital and temporal lobes to the frontal lobe. The uncinate fasciculus (black) connects the hippocampus and amygdala with the orbitofrontal cortex.

Source: http://www.wikipedia.org.

hemisphere to the other, and (3) association tracts connecting different gyri within the same hemisphere of the brain.

There are several long association tracts that convey key cognitive information between cortical regions. The inferior longitudinal fasciculus (ILF) is a long white matter tract that extends from the visual cortices anteriorly to the temporal lobe (Figure 2.22). This connection transfers visual information to both language and memory centers. There is an analog superior version of the ILF, the superior longitudinal fasciculus (SLF), which bidirectionally connects visual and temporal cortices to prefrontal regions (Figure 2.23). This tract has been further subdivided into four different bundles (SLF I, II, III, and arcuate fasciculus) that are engaged in a range of cognitive functions, including regulating motor behavior, spatial attention, language functions, working memory, and auditory processing.

The uncinate fasciculus connects the hippocampus and the amygdala with the orbitofrontal cortex (Figure 2.23). This foreshortened pathway obviates having to go around the Sylvian fissure to access the frontal lobe from the temporal lobe and has been implicated in memory functions and behavior (see Figure 2.23). The arcuate fasciculus is a much studied cortico-cortical connection in cognition because it is the primary white matter pathway involved in language as the connection between Wernicke's and Broca's areas (Figure 2.24). A lesion of the arcuate fasciculus leads to a disconnection of Wernicke's area from Broca's area and results in the aphasic syndrome of conduction aphasia, a condition known for a prominent deficit in the ability to repeat words.

The largest and most significant white matter bundle in the brain is the corpus callosum—a commissural tract connecting the two hemispheres (Figure 2.25). This tract provides extensive cross-hemispheric cortico-cortical communication that leads to synergistic communication and/or inhibition between hemispheres. Lesioning of the corpus callosum has occurred previously by transection of

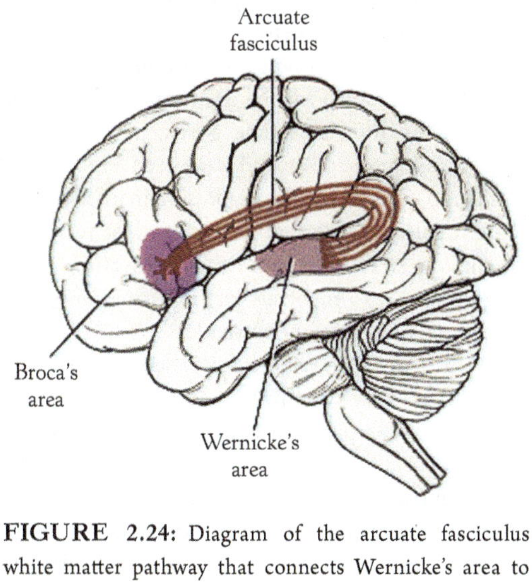

FIGURE 2.24: Diagram of the arcuate fasciculus white matter pathway that connects Wernicke's area to Broca's area.

Source: http://ztopics.com.

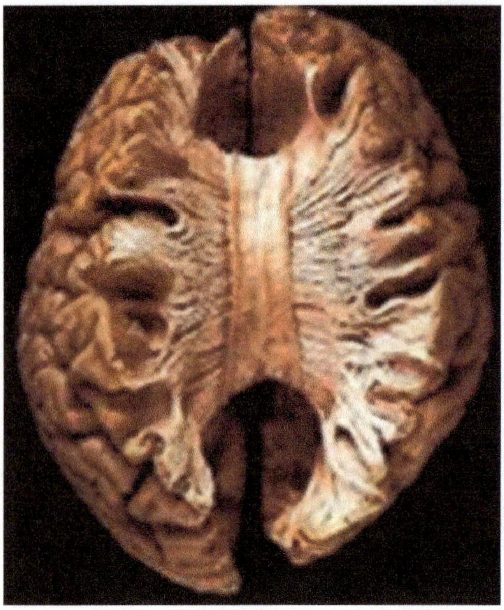

FIGURE 2.25: The corpus callosum white matter tract in a dissected brain specimen.

the anterior two-thirds as a treatment for intractable epilepsy. These patients developed multiple cognitive and behavioral dysfunctions, demonstrating how disconnection between the two hemispheres can disrupt coordination of cognitive operations.

LIMBIC SYSTEM

The limbic system is a collection of deep brain structures, referred to as the paleomammalian brain, that lies beneath the cerebral cortex. The structures include the olfactory bulb, hippocampus, amygdala, anterior thalamus, fornix, mammillary body, septum pellucidum, cingulate gyrus, parahippocampal gyrus, and upper midbrain (see Figures 2.18 and 2.26). These structures, present in many species of animals, are engaged in a variety of functions, including smell, emotion, and motivation. These regions are also involved in the formation of episodic and long-term memories.

Many of these regions have been described as part of the lobe or brain region where they reside (parahippocampal gyrus and hippocampus with the temporal lobe) or will be explained in detail in Chapter 6 as part of the Papez circuit. The existence is raised at this point to demonstrate the organization of these structures in one system and the evolutionary significance of this group of structures across species.

BRODMANN AREAS

In addition to the gyral/sulcal localization schema used traditionally for functional-anatomic assignment, there exist other organizational schema to classify brain locations, with the most popular being the use of Brodmann areas. Brodmann initially described this organization in 1909 based on characterization of different patterns of layers of neurons in the cerebral cortex. He numbered these areas by regions that had similar neuronal organization in the cortical layers. These areas crossed over boundaries of the traditional gyral/sulcal patterns (Figure 2.27). The effectiveness of this organization extends from the number of significant correlations of these Brodmann areas with specific cognitive and other brain functions.

Sensory cortices map effectively to the Brodmann area organization. BA 1–3 correspond to primary somatosensory cortices, BA 17 to primary visual cortex, BA 4 to primary motor cortex, and BA 41 and 42 are primary auditory cortices. Related association cortices include visual association cortex in areas 18 and 19 and somatosensory association cortices in area 7.

The following are other key Brodmann areas that are relevant to cognitive and behavioral functions:

- Frontal lobe
  - Premotor cortex and SMA are BA 6.
  - Frontal eye fields are BA 8.
  - DLPFC is BA 9 and 46.
  - Broca's area is BA 44 and 45.
  - Orbitofrontal cortex is BA 11 and 12.
  - Insular cortex is BA 13, 14 and 16.
  - Cingulate cortex in BA 24, 32, and 33 (anterior) and BA 23, 26, and 29–31 (posterior).
- Temporal lobe
  - Anterior temporal lobe is BA 15.
  - Superior temporal gyrus is BA 22 (Wernicke's area is part of BA 22).
  - Middle temporal gyrus is BA 21.
  - Inferior temporal gyrus is BA 20.
  - Anterior temporal pole is BA 38.
- Parietal lobe
  - Angular gyrus is BA 39 (part of which is Wernicke's area).
  - Supramarginal gyrus is BA 40 (also part of Wernicke's area).

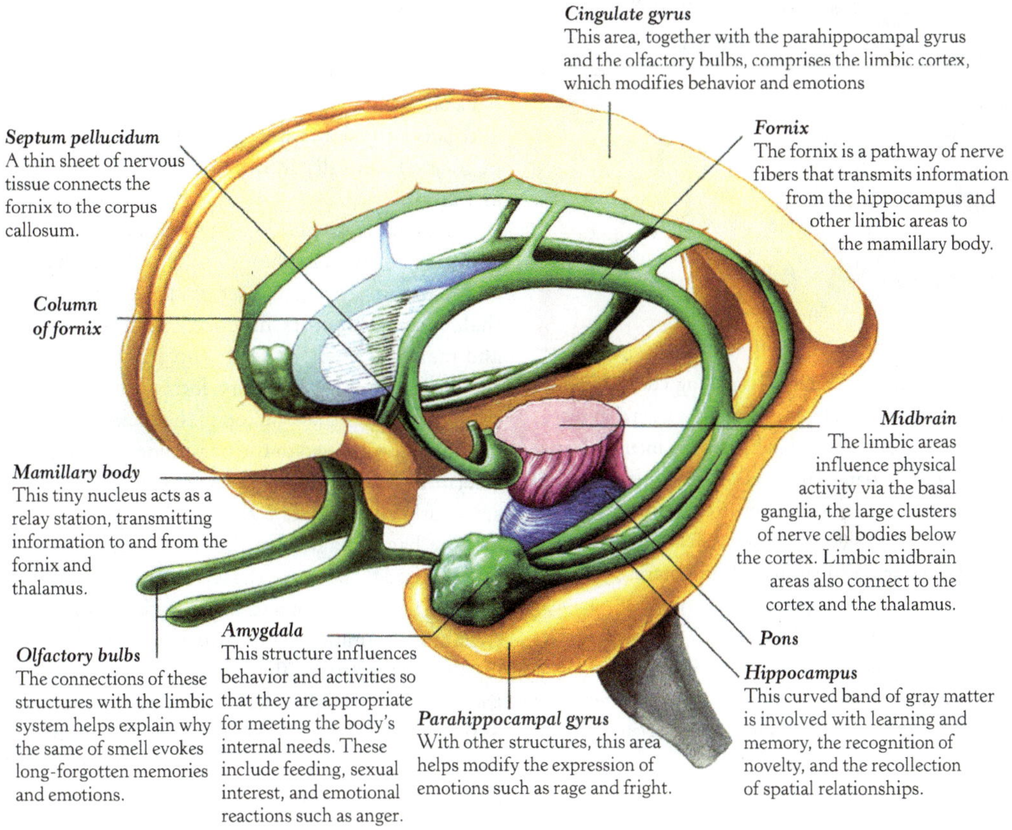

FIGURE 2.26: The limbic system structure with descriptions of anatomic locations and related functions.

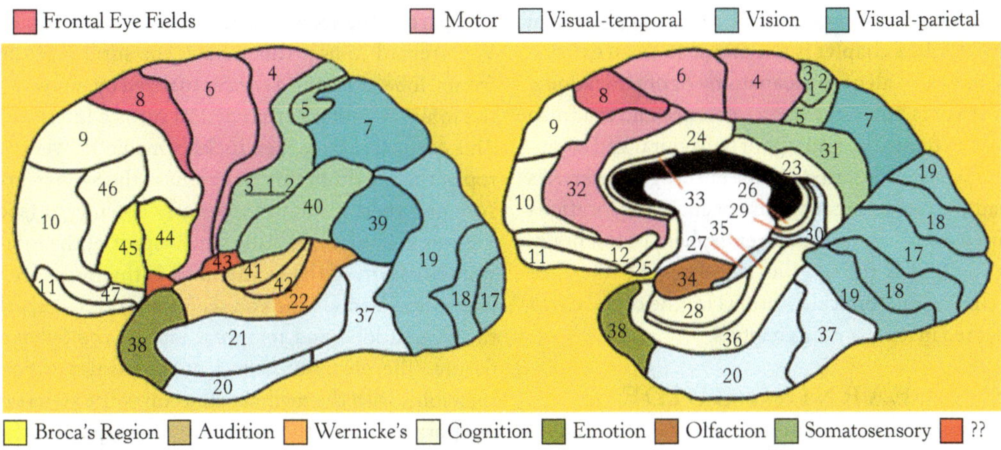

FIGURE 2.27: Schematic of Brodmann areas with the lateral view of the brain on the left and a medial view on the right.

Source: http://brainmaps.com (see also Brodmann areas in Wikipedia Commons).

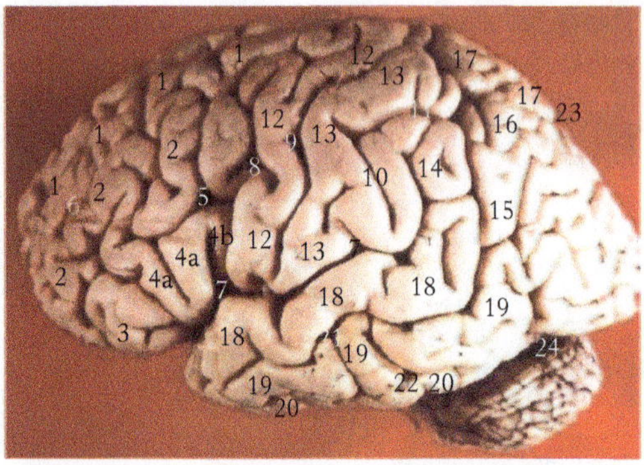

FIGURE 2.28: Numbers designating cortical regions on a lateral view of the brain: 1, superior frontal gyrus; 2, middle frontal gyrus; 3, orbital gyrus; 4, inferior frontal gyrus—(a) pars triangularis and (b) pars opercularis; 5, inferior frontal sulcus; 6, superior frontal sulcus; 7, lateral sulcus; 8, precentral sulcus; 9, central sulcus; 10, postcentral sulcus; 11, intraparietal sulcus; 12, precentral gyrus; 13, postcentral gyrus; 14, supramarginal gyrus; 15, angular gyrus; 16, inferior parietal lobule; 17, superior parietal lobule; 18, superior temporal gyrus; 19, middle temporal gyrus; 20, inferior temporal gyrus; 21, superior temporal sulcus; 22, middle temporal sulcus; 23, parieto-occipital sulcus; 24, preoccipital incisures.

Occipital lobe

Fusiform gyrus is BA 37.

All of the frameworks presented provide different perspectives on how to view the brain's anatomical divisions. Throughout investigations in neuroscience, studies are reported using the anatomic localization system that best fits reporting of the data. This chapter is not meant to be an exhaustive review of all of neuroanatomy or organizational frameworks but, rather, as a reference and roadmap to use to frame the findings of behavioral and cognitive correlates described in the ensuing chapters. As an additional summary figure of anatomic locations from a lateral view of one hemisphere of the brain, Figure 2.28 is included as a convenient reference for finding anatomical locations for the correlations reported in the ensuing chapters.

LEARNING GUIDE

For those learning neuroanatomy, as one adopts a conceptual framework of anatomical structures and their interrelationships in the brain, it is again recommended to have a 3-D model of the brain available, particularly one that allows for opening to see deep structures. One approach of a 3-D conceptualization of the brain is to start with the most deep and midline structures and build layers on top of them. That starting point is the thalamus, midline and deep in location. It is neurally efficient because the "relay station" connecting all cortical and subcortical brain regions (thalamus) would be located centrally in the brain (see Figures 2.19 and 2.20).

The next layer placed on top of the thalamus is the limbic system. Evolutionarily speaking, the limbic system is a primitive set of structures like the thalamus. It supports functions such as learning and memory, smell, and fear/threat. One can take the amygdala, hippocampus, fornix, and mammillary body and sit them on top of the thalamus. These can then be wrapped in the parahippocampal gyrus inferiorly and the cingulate gyrus posteriorly and superiorly (see Figures 2.18 and 2.26).

The basal ganglia are the next layer to overlay on the model. Because these structures modulate cortical to brain stem and in some cases cortical to thalamic communications, this is an ideal location for these structures. The globus pallidus and then the putamen are laid laterally around our building brain with the caudate head placed superiorly and anteriorly by the lateral ventricle, with the body and tail extending posteriorly and curving inferiorly to complete the basal ganglia structure overlay (see Figure 2.19).

The last layer is the cortices of the frontal, parietal, temporal, and occipital lobes. The area that can be confusing among the cortical regions is the area underneath the temporal lobe that is the inferior part of the frontal lobe containing the insula. With regard to how this follows the surface of the frontal lobe, this is best conceptualized by following the inferior frontal gyrus cortical surface inferiorly. This cortical surface then tucks in medially over the top of the superior temporal gyrus at the Sylvian fissure and then continues inferiorly downward (see Figures 2.4 and 2.19). This latter aspect of the inferior extension of the frontal lobe is the insula, the part of the frontal lobe you see when you pull apart the frontal lobe and temporal lobe at the Sylvian fissure. The posterior aspect of the insular region then joins with the medial extension of the superior temporal gyrus in the most posterior aspect of the frontal and temporal lobes. This is best seen in the coronal view of the brain in Figure 2.19.

Again, this is one formulation to conceptualize the brain structure and interrelationships. It is left to each individual to best develop a framework that is most effective for his or her use.

REFERENCES

Başar, E., Başar-Eroğlu, C., Güntekin, B., & Yener, G. (2013). Brain's alpha, beta, gamma, delta, and theta oscillations in neuropsychiatric diseases: Proposal for biomarker strategies. *Supplements to Clinical Neurophysiology, 62*, 19–54.

Buckner, R., Krienen, F., & Yeo, B. (2013). Opportunities and limitations of intrinsic functional connectivity MRI. *Nature Neuroscience, 16*(7), 832–837.

Cieslik, E., Zilles, K., Caspers, S., Roski, C., Kellermann, T., Jakobs, O., et al. (2013). Is there "one" DLPFC in cognitive action control? Evidence for heterogeneity from co-activation-based parcellation. *Cerebral Cortex*, 23(11), 2677–2689.

Griessenberger, H., Hoedlmoser, K., Heib, D., Lechinger, J., Klimesch, W., & Schabus, M. (2012). Consolidation of temporal order in episodic memories. *Biological Psychology, 91*(1), 150–155.

Hart, J., Anand, R., Zoccoli, S., Maguire, M., Gamino, J., Tillman, G., et al. (2007). Neural substrates of semantic memory. *Journal of the International Neuropsychological Society, 13*(5), 865–880.

Hart, J., Maguire, M., Motes, M., Mudar, R., Chiang, H.-S., Womack, K., et al. (2013). Semantic memory retrieval circuit: Role of BA6 and thalamus. *Brain and Language, 126*(1), 89–98.

3

Classic Aphasia Syndromes

This was chosen as the first chapter on specific brain–behavior correlations for historical reasons. The approach used for language-related brain correlations extends back for years and in essence was the first domain that was mapped extensively for brain–behavior correlations. The cognitive units described for classification of language disorders were not based on a cognitive–anatomic units type of approach. Nor was the approach to describing language based on cognitive units but, rather, on how groups of cognitive units regularly co-occur in what are referred to as aphasic syndromes. Because this was historically the first domain to be explored, starting with this classical description of language syndromes allows for one to see from the following chapters the refinement of the approach to brain–behavior correlations.

Aphasic syndromes are language disorders that develop after a brain lesion. Acquired language disorders were one of the first types of dysfunctions investigated for brain–behavior correlations; however, it is unclear why language disorders were the first to be characterized. This early interest has been suggested to stem from the intrinsic interest in language because it is so highly linked to the process of thought, which has intrigued neuroscientists for years, or from the shear frequency of occurrence of these types of cognitive deficits after a stroke.

The first delineation of these aphasic syndromes with neuroanatomic correlates dates back to studies performed in the late 1800s by Paul Broca (Broca, 1865) and Carl Wernicke (Wernicke, 1874). The famous cases of Broca's and Wernicke's aphasia were described by their namesakes using the approach of examining their patients extensively after the patients had experienced a stroke and describing in great detail the intact performance of their patients in multiple cognitive domains, including language, for both their intact and impaired performance. Then, after the patients died, each examined their patients' brains at autopsy to correlate the location of their respective brain lesion with the specific language functions that were disrupted for those patients while they were alive.

Lichtheim (1885) introduced a model of language function that consisted of centers and connections that were hypothesized to represent the language system both functionally and anatomically (Figure 3.1). This framework emphasized functions more than exact anatomic locations, as would be expected with the techniques available at the time. The centers were purported to represent stores of information located in specific cortical regions. The connections served to transfer information between centers. This approach of localized centers of brain functions, along with the work of Broca and Wernicke, led to a localizationist movement to cognition and behavior.

Subsequently, multiple cases of aphasic behavior were correlated with careful autopsy localization of the corresponding brain lesions. A compendium of aphasic syndromes along with a theoretical framework to account for their behavioral–anatomic correlations was summarized in a classic article titled "Disconnection Syndromes in Animals and Man" by Norman Geschwind (1965). This publication in essence solidified the movement toward the establishment of the field of behavioral neurology. Not only did Geschwind's work spawn the field but also his trainees became the next generation of behavioral neurologists who have further carried on his tradition to the present time. His disconnection theory of cognition and particularly language built on the work of Wernicke, Lichtheim, and others and formalized a testable set of hypotheses as well as a clinically applicable model for localizing lesions in patients. Lost in recent studies is that Geschwind's disconnection model represents one of the first modern *network* models of cognition and has spawned a host of more recent, varied network models of cognition.

Unfortunately, it has been estimated that only 20–30% of all patients with aphasia will fit neatly

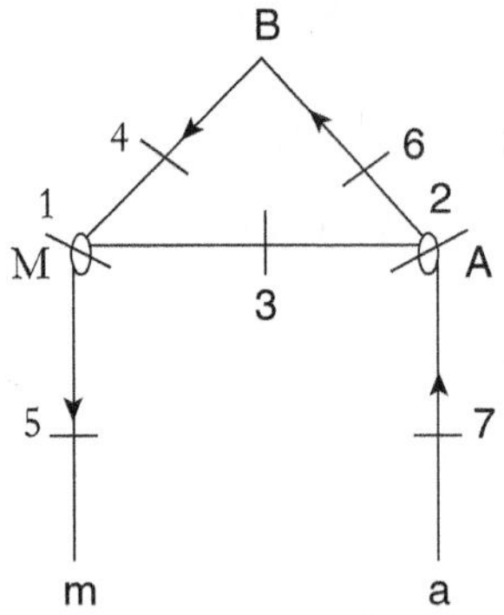

FIGURE 3.1: One of the figures that Lichtheim proposed as a model of language. Word representations are purported to reside in Center A, which is connected to Center M, where coordinated motor images to say the words are stored. Center B provides the conceptual meaning to the words. Arrows designate the directional flow of information in the model.

into one of the classically described aphasic syndromes in the disconnection model (Albert et al., 1991). Despite the limited number of aphasic patients accounted for by the model, the clinical utility of the classic aphasia syndromes described with the model has been quite useful and has led to a framework to describe cognitive disorders with an accompanying anatomic underpinning to account for patients' impairments.

As such, the assumption has been that the aphasic syndromes described were associated with a certain degree of anatomical predictability, which allowed the clinician to infer lesion location, etiology, and prognosis (Albert et al., 1991). In the absence of a better system for characterizing clinical aphasia subtypes, the organization of patients into classical aphasic syndromes, if they fit the profile, has persisted to the present. This system of classifying aphasia by these syndromes is thus described in this Chapter.

One commonly used alternative to this classic aphasia taxonomy is to dichotomize patients on the basis of speech fluency. Fluency refers to the flow with which sounds, syllables, words, and phrases are joined together when speaking. Fluency is based largely on the flow of continuous speech and thus can best be rated on the basis of conversational speech. One of the standard aphasia evaluation tools, the Boston Diagnostic Aphasia Examination (BDAE; Goodglass & Kaplan, 1983), provides a schema for evaluating speech fluency. The BDAE is a comprehensive test battery designed to evaluate a broad range of language functions from a variety of modalities (auditory, visual, and gestural) and response modalities (writing, articulation, and manipulation). The BDAE criteria for fluency are based on the "longest occasional uninterrupted string of words" that the patient is able to produce. The speech of nonfluent patients may range from complete mutism to slow, halting, and effortful production of individual words. Mutism is a rare finding in aphasia and most often occurs as a transient initial sign. Nonfluent speech is often associated with articulatory problems, referred to as dysarthria. Dysarthria is a motor speech disorder, not a language disorder, and is characterized by poor articulation of sounds secondary to the muscles of the speech system not working effectively to pronounce words correctly. It is typically due to damage in the central or peripheral nervous system that results in weakness or a lack of coordination of muscles of speech (respiration, throat, oropharynx, tongue, and lips). This leads to speech that can be slurred, unintelligible, and/or inaudible.

Some nonfluent aphasics have normal articulation. For example, a subset of nonfluent patients have a tendency to omit grammatical words from their speech, resulting in speech output that sounds like a telegraph message with all words other than the nouns and verbs missing from the utterance.

The speech of patients with fluent aphasia resembles normal speech in terms of rate of word production and phrase length. They may use random or invented words (called neologisms), substitute the wrong sound in a word for another sound ("slair" for "chair"), incorrectly substitute one word for another, and/or utter sentences that do not make sense.

Speech fluency provides an approximate guide to lesion location in that nonfluent aphasia is most commonly associated with lesions that include anterior regions of the perisylvian language areas, whereas fluent aphasia is frequently associated with posterior perisylvian lesions. This classification by itself does not necessarily mean much in terms of prognostic implications, although patients who remain nonfluent at 1 month after stroke are not likely to show substantial future improvement in fluency (Knopman et al., 1983).

Fluency has been suggested to be the parameter by which to group aphasic disorders: fluent versus nonfluent. Overall, impaired fluency can be indicative of either a language or a speech dysfunction. Also, no single language symptom can adequately capture the nature of observed language disorders or provide adequate anatomic specificity to allow for an anatomic classification of aphasic disorders. Nor at this point does any one language symptom provide a clear theoretical framework to account for what a particular brain region "subserves" (e.g., there is no brain region that specifically performs a function such as "fluency" or "comprehension"). Thus, clinicians have been faced with performing a systematic evaluation of aphasia by characterizing a group of standard language functions (e.g., speech, comprehension, naming, and repetition) and the aphasic symptoms that would occur if one or more of these functions were disrupted. As a consequence, the initial investigations of language impairment were based on language functions that were common to daily communication performance of the patients, not more finely grained cognitive operations (lexical search, semantic match, etc.). The initial framework of assessing the pattern of impaired performance on language functions, and inferring anatomic localization resulting in these deficits from these patterns, was based on daily language functions (e.g., naming) that were composed of multiple cognitive operations (for naming, visual object recognition, semantic processing, semantic to phonological access, output phonology, and speech). This framework based on aphasic symptoms of daily language functions is delineated in this chapter, as is the way in which these symptoms are used to classify aphasic syndromes. This discussion begins with the outline of the signs and symptoms of aphasia associated with these functions and syndromes.

SIGNS AND SYMPTOMS OF APHASIA

Most cases of aphasia are secondary to stroke, and the abrupt onset of change in language-related functions may be the most reliable indicator that the symptoms stem from an aphasia due to a lesion such as a stroke. Very few language impairment symptoms are by themselves unique or diagnostic of aphasia. Inability to name or making speech/language output errors such as word substitution may occur in neurologically intact individuals. Therefore, it may be difficult to diagnose cases of aphasia due to causes other than stroke, where the symptoms all occur at once. Thus, the timing of the onset of symptoms is key to diagnosing an aphasic syndrome and its etiology.

The symptoms of language dysfunction within this framework are assessed for in the functions of spontaneous speech, comprehension, naming, repetition, writing, and reading. As noted previously, these functions are not based on specific brain centers associated with each function or specific cognitive operations but, rather, on major language functions used in daily communication. The following details this standard approach to assessing these symptoms.

BEDSIDE LANGUAGE EXAMINATION

The bedside evaluation occurs usually after an acute neurological event, although it can occur at any time when a patient presents with a language or speech problem. The studies in aphasia mostly emanated from investigators following patients who had recently had a stroke.

A *stroke* can be defined in its simplest terms as a disruption in blood flow to the brain, resulting in cell death (including neurons) in the region to which the blocked part of the artery had previously supplied blood. Strokes occur from several different etiologies. A blockage of an artery can occur from a clot that is delivered from a distant source (the heart, carotid artery, etc.) and travel until it is too large to pass any further. Blood is blocked from traveling any further than where the clot lodges, and thus the brain regions that were supplied by the part of the artery beyond the clot no longer receive blood and eventually the cells there die. This type of stroke is called an embolic stroke, and it is important in aphasia in that Wernicke's aphasia typically occurs as the result of embolic strokes. A clot can also form in the artery in the blood vessels in the brain and grow until it blocks the artery. This is referred to as a thrombotic stroke. Thrombotic strokes appear to recover less completely from their acute presentation than do embolic strokes. A third type of stroke is a hemorrhage where a blood vessel ruptures due to a hole/tear forming in the vessel wall. If the blood vessel is in the brain, then the hemorrhage is referred to as an intracerebral hemorrhage. The shearing of the brain due to the rupture of the vessel and blood extrusion, blood pushing on brain parenchyma, and the lack of blood to the rest of the artery beyond the spot of the hemorrhage are the causes of cell death from a hemorrhage. If the blood vessel hemorrhaging is not in the brain but on the outside or occurs prior to the blood vessels entering the brain, this is referred to as a subarachnoid hemorrhage. These hemorrhages can cause cell death to the brain by a lack of blood to the brain at the time of hemorrhage. In addition, several days later there is a breakdown of the hemorrhaged blood in the area around the brain that can lead to the arteries going into spasm, which results in a lack of blood to the brain due to what is referred to as a secondary stroke that occurs after a hemorrhage. The last type of stroke to be discussed is a "watershed" stroke that is somewhat different from the normal blockage or hemorrhage. In this type of stroke, there is typically a lack of blood flowing from the heart to the brain for a short period of time (e.g., heart attack with heart pump failure and then recovery). The parts of the brain fed by the end (distal) aspects of arteries lose blood supply and their cells die. When the pump starts working again and blood flow returns, the parts of the brain supplied by the root or beginning of the artery remain intact, but the brain regions supplied by the end regions of the artery are damaged. For example, Broca's area is fed off the beginning of a branch of artery, whereas its surrounding area is supplied by the end of the artery and is in danger of being damaged by a watershed lesion. Areas most at risk are those that are supplied by the ends of one or several arteries (e.g., regions fed by the end of arteries off of the middle cerebral and posterior cerebral arteries). These strokes are important in aphasia classification because the transcortical aphasias typically result from watershed strokes.

At a minimum, the bedside language examination should include the basic elements listed in Box 3.1. Information about the quality of *speech fluency* and the ability to comprehend conversational speech can be partially obtained from a clinical interview. Further characterization of spontaneous speech abilities can be assessed using standard automatic sequences, such as asking the patient to count from 1 to 10 and reciting the letters of the alphabet, days of the week, or months of the year. Assessing the quality of the responses to these requests can be helpful in eliciting enough speech to allow assessment of articulation and fluency. The critical elements in assessing spontaneous speech include articulation, fluency, melodic line (defined later but referred to as prosody), grammatical form (syntax of the utterances), paraphasic (substitution of one wrong sound for the correct sound in a word) errors, and word-finding errors. Another manner to obtain a speech sample to assess fluency is to have a patient describe a complex scene in a picture (e.g., the Cookie Theft Picture from the BDAE). In patients with no verbal output after using all of these approaches, assessment of writing can help differentiate between aphasia, which affects all language output, and aphonia, in which writing is intact but a patient cannot speak.

BOX 3.1
LANGUAGE EXAM

Spontaneous speech
- **Picture description**

Auditory comprehension
- **Single word; sentences (commands)**

Naming
- **Objects, body parts, colors**

Repetition
- **Single words and sentences**

Writing
- **Spontaneous; dictation; copying**

Reading
- **Aloud; comprehension**

Auditory comprehension for individual words can be tested by asking the patient to point to body parts, everyday objects, or items in the room. Single word comprehension may be the best index of initial aphasia severity and thus carries potential prognostic implications (Selnes et al., 1984). The more severe single word comprehension is, the poorer functional long-term outcome, in general. Sentence comprehension can be assessed by asking the patient to perform single or multistep commands. The ability to comprehend more complex syntactical relationships can be probed by the use of so-called syntactically reversible sentences. For example, in response to a sentence such as "The lion was killed by the tiger," some patients have difficulty answering the question, "Which animal died?"

The easiest commands for a patient to follow, regardless of the severity of the aphasia, are those that involve the body axis, such as "Look up, look down, stand up, lean forward" (Albert et al., 1991). These types of commands can be used when the patient cannot perform the previous listed commands to assess for only low-level comprehension. A formal test used to assess comprehension in a systematic manner is the Token Test (De Renzi & Faglioni, 1978), which can be used when a metric is desired to follow objectively changes in comprehension.

Naming can be assessed by asking the patient to name objects, body parts, or colors that are presented visually. For more detailed assessment, quantitative tests such as the Boston Naming Test are recommended (Kaplan et al., 1983). *Repetition* can be screened with sentences such as "no ifs, ands, or buts." Patients who are able to repeat this sentence generally have grossly intact repetition. The reason for using this phrase is that words without a concrete, real-world reference (e.g., concrete → ball, car, elephant) are most affected in aphasia, including being the most difficult to repeat. If the patient does not repeat this sentence correctly, however, additional testing of repetition with single words and simpler sentences should be performed. *Writing* can be assessed by asking the patient to write a sentence spontaneously. Patients who are unable to write a sentence should be asked to attempt to copy single words or sentences. In patients with severe motor deficits, testing oral spelling can be useful. *Reading* aloud of single words, sentences, and paragraphs should also be assessed. Most patients with problems in reading comprehension also have problems when reading aloud, but the converse is not always true. A selective deficit of reading words that do not conform to standard sound-to-print rules, such as "lieutenant, beautiful, steak," is at times observed more often in aphasia than a deficit of "regular" words such as "stand, gave, napkin."

The type or pattern of errors in these tasks can at times reveal a great deal about the underlying aphasic impairment of the patient. In particular, the errors in speech/language production (spontaneous speech, naming, repetition, reading, and writing) can be quite varied and provide useful insights into the underlying dysfunctional language components. The following discussion delineates characterizations of the type of abnormalities of speech/language production in the previous tests that provide useful descriptions of the behavior and in some cases localizing value provided by their analysis.

Of the variety of symptoms associated with aphasia, none is more ubiquitous than anomia. *Anomia* is a disorder of word finding or word retrieval and is present in all types of aphasia. In most cases, word-finding difficulties are readily apparent in the patient's attempts at conversational speech. In milder cases, formal testing with confrontation naming tasks may be required to document the anomia. Anomia in the absence of significant impairment in other aspects of speech and language does not appear to carry any specific localizing value, and one must consider if the patient has an aphasic disorder at all because conditions other than aphasia from a neurological insult can cause word-finding and naming deficits.

Paraphasias refer to unintended substitutions at the level of individual sounds or words and are common in all types of aphasia and rare in other disorders. The principal subtypes of verbal substitutions are phonemic, semantic, and neologistic. Phonemic paraphasias refer to substitutions of one *sound* (or phoneme) for another, such as saying "tork" instead of "fork." Phonemic paraphasias are common to most subtypes of aphasia, but they are particularly abundant in fluent aphasias secondary to lesions of the posterior language areas. Semantic paraphasias are substitutions of a word related in meaning to an intended target word (e.g., "table" for "chair"). Neologisms are substitutions that are far removed from the intended target word and are actually not English words (e.g., "slairket").

Verbal *perseverations* are the unintended repetition of a preceding response (e.g., answering every subsequent question with the same answer as that to the first question on a test). These are common during the early stages of any acute aphasia syndrome, but they occur in non-aphasic brain-injured patients as well.

Echolalia refers to unsolicited, compulsive repetition (echoing) of verbal stimuli. Patients with echolalia do not echo everything they hear, only utterances directed toward them. It is typically associated with poor comprehension.

Stereotypical utterances occur when the speech of patients with severe nonfluent aphasia is limited to only one or two utterances, repeated in succession. These utterances may be real words or meaningless nonsense syllables.

TRADITIONAL APHASIC SYNDROMES

The perisylvian area (frontal and temporal lobe regions surrounding the Sylvian fissure) has been referred to as the classic language area (Figure 3.2). The key regions include Wernicke's area in the posterior aspect of the left superior temporal gyrus; Broca's area at the posterior aspect of the left inferior frontal gyrus; and the arcuate fasciculus, which is the white matter tract connecting Wernicke's area to Broca's area (Figure 3.2). Lesions in these regions have led to what are referred to as the classic aphasic syndromes (Geschwind, 1965), which are described next.

Broca's Aphasia

These patients are noted to have halting, nonfluent speech, which is the hallmark feature of this

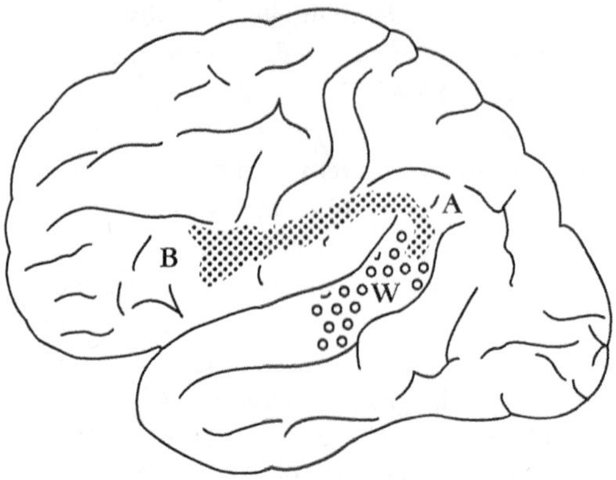

FIGURE 3.2: Schematic of the major perisylvian brain regions associated with language function. A, angular gyrus; B, Broca's area; W, Wernicke's area. The dotted region represents the arcuate fasciculus white matter tract connecting Wernicke's and Broca's areas.

aphasia (see Video 3.1). Their speech is reduced in output with short utterances, which are laborious and choppy. They produce mostly nouns and verbs in their speech, but they do not produce function words (grammatical markers such as "the," "by," "through," and "with"). These speech characteristics are also paralleled in the patient's repetition and writing. Naming is impaired with the same halting, effortful production as well as other anomic errors. Comprehension is intact in comparison to speech fluency, except that patients can have difficulty comprehending syntactically complex sentences. This selective syntactic comprehension deficit and lack of production of function words has led to these patients being referred to as agrammatic.

The lesion required to produce Broca's aphasia is more extensive than just Broca's area and is a relatively large left perisylvian lesion that includes the left inferior frontal gyrus, insula, and surrounding white matter (Figures 3.3 and 3.4).

Wernicke's Aphasia

Patients with Wernicke's aphasia have fluent connected speech; however, the words and sentences that are produced do not make sense (see Video 3.2). The patients have normal sentence length and intonation, but the sentences are devoid of meaning. This is due to the patients first making errors in word production that are classified as paraphasic speech. This consists of substituting the wrong letters/sounds in a word to form a phonemic paraphasic error (saying "slair" for "chair") or substituting a word of similar but incorrect meaning (saying "table" when a patient means to say "chair"). In addition to substituting sounds, Wernicke's aphasia patients will substitute the wrong words or add or delete words that belong in a sentence. As a consequence, the patient's speech is incomprehensible. The most characteristic aspect of Wernicke's aphasia patients' speech, however, is neologisms, which are nonsense words that the patients produce (e.g., saying the word "slitch"). The other hallmark feature of Wernicke's aphasia is markedly poor comprehension. Naming and repetition can have the same semantic or phonemic paraphasias and neologisms as heard in their spontaneous speech. Due largely to the impaired comprehension, these patients are quite dysfunctional. Fortunately, in most cases, Wernicke's aphasia is a fairly transient state that occurs acutely after a stroke and quickly evolves into anomic aphasia.

The lesions that result in Wernicke's aphasia involve the left posterior superior temporal gyrus that includes Wernicke's area (Figure 3.5). Partial lesions that are less than 50% of this region appear to have a better long-term outcome than more complete lesions of the region.

Conduction Aphasia

Although this aphasia occurs uncommonly, it is of great theoretical importance to the Geschwind disconnection model. These patients have a relatively more severe impairment in repetition compared to spontaneous speech (see Video 3.3). In all the other aphasic disorders, the type and severity of spontaneous speech impairment are comparable to the deficit in repetition, except in the case of conduction aphasia. Conduction aphasics have intact comprehension and fluent but paraphasic speech with substitution or transposition of sounds. The hallmark of this aphasia is that although patients are capable of understanding a sentence, they are unable to repeat that same sentence.

The lesion proposed to produce this aphasic syndrome is disruption of the white matter connection, the left arcuate fasciculus, between Wernicke's and Broca's area (Figure 3.6). However, recent studies show that lesions in the arcuate fasciculus are neither necessary nor sufficient for conduction aphasia. It has been found that a lesion is needed only to the most posterior area of the superior temporal lobe that projects to Broca's area to result in conduction aphasia.

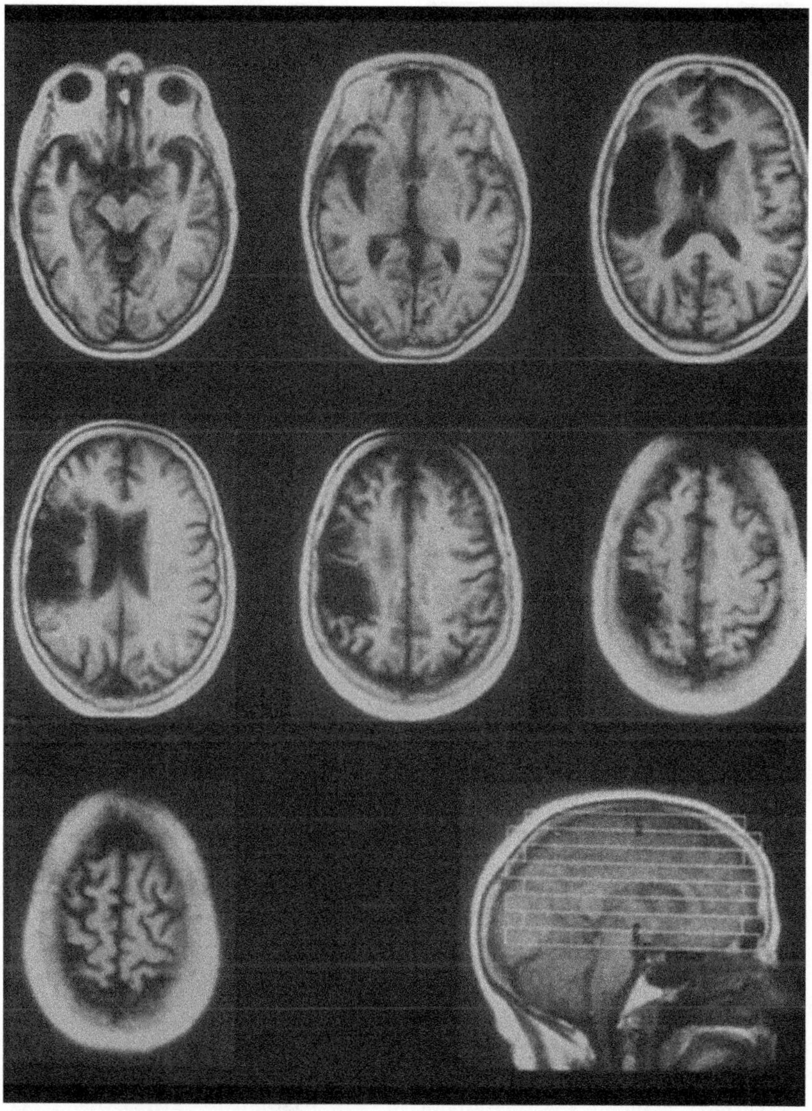

FIGURE 3.3: Lesion in the posterior aspect of the left inferior frontal gyrus plus deeper structures such as the insula that results in the syndrome of Broca's aphasia (right is left in this radiological organization).

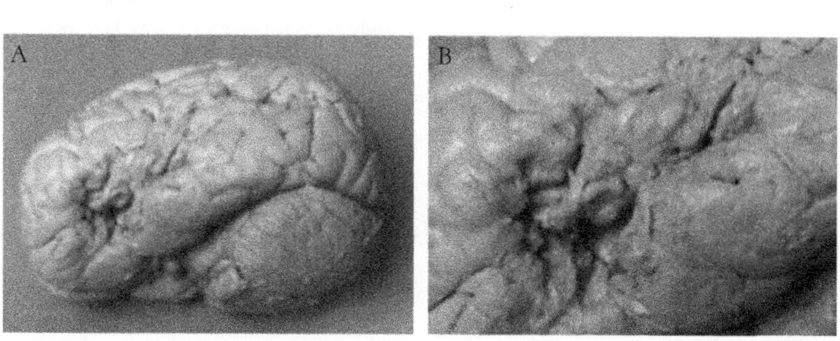

FIGURE 3.4: The brain of Broca's patient "Tan" was re-examined by Dronkers and colleagues, and this lateral view demonstrates the damaged area in the left inferior frontal gyrus.

Source: Dronkers et al. (2007).

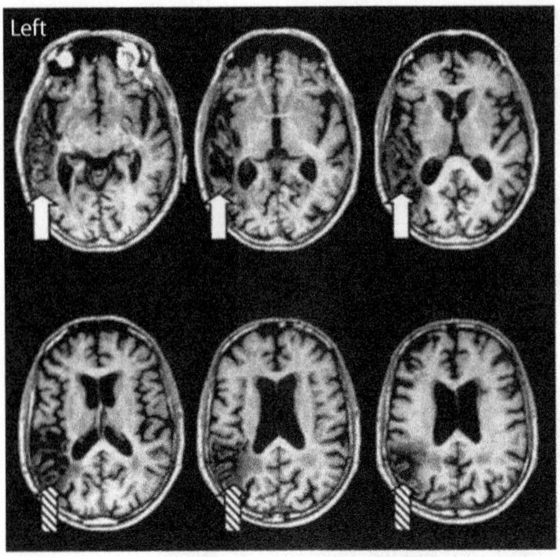

FIGURE 3.5: Lesion in the posterior aspect of the left superior temporal gyrus (arrows) that results in the syndrome of Wernicke's aphasia (right is left in this radiological organization).

Anomic Aphasia

This aphasia is characterized by fluent speech notable for substituting incorrect words for target words, making semantic and occasionally phonemic paraphasic errors, and by circumlocutions (see Video 3.4). Circumlocutions refer to speaking around the target word, including at times the description of the target object, without saying the actual name. Patients' spontaneous speech has few specific content words and thus at times is referred to as empty speech. These patients have only mild comprehension and repetition dysfunction. Their naming performance mirrors that of their spontaneous speech.

The lesions that result in anomic aphasia are more varied than those of the other aphasic syndromes, but they typically include the left supramarginal and/or angular gyrus, or just minimal involvement of posterior superior temporal gyrus (Figure 3.7).

Global Aphasia

This devastating aphasia consists of impairments in all language domains. There typically is nonfluent speech with impairment in comprehension as well as repetition and naming.

This is typically the result of an extensive lesion throughout the entire left perisylvian area, including the posterior inferior frontal region, the insula, the underlying white matter, the inferior parietal lobe, and the posterior superior temporal gyrus (Figure 3.8).

Transcortical Motor Aphasia

This uncommon aphasia is characterized by impaired fluency and naming; with intact comprehension and repetition. Patients' speech is nonfluent and effortful with short utterances similar to the speech of a Broca's aphasic. Their comprehension and naming performance is also similar to that of a Broca's aphasic. The only difference between these patients and a Broca's aphasic is that the transcortical motor aphasic patient has intact repetition.

The lesion is more anterior and superior than a Broca's aphasic's lesion. It is typically a "watershed" lesion surrounding Broca's area but sparing the arcuate fasciculus (thus leaving repetition intact; Figure 3.9).

Transcortical Sensory Aphasia

This other uncommon aphasia has been referred to as Wernicke's aphasia with intact repetition. These patients have impaired comprehension and naming, with intact repetition. Their fluency and spontaneous speech characteristics are similar to those of Wernicke's aphasics, with fluent speech, paraphasic errors, and neologisms.

The lesions that produce transcortical sensory aphasia are located posterior and inferior to Wernicke's area. The involvement is typically located in the most posterior aspects of the left middle and inferior temporal gyri while sparing the arcuate fasciculus (again sparing repetition performance; Figure 3.10).

Mixed Transcortical Aphasia or Isolation of the Speech Area

This is the least common of the aphasic syndromes. These patients only have preserved repetition, with all other functions impaired. The chief characteristic of these patients is echolalia, where they continuously repeat the same word or utterance.

The lesion resulting in this syndrome surrounds the perisylvian area, sparing Broca's area, Wernicke's area, and the arcuate fasciculus. This type of lesion typically involves having both anterior cerebral artery–middle cerebral artery and middle cerebral artery–posterior cerebral artery watershed infarcts (Figure 3.11; Maeshima et al., 2002) that typically result from heart pump failure.

Table 3.1 details the symptoms associated with each of the classical aphasic disorders.

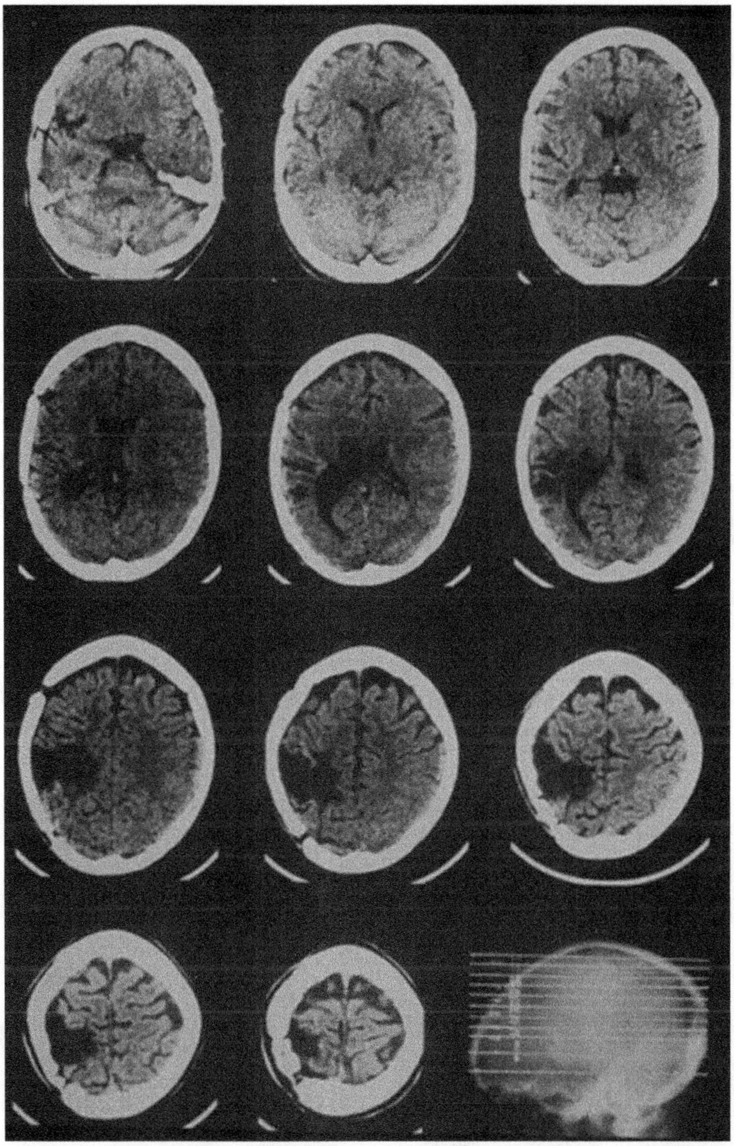

FIGURE 3.6: Lesion in the most posterior area of the superior temporal lobe that projects to Broca's area, including aspects of the arcuate fasciculus, that results in the syndrome of conduction aphasia (right is left in this radiological organization).

ANATOMIC AREAS ASSOCIATED WITH APHASIA—UPDATED IN THE MODEL NOT BY SYNDROME

Our understanding of the anatomy of the left hemisphere language system, like most cognitive systems, has been constrained by a bias in patient investigation: Only patients with symptoms of aphasia were investigated. Patients with left hemisphere lesions but no aphasia were rarely subjected to systematic study (but see Basso et al., 1985). Consequently, this resulted in a somewhat biased and restricted view. Advances in neuroimaging technologies during the past several decades have resulted in several modifications of the disconnection model of the left hemisphere language system. Although contemporary textbooks still feature the standard model of Wernicke's and Broca's areas interconnected by

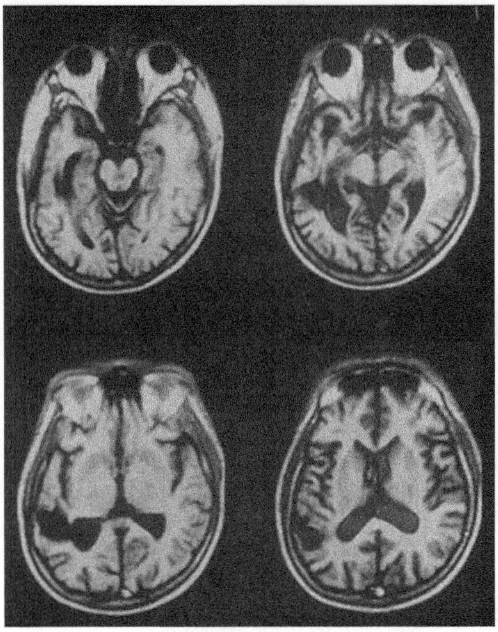

FIGURE 3.7: Lesion in the left supramarginal and angular gyrus that results in the syndrome of anomic aphasia (right is left in this radiological organization).

the arcuate fasciculus, evidence from several different lines of inquiry is now accumulating that this model is an oversimplification, as updated in the examples discussed previously. There have been three major trends. First, it is now appreciated that lesions restricted to the traditional language areas of Broca and Wernicke are neither necessary nor sufficient to produce the classical syndromes. Second, it is now commonly accepted that multiple left hemisphere regions other than Broca's and Wernicke's areas appear to participate in language functions. Third, there is variability in the lesion correlates of the traditional syndromes, and this needs to be considered in localization (Basso et al., 1985; Vignolo et al., 1986). The following discussion describes by area—not syndrome—the brain regions and their contribution to language processing.

Broca's Area (Brodmann's Area 44/45)

The first major revision to standard teaching about the role of Broca's area in language came with the studies of J. P. Mohr, who showed that a lesion restricted to Broca's area did not produce the

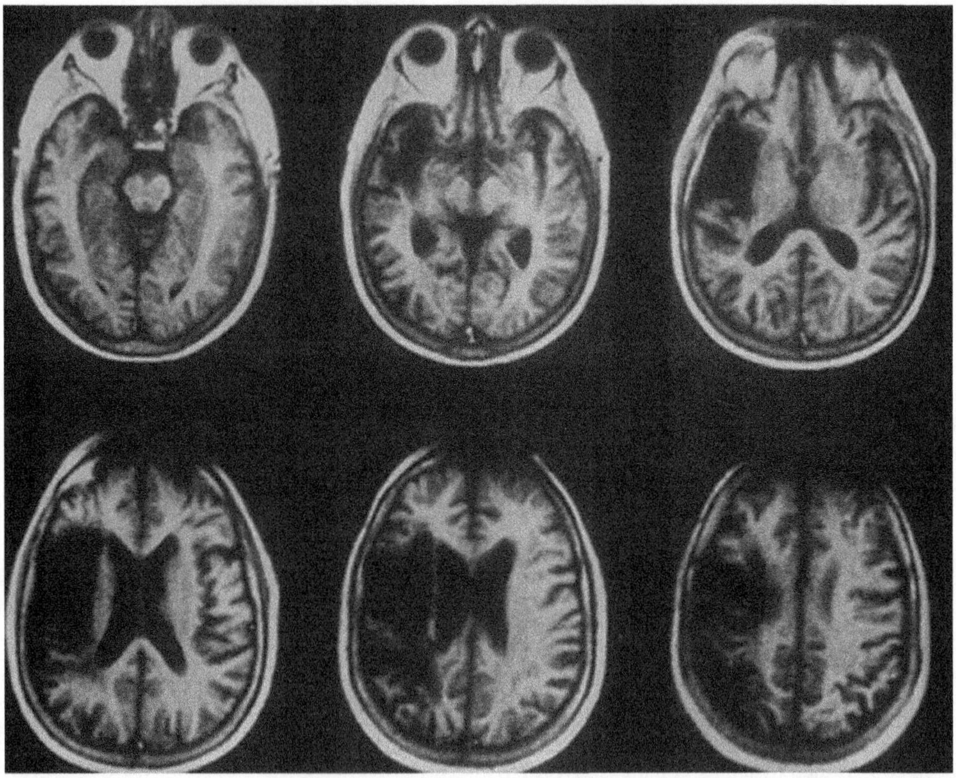

FIGURE 3.8: Lesion in the posterior inferior frontal, the insula, the underlying white matter, the inferior parietal lobe, and the posterior superior temporal gyrus that results in the syndrome of global aphasia (right is left in this radiological organization).

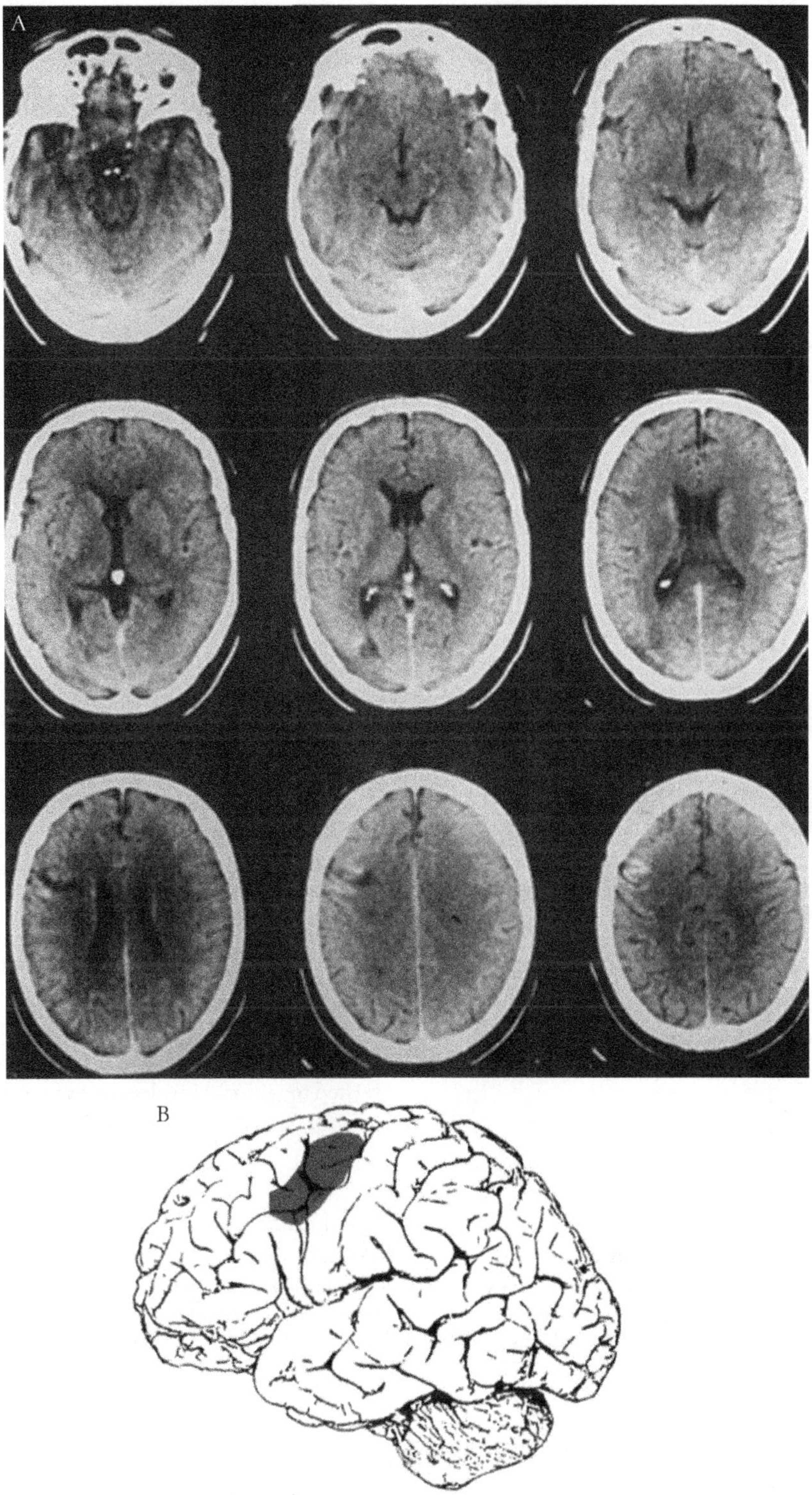

FIGURE 3.9: (Top) Lesion that is anterior and superior to Broca's area (sparing the arcuate fasciculus) that results in the syndrome of transcortical motor aphasia (right is left in this radiological organization). (Bottom) A schematic of the typical type of lesion associated with transcortical motor aphasia in the left frontal lobe.

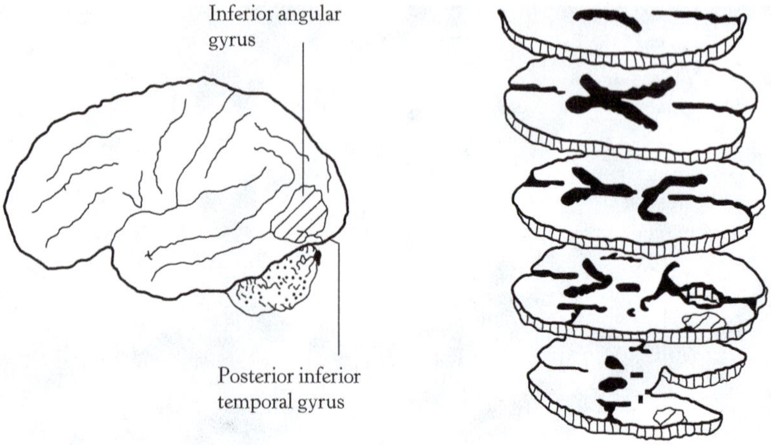

FIGURE 3.10: Schematic of the lesion in the most posterior aspects of the left middle and inferior temporal gyri while sparing the arcuate fasciculus (again sparing repetition performance) that results in the syndrome of transcortical sensory aphasia.

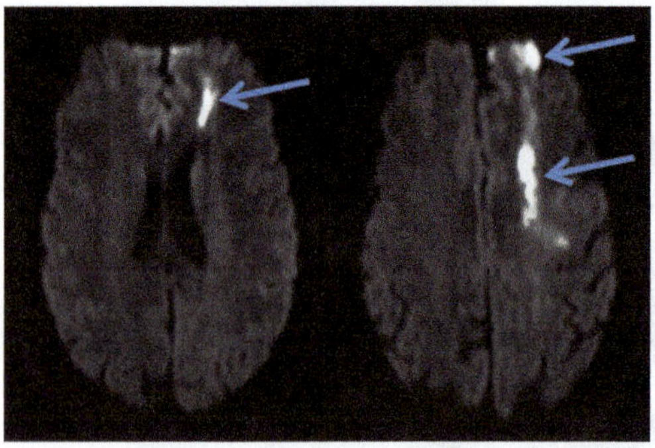

FIGURE 3.11: MRI of the brain revealed the left frontal and subcortical infarct in a patient with mixed transcortical aphasia. The blue arrows point to the lesion.

Source: http://galleryhip.com.

clinical syndrome of Broca's aphasia (Mohr et al., 1999). According to Mohr, the lesion responsible for the clinical picture of Broca's aphasia is a large infarct in the perisylvian area, which includes the posterior inferior frontal gyrus, the insula, and the surrounding deep white matter. Others have shown that although the anterior insula is consistently involved, Broca's area proper need not be part of the lesion (Blunk et al., 1981; Knopman et al., 1983). Thus, a lesion of Broca's area is neither sufficient nor necessary for producing the syndrome of persistent nonfluent Broca's aphasia. More detailed analysis suggests that components of the syndrome of Broca's aphasia, such as impaired articulation, delayed initiation of speech, and aprosody, can be related to regional involvement of just the posterior inferior frontal gyrus (Alexander et al., 1990).

TABLE 3.1: SYMPTOMS ASSOCIATED WITH EACH OF THE CLASSICAL APHASIC DISORDERS

	Fluency	Comprehension	Repetition	Naming
Broca's	↓↓↓	↑	↓↓	↓↓
Wernicke's	↑	↓↓↓	↓↓	↓↓
Conduction	↑	↓	↓↓↓	↓
Anomic	↑	↓	↑	↓↓↓
Global	↓↓↓	↓↓↓	↓↓↓	↓↓↓
TMA	↓↓↓	↑	↑	↓↓
TSA	↑	↓↓↓	↑	↓↓
ISA	↓↓↓	↓↓↓	↑	↓↓↓

Wernicke's Area

The anatomical boundaries of the part of the posterior superior temporal lobe that constitutes Wernicke's region have never been specified because there are no specific cytoarchitectonic or other criteria for supporting such a definition (Bogen & Bogen, 1976). A lesion of the posterior superior temporal lobe typically is associated with fluent, paraphasic speech and poor comprehension. It has also been demonstrated that the degree of destruction of the posterior superior temporal lobe is correlated with long-term aphasic outcome. Partial lesions of the region are associated with favorable outcomes, whereas lesions that include more than 50% of the region are associated with poor outcomes (Selnes et al., 1984). If the lesion is limited to the posterior superior temporal lobe, prognosis for improvement to anomic aphasia is good, but if the lesion includes anterior extensions, prognosis for recovery is poor (Naeser et al., 1987).

Planum Temporale

The planum temporale is a triangular structure located on the superior plane of the temporal lobe within the Sylvian fissure. The normal anatomy of this region is quite variable, but cytoarchitectonically it consists of auditory association cortex. It has attracted considerable research attention following the discovery by Geschwind and Levitsky (1968) that this particular region of the brain tends to be larger in the left hemisphere. Although the distribution of the anatomical asymmetry (left larger in 64% of brains) did not exactly fit with estimates of left hemisphere language dominance, the assumption was made that the asymmetry somehow reflected the important role of the posterior superior temporal lobe in language. However, a specific role of this area in language, if any, has not been demonstrated (Binder et al., 1996).

Insula

The anterior insula is almost always implicated in patients with persistent nonfluent aphasia. In addition, its involvement in a lesion has been shown to be necessary to develop Broca's aphasia (Dronkers et al., 2007).

Angular/Supramarginal Gyri

The angular and supramarginal gyri are part of the inferior parietal lobule, and they are strategically located for multimodal association of vision, touch, and hearing. Lesions of this region have been shown to be associated with anomic aphasia. In addition, these regions have been implicated in the syndrome of alexia with agraphia; the lesions responsible for this syndrome typically include other structures as well (Sakurai et al., 2000; see Chapter 4). Gerstmann syndrome has also been shown to be associated with larger lesions that include the angular gyrus but not restricted to this area (Benton, 1992). This region is discussed more extensively in Chapter 4 with regard to its association with specific cognitive operations.

Arcuate Fasciculus

The long white matter tract known as the arcuate fasciculus has traditionally been conceptualized as the direct pathway between the posterior and anterior language areas. Lesions of the arcuate fasciculus have been thought to be responsible for the repetition deficit observed in patients with conduction aphasia. Other findings have suggested that a lesion of the arcuate fasciculus is neither necessary nor sufficient for the production of the syndrome of conduction aphasia (Anderson et al., 1999; Brown, 1975; Damasio & Damasio, 1980; Selnes et al., 1985; Shuren et al., 1995). Recent anatomical studies propose that it is only the most posterior areas of the superior temporal lobe that project to anterior speech areas via the arcuate fasciculus that need be damaged to cause conduction aphasia. Thus, there is no clear evidence for a specific role of the arcuate fasciculus in repetition. The arcuate fasciculus and its role in cognition are discussed in more detail in Chapter 12.

Basal Temporal Language Area

Functional localization of language-relevant cortex by using electrical stimulation has become routine in patients who are candidates for epilepsy surgery (Lesser et al., 1986; Schäffler, Lüders, Dinner, Lesser, & Chelune, 1993). This methodology has revealed evidence of interference with language functions in areas outside the classical language areas. Electrical stimulation of the dominant basal temporal area has been shown to produce problems in both comprehension and production in some patients (Luders et al., 1986, 1991). Surgical resection of this area does not produce any lasting language deficits in most patients, but some patients have persistent dysnomia (Krauss et al., 1996). Currently, the specific role that this region subsumes in language functions is unclear.

Supplementary Motor Area and Presupplementary Motor Area

The anterior part of area 6 on the medial surface of the cerebral hemisphere, the supplementary motor area, has been implicated in speech functions since the work of Penfield and Roberts (1959), but its specific functions are still poorly understood. Stimulation of the supplementary motor area most commonly results in speech arrest (Fried et al., 1991). Surgical lesions of the dominant supplementary motor area may produce moderate to severe initial deficits, but significant lasting speech changes are uncommon (Rostomily et al., 1991). This region is also discussed further in Chapter 4.

Summary

The basic disconnection model of the anatomy of language has thus undergone considerable evolution during the past several decades. Chapter 4 extends this concept of language localization to more specific units of cognitive operations.

REFERENCES

Albert, M., Goodglass, H., Helm, N., Rubens, A., & Alexander, M. (1991). *Clinical aspects of dysphasia*. New York, NY: Springer-Verlag.

Alexander, M., Naeser, M., & Palumbo, C. (1990). Broca's area aphasia: Aphasia after lesions including the frontal operculum. *Neurology, 40*, 353–362.

Anderson, J., Gilmore, R., Roper, S., Crosson, B., Bauer, R., Nadeau, S., et al. (1999). Conduction aphasia and the arcuate fasciculus: A reexamination of the Wernicke–Geschwind model. *Brain and Language, 70*, 1–12.

Basso, A., Lecours, A., Moraschini, S., & Vanier, M. (1985). Anatomoclinical correlations of the aphasias as defined through computerized tomography: Exceptions. *Brain and Language, 26*, 201–229.

Benton, A. (1992). Gerstmann's syndrome. *Archives of Neurology, 49*, 445–447.

Binder, J., Frost, J., Hammeke, T., Rao, S., & Cox, R. (1996). Function of the left planum temporale in auditory and linguistic processing. *Brain, 119*, 1239–1247.

Blunk, R., De Bleser, R., Willmes, K., & Zeumer, H. (1981). A refined method to relate morphological and functional aspects of aphasia. *European Neurology, 20*, 69–79.

Bogen, J., & Bogen, G. (1976). Wernicke's region: Where is it? *Annals of the New York Academy of Sciences, 280*, 834–843.

Broca, P. (1865). Sur la faculte´ du language article. *Bulletin de la Socie´te´ d'Anthropologie Paris, 6*, 337–393.

Brown, J. (1975). The problem of repetition: A study of "conduction" aphasia and the "isolation" syndrome. *Cortex, 11*, 37–52.

Damasio, H., & Damasio, A. (1980). The anatomical basis of conduction aphasia. *Brain, 103*(2), 337–350.

De Renzi, E., & Faglioni, P. (1978). Normative data and screening power of a shortened version of the Token test. *Cortex, 14*, 41–49.

Dronkers, N., Plaisant, O., Iba-Zizen, M., & Cabanis, E. (2007). Paul Broca's historic cases: High resolution MR imaging of the brains of Leborgne and Lelong. *Brain, 130*(Pt. 5), 1432–1441.

Fried, I., Katz, A., McCarthy, G., Sass, K., Williamson, P., Spencer, S., et al. (1991). Functional organization of human supplementary motor cortex studied by electrical stimulation. *Journal of Neuroscience, 11*, 3656–3666.

Geschwind, N. (1965). Disconnexion syndromes in animals and man. *Brain, 88*, 237–294, 585–644.

Geschwind, N., & Levitsky, W. (1968). Human brain: Left–right asymmetries in temporal speech region. *Science, 161*, 186–187.

Goodglass, H., & Kaplan, E. (1983). *The Boston Diagnostic Aphasia Examination*. Philadelphia, PA: Lea & Febiger.

Kaplan, E., Goodglass, H., & Weintraub, S. (1983). *The Boston Naming Test* (2nd ed.). Philadelphia, PA: Lea & Febiger.

Knopman, D., Selnes, O., Niccum, N., Rubens, A., Yock, D., & Larson, D. (1983). A longitudinal study of speech fluency in aphasia: CT correlates of recovery and persistent nonfluency. *Neurology, 33*, 1170–1178.

Krauss, G., Fisher, R., Plate, C., Hart, J., Uematsu, S., Gordon, B., et al. (1996). Cognitive effects of resecting basal temporal language areas. *Epilepsia, 37*, 476–483.

Lesser, R., Luders, H., Morris, H., Dinner, D., Klem, G., Hahn, J., et al. (1986). Electrical stimulation of Wernicke's area interferes with comprehension. *Neurology, 36*, 658–663.

Lichtheim, L. (1885). On aphasia. *Brain, 7*, 433–484.

Luders, H., Lesser, R., Hahn, J., Dinner, D., Morris, H., Resor, S., et al. (1986). Basal temporal language area demonstrated by electrical stimulation. *Neurology, 36*, 505–510.

Luders, H., Lesser, R., Hahn, J., Dinner, D., Morris, H., Wyllie, E., et al. Basal temporal language area. *Brain, 114*, 743–754.

Maeshima, S., Toshiro, H., Sekiguchi, E., Okita, R., Yamaga, H., Ozaki, F., et al. (2002). Transcortical mixed aphasia due to cerebral infarction in left inferior frontal lobe and temporo-parietal lobe. *Neuroradiology, 44*(2), 133–137.

Mohr, J., Pessin, M., Finkelstein, S., Funkenstein, H., Duncan, G., & Davis, K. (1999). Broca aphasia: Pathologic and clinical. *Neurology, 28*, 311–324.

Naeser, M., Helm-Estabrooks, N., Haas, G., Auerbach, S., & Srinivasan, M. (1987). Relationship between lesion extent in "Wernicke's area" on computed tomographic scan and predicting recovery of comprehension in Wernicke's aphasia. *Archives of Neurology, 44*, 73–82.

Penfield, W., & Roberts, L. (1959). *Speech and brain mechanisms*. Princeton, NJ: Princeton University Press.

Rostomily, R., Berger, M., Ojemann, G., & Lettich, E. (1991). Postoperative deficits and functional recovery following removal of tumors involving the dominant hemisphere supplementary motor area. *Journal of Neurosurgery, 75*, 62–68.

Sakurai, Y., Takeuchi, S., Takada, T., Horiuchi, E., Nakase, H., & Sakuta, M. (2000). Alexia caused by a fusiform or posterior inferior temporal lesion. *Journal of the Neurological Sciences, 178*, 42–51.

Schäffler, L., Lüders, H., Dinner, D., Lesser, R., & Chelune, G. (1993). Comprehension deficits elicited by electrical stimulation of Broca's area. *Brain, 116*(Pt. 3), 695–715.

Selnes, O., Knopman, D., Niccum, N., & Rubens, A. (1985). The critical role of Wernicke's area in sentence repetition. *Annals of Neurology, 17*, 549–557.

Selnes, O., Niccum, N., Knopman, D., & Rubens, A. (1984). Recovery of single word comprehension: CT-scan correlates. *Brain and Language, 21*, 72–84.

Shuren, J., Schefft, B., Yeh, H., Privitera, M., Cahill, W., & Houston, W. (1995). Repetition and the arcuate fasciculus. *Journal of Neurology, 242*, 596–598.

Vignolo, L., Boccardi, E., & Caverni, L. (1986). Unexpected CT-scan findings in global aphasia. *Cortex, 22*, 55–69.

Wernicke, C. (1874). *Der Aphasische Symptomencomplex. Ein psychologische studie auf anatomischer Basis.* Breslau, Germany: Cohn & Weigert.

4

Integrated Cognitive Neuroscience Approach to the Neural Basis of Language

The classical disconnection model has utility in clinical settings; however, dissatisfaction with the classical taxonomy of aphasia was first expressed by researchers in the field of aphasia, particularly psycholinguists and cognitive psychologists (Schwartz, 1984). One major concern was that the classical model does not necessarily generate meaningful insights into the organization of language in the brain, as opposed to its accounting for a set of observed aphasic symptoms. Some have argued that the classical aphasia syndromes do not meet standard criteria for a syndrome in that none of the syndromes can be characterized in terms of invariant features that are shared by all patients given a certain classification and are absent in patients with a different classification (Caramazza, 1984).

Of paramount importance, however, were claims by clinicians that the aphasia syndromes described too few patients (Basso et al., 1985; Vignolo et al., 1986; Willmes & Poeck, 1993). A study assessing patients 1 year after their stroke demonstrated that the frequencies of aphasias were as follows: global, 7%; Broca's, 13%; isolation, 0%; transcortical motor, 1%; Wernicke's, 5%; transcortical sensory, 0%; conduction, 6%; and anomic, 29% (Pedersen et al., 2004). Even with this limited number of patients being classified by the disconnection model, the clinical use of the classical syndrome classification as a basis for diagnosis has continued.

The evidence that classic aphasia syndromes carry prognostic implications was also not compelling. The Boston Diagnostic Aphasia Examination diagnostic classifications were somewhat predictive of outcome for syndromes characterized by mild impairment, such as anomic and conduction aphasia, and for those characterized by severe syndromes, such as global aphasia. This was consistent with the findings from several studies showing that one of the best prognostic indicators for recovery from aphasia is initial degree of severity (Pedersen et al., 1995). Syndromes that were characterized by a greater range in severity, such as Broca's and Wernicke's aphasia, are not predictive of outcomes (Kertesz & McCabe, 1977). One of the most compelling reasons to expand upon, not replace, the classical disconnection model is the fact that the disconnection approach accounts for so few aphasic patients.

The field of cognitive brain localization grew out of the studies of language syndromes and their associated brain lesions. Rapid developments in cognitive neuroscience and neuroimaging since the 1990s have allowed for the proposal of a cognitive neuroscience model that describes how the brain encodes language operations and explains aphasic behavior. The advantages of these types of models are that they (1) attempted to account for all observed aphasic language symptoms, (2) provided more theoretically and clinically relevant language components that correlate with specific brain regions, and (3) took advantage of the multitude of activation studies conducted in control subjects to understand how the normal brain performs language functions. This last point raised the important issue that an integrated account of language and aphasia was required to reconcile the findings of activation and lesion studies in describing how the brain performs language operations.

The basic language operations assessed previously for the classical disconnection approach are still correlated with their associated anatomic regions within this new framework. The cognitive neuroscience approach supplemented the classical approach by assessing the brain regions associated with representation and access to the language components of lexical semantics, orthography, phonology, and syntax (Figure 4.1). These components are most useful for developing both theoretical and practical explanations for normal and aphasic language function. These language components have

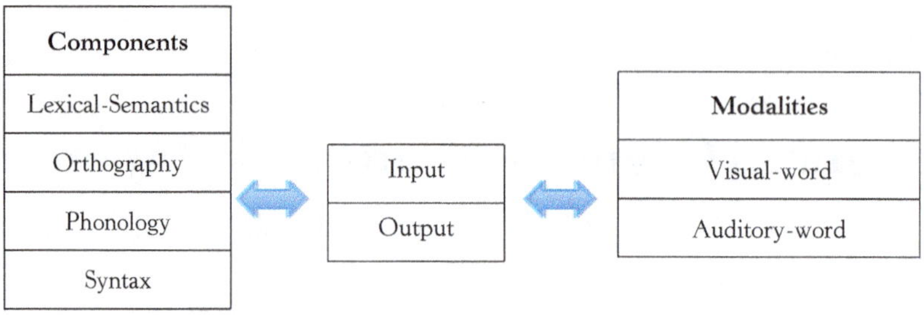

FIGURE 4.1: The four major language components are defined as follows: (1) lexical semantics, which refers to stores encoding for the meaning and associated meaning-based relationships of words; (2) orthography, which refers to the organization of written word representations in language; (3) phonology, which represents the systematic organization of the sound system in a language; and (4) syntax, which refers to the rules governing word order by which sentences are constructed in a language. These components can receive input and/or send output to each other. More important, input and output to each of these components can be in visual word or auditory word modalities.

additional subcomponents that engage various combinations of brain regions subserving representation of language units (e.g., words, letters, and sounds), some of which may be encoded in spatially distributed representations (Hinton, 1981), and processing of these representations.

The four major language components are defined as follows:

1. Lexical semantics, which refers to stores encoding for the meaning and associated meaning-based relationships of words
2. Orthography, which refers to the organization of written word representations in language
3. Phonology, which represents the systematic organization of the sound system in a language
4. Syntax, which refers to the rules governing word order by which sentences are constructed in a language

These components can receive input and/or send output to each other. More important, input and output to each of these components can be in visual word or auditory word modalities (see Figure 4.1). A clear example to demonstrate this is that recognition of a visual word input to the orthographic system is the function of reading, whereas output from that system is spelling, which can be either in auditory or in written word (oral spelling and written spelling, respectively). As each of these components is discussed, the input and output pathways need to be considered when assigning any cognitive–anatomic correlations.

The tests for assessing each of these language components can be similar to those outlined for the disconnection model; the results are interpreted and framed in terms of language and cognitive units. As a result, the cognitive–brain correlations described in this chapter are now framed not in terms of aphasic syndromes as in Chapter 3 but, rather, by the specific cognitive language components and correlated cognitive anatomic units (CAUs) when isolatable. The following outlines a framework for this integrated cognitive neuroscience approach to language in the brain and its application to explaining aphasic behavior. As further studies are completed, clarification and expansion of the framework will provide a more detailed account of the regions involved.

In most of the following chapters, there is a summary table of the brain lesions and correlated cognitive units. These tables are included for ease of reference and to find main points more easily.

LEXICAL SEMANTICS (STORES ENCODING THE MEANING AND ASSOCIATED MEANING-BASED RELATIONSHIPS OF WORDS)

The term "semantics" has many meanings in cognitive neuroscience, which has led to much confusion throughout the years (Shallice, 1993). Semantics in the context of this text refers to stores of knowledge. Hart and Gordon (1992) demonstrated the difference between semantic knowledge in the visual system (e.g., visual semantics) and semantic knowledge in the language system (e.g., lexical semantics). Because we are concerned here with the language system, we concentrate on the lexical semantic system encoding the knowledge and meaning of words and the interrelationships between these words based on their meanings and associations.

This component is usually assessed by patient performance on comprehension testing questions (e.g., "Do birds have wings?"), comprehension of single words, confrontation naming, and the output of spontaneous speech (e.g., error patterns and semantic substitutions). The pattern of performance across these types of tasks can indicate deficits in the lexical semantic system. For example, a patient with a lexical semantic impairment may present with fluent speech but notable for semantic paraphasias, impaired naming with circumlocutions and occasional semantic errors in naming, and impaired comprehension.

Studies on clinical patients and functional imaging activation studies have both demonstrated cognitive and anatomical aspects associated with the *organization* of lexical semantics and possible associated *processing* regions (see Hart et al., 2007; Binder & Desai, 2011). The organization term refers to the CAUs by which lexical semantic knowledge is organized, whereas processing refers to operations that are performed to this knowledge. These correlates are described next.

Lexical Semantic Representational Organization

Evidence from focal brain lesions and from degenerative brain conditions has shown that aspects of the lexical semantic system may be organized by semantic category (Caramazza & Shelton, 1998) because categories can be differentially affected by these neural injuries. Nielsen (1946) was the first to describe a double dissociation between the ability to name living things and the ability to name nonliving things (with opposite patterns of preservation or impairment across different patients). Hart et al. (1985) made the proposition from a case of anomia for fruits and vegetables that the lexical semantic system is organized by categories. Since then, there have been many individual and group reports of such dissociations for a variety of categories, including living things, animals, plants, food, fruits and vegetables, body parts, countries, emotional facial expressions, small manipulable objects, shapes, colors, letters, numbers, action names, verbs, case marking prepositions and tense, girl and boy names, family and friends, famous people, proper names, cities, rivers, countries, and mountains (Berndt, 1988; Cappa et al., 1998; Damasio, 1990; Damasio et al., 1990, 1996; Farah, 1989; Farah & Wallace, 1992; Farah et al., 1991, 1996; Ferreira et al., 1997; Funnell & Sheridan, 1992; Gainotti et al., 1995; Garrard et al., 1998; Goodglass et al., 1966, 1986; Hart & Gordon, 1992; Hillis & Caramazza, 1991; Humphreys & Riddoch, 1987; Mauri et al., 1994; McCarthy & Warrington, 1988; Rapcsak et al., 1989, 1993; Robinson et al., 1996; Sacchett & Humphreys, 1992; Sartori & Job, 1988; Sartori et al., 1993; Semenza & Zettin, 1988, 1989; Silveri & Gainotti, 1988; Silveri et al., 1991; Temple, 1986; Tippett et al., 1996; Warrington & McCarthy, 1983, 1987; Warrington & Shallice, 1984; for similar issues in degenerative conditions, see Grossman et al., 1998). In addition, functional imaging studies of the picture-naming task have suggested that aspects of this categorical organization may be localized to specific brain regions. Animals selectively activate the left medial occipital lobe and tools selectively activate the left middle temporal gyrus and the left premotor region (Martin et al., 1996), or animals associate with activation of the left inferior temporal gyri and naming of tools is associated with activation of the left middle and inferior temporal gyri (Damasio et al., 1996). These distinctions have not yet been fully reconciled (see Spitzer et al., 1995; Moore & Price, 1999). However, lesions in these regions do not result consistently in deficits specific to these categories of stimuli. Another lexical semantic organizational unit, the category by feature interaction (visual perceptual properties of the category animals), has been isolated several times behaviorally after lesions have occurred; however, anatomic correlates for these units have not been clearly identified (Hart & Gordon, 1992; Sartori & Job, 1988; Silveri & Gainotti, 1988). Taking into consideration both the functional imaging and lesion data, there appears to be clearly definable and dissociable cognitive units; however, there is not a sufficiently consistent anatomic correlate to identify a CAU.

Whereas there is no clear anatomic unit that designates the localization of a category of lexical semantic knowledge, there is less evidence for a localizable anatomic region for individual specific entities/items. In fact, to the author's knowledge, an anatomic correlate for loss of a single word or word meaning has not been identified. It is obvious that individual words, or word meanings in the case of lexical semantics, are stored in the brain, but the manner by which they are stored is clearly not a CAU as these units have been defined. With the smallest cognitive unit delineated being a category or category feature interaction (e.g., visual perceptual features of animals; Hart & Gordon, 1992), and

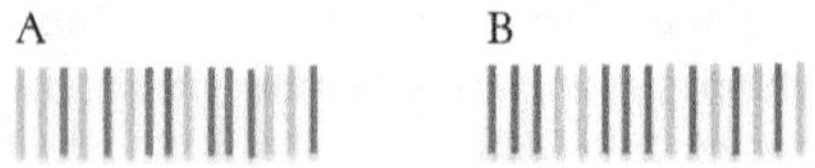

FIGURE 4.2: In this schematic, each line represents a neuron (or group/network of neurons), with each one being located in various parts of the brain. Although they appear as a bar code in this schematic, the neuron/neurons signified by each line are referred to as a neural unit and are spatially distinct and likely not neighboring each other. At a given time, these neural units will be active (green signifying "on") or not active (red signifying "off"). The pattern of all the "on" and "off" neural units taken together signifies a specific semantic entity (e.g., pattern A is the word "cup"). The same neural units, but more likely each neural unit is involved in different groupings for each specific semantic entity, firing in a different pattern (e.g., pattern B) would signify another distinct entity (e.g., bison). This different firing pattern will likely occur at a different time. (One could propose that if both patterns are activated at the same time, then both entities would be activated and thus be somewhat conflicting, with less conflict if both entities are semantically related). In this manner, one can encode an extremely large number of unique entities with many fewer neurons than entities. Also, by being in spatially different locations, this type of coding protects against losing individual entities when there is focal brain damage.

Source: Hinton (1981) and Hart and Kraut (2007).

this without a circumscribed anatomic correlate, the neural organization of individual items can only be speculative.

Given the importance and interest in how individual units of knowledge may be encoded in the brain, multiple theories have been proposed. One theory proposes that an extensive amount of semantic knowledge is encoded in a spatially distributed manner (for details, see Figure 4.2). This is delineated in the neural hybrid model of semantic memory (Hart & Kraut, 2007; Hart et al., 2013) and is based on a "coarse coding" model of semantic organization proposed by Hinton (1981). In this type of schema, relevant neurons (or groups of neurons) that encode for units of semantic knowledge are located in spatially different locations. The firing pattern of all the relevant neurons for a unit of knowledge, the "on" and "off" of all of the neurons taken together at a given time, signifies a specific entity (e.g., in Figure 4.2, pattern A is the word "cup"). Neurons can be associated with a variety of groups of other neurons so that when firing in different "on" and "off" patterns, each time they signify a different specific semantic entity (e.g., Figure 4.2, pattern B is another, different word). This proposed, hypothetical schema allows for the capacity to encode for large amounts of information, and the multiple neurons involved in encoding a single entity (and located in different locations) protect against damage causing loss of individual entities, all of which is consistent with observed behavior.

The following section delineates processing units that can detect, access, manipulate, and interact with these entities when engaging the lexical semantic system.

Lexical Semantic Processing

Distinct brain regions have been associated in both activation and lesion studies with aspects of semantic processing, including the following:

1. Left inferior parietal–posterior superior temporal region (IP-ST) for categorization, synonymity, and property judgments for objects/items (Figure 4.3) (Hart & Gordon, 1990; Vandenberghe et al., 1996), as well as thematic or what–where processing for sentence comprehension (Dronkers et al., 2004; Thothathiri et al., 2012; and see Race et al., 2012). This region is imputed to be associated with semantic processing in general, with the likely major function of the region being multimodal integration of semantic knowledge from multiple semantic memory subsystems (e.g., visual, auditory, and tactile). Further evidence of the role that this region plays in integration of knowledge from multiple semantic subsystems in humans extends from nonlinguistic electrophysiological studies in nonhuman primates demonstrating multimodal integration occurring at this site.
2. Left fusiform gyri (Abdullaev & Posner, 1998; Hart et al., 1998; Nobre et al., 1994) with categorization, synonymity, and property judgment of objects/items. This also appears to be a multimodality integration region (Figure 4.4), particularly in integrating visual semantic information with other modalities supporting semantics and processing that information. Another function that this region may perform is as an interface between visual semantic and episodic memory (Levy et al., 2004).

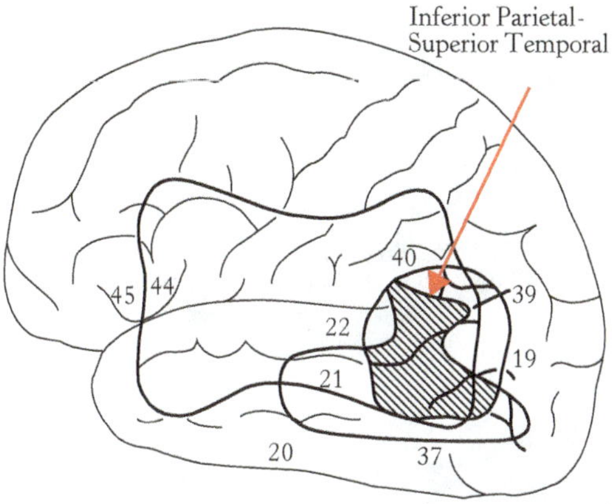

FIGURE 4.3: The diagonally lined region represents the area of overlap between lesions of patients who had experienced strokes and exhibited lexical semantic deficits. This identifies that an inferior parietal superior temporal region as designated.

Source: Hart and Gordon (1990).

3. Left presupplementary motor area (pre-SMA) with semantic cued generation and selection of targets for semantic retrieval of single words (Crosson et al., 1999; but see also Alexander & Benson, 1993; Binder et al., 2009; Kraut et al., 2002). This region has also been proposed to engage in identifying/selecting a target item from semantic memory as part of the search process (Figure 4.5). In fact, this CAU's cognitive unit of search/identification with this brain region may also be engaged by other cognitive domains (see the "energization" section in Chapter 9) and thus represents a domain-general function. The region has been found to be lesioned in patients with transcortical motor aphasia who have decreased spontaneous speech, which requires conducting a semantic search for words to string together for cogent speech. These patients have relatively intact repetition, where searching is not required because the words to say are presented to the patient aurally to repeat. Thus, the finding of disruption of this cognitive unit best explains the symptoms of the aphasic syndrome.
4. Left inferior frontal gyrus with selection between multiple semantic stimuli (Demb et al., 1995; Demonet et al., 1992; Kapur et al., 1994; Petersen et al., 1988, 1990; Posner et al., 1988; Ricci et al., 1999; Thompson-Schill et al., 1997). This function was most notable during effortful selection of semantic information when many alternative responses are possible or there may be competing semantic representations. This region may not be specific to just selecting semantic stimuli but, rather, could be

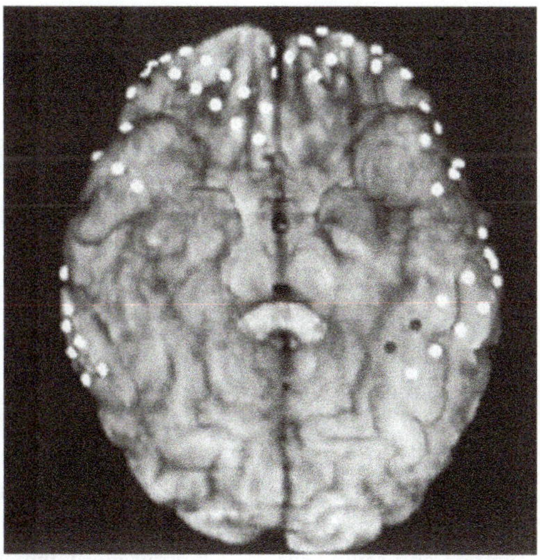

FIGURE 4.4: Co-registration of CT scan of subdural electrodes with 3-D reconstruction of subject's brain MRI. The perspective is a basal brain view with electrode locations represented by the circles. The pair of dark circles in the left lingual gyrus (anterior aspect) represents the electrode pair. Electrical stimulation at the dark pair of electrodes resulted in a semantic deficit in the functions of categorization, synonymity, and property judgments for objects.

Source: Hart et al. (1998).

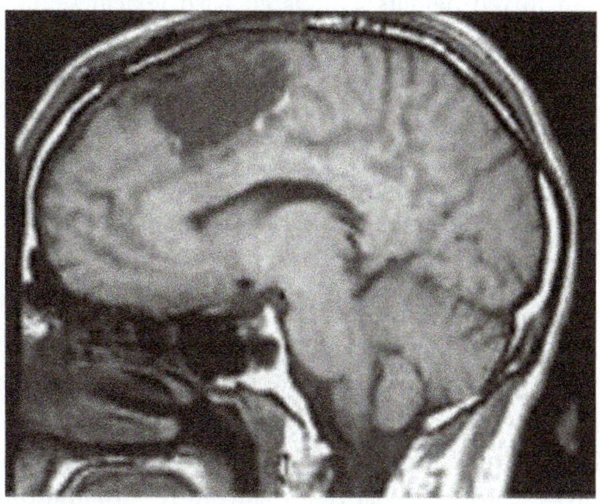

FIGURE 4.5: Medial frontal lobe (supplementary and presupplementary motor area) lesion associated with decreased verbal output.

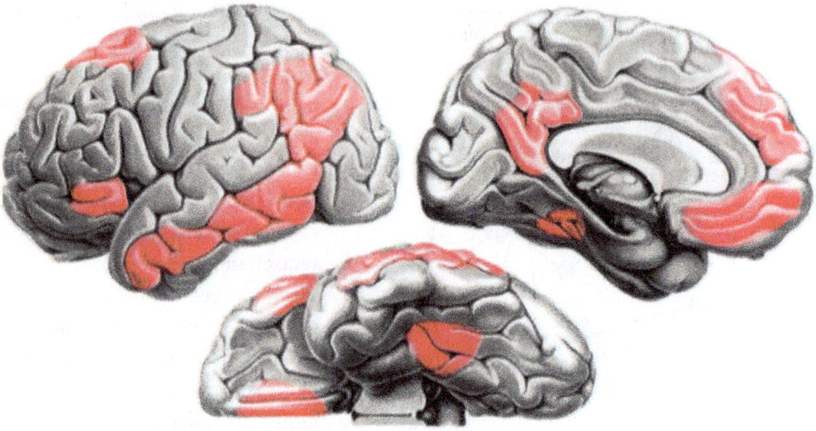

FIGURE 4.6: Summary diagram of regions involved in semantic operations in the brain.
Source: Binder et al. (2009).

a "cognitive domain general" processing region involved in item selection in other cognitive domains in addition to semantics and language.

The previously mentioned regions have each been associated with deficits in lexical semantic processing in both activation and lesion studies by independent lesions affecting only the brain region noted. The group of regions involved is summarized in Figure 4.6.

As investigative techniques provide greater resolution, and further regions involved in the lexical semantic network are identified with their associated functions (more CAUs), the group of regions supporting the lexical semantic system will be further defined, resulting in descriptions of pure and mixed deficits associated with lexical semantics, in addition to the already reported semantic impairments seen in semantic aphasia and semantic dementia (Hodges et al., 1992).

ORTHOGRAPHY (ORGANIZATION OF WRITTEN WORD REPRESENTATIONS)

The orthographic lexicon is the store of written word representations in the brain. Localization of aspects of orthography has been a controversial issue in functional imaging studies. Whereas some investigators suspect that the word representations or stores themselves are encoded in a spatially distributed manner (Hart et al., 2000), others have suggested a more focal circumscribed localization (Petersen et al., 1988), including a proposed fusiform gyrus word area. These localizations demonstrated with functional imaging studies, however, have not always been correlated with disruption to aspects of orthography in lesion studies.

The most efficacious method of assessing these components is to have the patient write, read, or perform a task referred to as the lexical decision task. The lexical decision task consists of presenting a letter string visually for the subject to decide if the letter string is a word or a nonword (e.g., "trest" vs. "treat"). This test readily assesses the integrity of an orthographic store of word representations as well as access to this store.

Extensive studies of patients with reading disorders have delineated several plausible pathways involved in the routes to reading. One of the proposed methods by which individuals read aloud, considered to be the method used by most individuals to learn to read, is referred to as orthographic-to-phonological conversion. In this method, a letter string is analyzed visually to identify the letters presented, followed by taking the letters and "sounding them out," putting the sounds together, and saying the sounded-out word, which also activates access to the orthographic lexicon at some point along this processing stream. A second pathway to reading is referred to as the direct access route to an orthographic lexicon. In this route, the subject can directly access the representation of the written word in the orthographic word store without sounding the word out. This is the way adults typically read and is referred to as sight word reading. Investigators have theorized that initially children learn to read using the orthographic-to-phonological conversion pathway, and continual repetition of reading a word in this manner leads to conversion to sight recognition of the word and thus use of direct access to the orthographic lexicon pathway upon seeing the word visually. The third proposed system for reading a word is a pathway purporting that word recognition via the orthographic lexicon can be accessed by first accessing the meaning of the word, referred to as the direct access to word recognition via semantics. This pathway is not well understood, and it is also unclear how frequently it is utilized.

Localizations based on reading impairments signifying disruption of the orthographic lexicon and/or access to it are interpreted within the context of these three mechanisms of reading (Coltheart et al., 1980; Coslett, 2000; Hillis et al., 1999; Patterson et al., 1985). The localizations that appear to be the most consistent with these orthographic constructs were first described in the 19th century. Dejerine and colleagues (1891, 1892) initially suggested from cases of alexia with concomitant agraphia that the *left angular gyrus* was a region that could be essential for a single orthographic lexicon or access to it. A second key region associated with the orthographic lexicon is the *left ventromedial occipital lobe* (including white matter areas), where lesions can produce pure alexia (without agraphia) by interfering with transmission of visual information to left hemisphere language areas (Dejerine, 1892). This localization suggests lesions to this region disrupt the visual pathway access to the orthographic lexicon or disrupt a distinct visual input orthographic lexicon or access to it. This is the classic lesion that affects both the left hemisphere occipital cortical area and underlying white matter regions to the extent that it blocks visual letter information from reaching the orthographic lexicon. This occurs by disrupting the left visual cortex processing of letter information and blocking transfer of visual letter information from crossing the posterior corpus callosum from the right hemisphere visual regions to reach the left hemisphere orthographic lexicon.

Extension of lesions in this region to include the left posterior inferior temporal cortex (PITC; fusiform and inferior temporal gyri (Brodmann areas 37/20)) results in those with alexia as well as agraphia and spelling difficulties (Bowers et al., 1996; Friedman & Hadley, 1992; Rapcsak & Beeson, 2004; Rapcsak et al., 1990). This suggests that the left PITC may play a more dominant role in the output from the orthographic lexicon (Figure 4.7). Further studies supportive of this finding are needed to consider this a consistent localization, particularly given the number of other operations other than orthographic processing associated with this region.

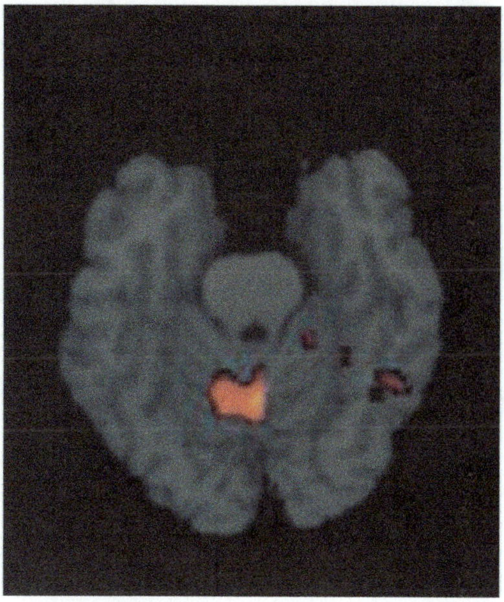

FIGURE 4.7: Composite lesion map of the overlap of lesions in patients with output from the orthographic lexicon dysfunction.

Source: Rapcsak and Beeson (2004).

PHONOLOGY (ORGANIZATION OF THE SOUND SYSTEM IN A LANGUAGE)

Phonology represents the systematic organization of the sound system in a language. This concept can be confused with phonemes and phonetics. *Phonemes* refer to the basic units of sounds in phonology and are defined as the "smallest linguistic unit that can change the meaning of a word." The neural instantiation of phonology and the phonological lexicon in the brain must account for encoding of the system of phonemes (which can also be defined as the abstract representation of sounds in the brain) and the combination of these phonemes to the point of making words. (*Phonetics* refers to the actual physical production (acoustic output) of speech sounds and perception of these speech sounds.)

Assessment of the phonological system and access to it are typically performed with the tasks of speech discrimination, repetition, and analysis of spontaneous speech. Phonemic paraphasic errors in speech production have been considered a hallmark feature of damage to the phonological lexicon or output from it. It is also clear that the inability to discriminate speech sounds can reflect impairment of input to the phonological lexicon or damage to the lexicon. This last point was demonstrated behaviorally in the description of those with pure word deafness (inability to understand speech or repeat words but able to recognize nonverbal sounds, speak, read, and write) that was shown to stem from a disruption related to the phonological lexical system (Caramazza et al., 1983).

It appears that there are at least several different access routes to the phonological system that can be dissociated, depending on whether it is input or output to phonology (Bub & Kertesz, 1982). Regions associated with access to phonology from speech input have been identified by focal, circumscribed temporary, reversible lesions produced by cortical electrical interference in the left posterior superior temporal gyrus during speech discrimination tasks (Boatman et al., 1995, 1997; Figure 4.8). These regions bordered the primary auditory cortex but were spatially distinct from it. Also, the left posterior superior temporal gyrus has been suggested to participate in phonemic aspects of speech production, in addition to its previously described role in speech perception (Hickok et al., 2000). Distinguishing between the cognitive roles that each region plays, if they do function independently, is left to future studies.

Blumstein (2009) reviewed the neural correlates of auditory word recognition in functional neuroimaging and lesion studies in the manner that is done in this text. The conclusions from that review are that auditory word recognition proceeds through stages via cascade processing (see Chapter 1). Information passes through regions encoding distinct stages of processing: acoustic–phonetic processing in superior temporal areas; the supramarginal gyrus (which could also be the bilateral supramarginal gyri; see Hartwigsen et al., 2010) functioning in discriminating words distinguished by close phonological contrasts and proposed to be engaged in mapping sound onto phonological lexical entities; and lexical selection (among lexical competitors) in the inferior frontal gyrus (see Thompson-Schill et al., 1997 and also selection in lexical semantics, suggesting that this region may be cognitive domain general and not specific to a given cognitive operation in one domain) (Blumstein, 2009).

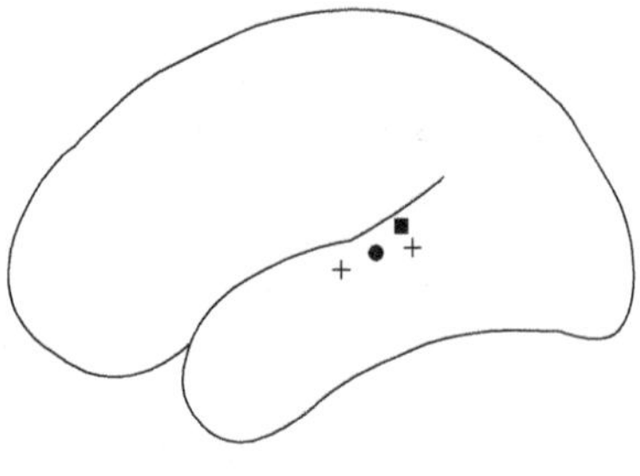

FIGURE 4.8: Electrode location on a Tailarach map from a patient who had disruption of access to phonology from speech as seen in disruption of a speech discrimination task.

Source: Boatman et al. (1995).

Hickok and Poeppel (2004) proposed a cognitive neuroscience model to account for processing auditory linguistic information—a dorsal stream for auditory–motor integration that traverses the posterior Sylvian fissure from the parietal–temporal boundary, an area that they designated Sylvian–parietal–temporal (Spt). Over this dorsal stream, information flows bidirectionally between auditory–phonological representations located in the posterior temporal cortex and articulatory–motor speech representations located in prefrontal speech regions (Schwartz et al., 2012). These prefrontal regions supporting motor speech output include the supplementary motor area, inferior premotor cortex (Broca's area), anterior insula, the mouth representation in the primary motor cortex, and the cerebellum (Fox et al., 2000).

Given this framework, the third region that appears to represent a CAU associated with phonological processing and is to be more clearly delineated in terms of cognitive operations is the left posterior inferior frontal gyrus. Damage to this region in Broca's area leads to the inability to transform word representations into the corresponding articulatory sequences (Price, 1998). This has been demonstrated in phonological errors in repetition with lesions in this region, showing that this impaired transformation of word representations includes when the input to be transformed originates in the phonological lexical system. In addition, studies have shown that impairment in this function may extend from spontaneous speech to other tasks such as reading, implying that this region is engaged in transforming word representations from both the phonological and the orthographic

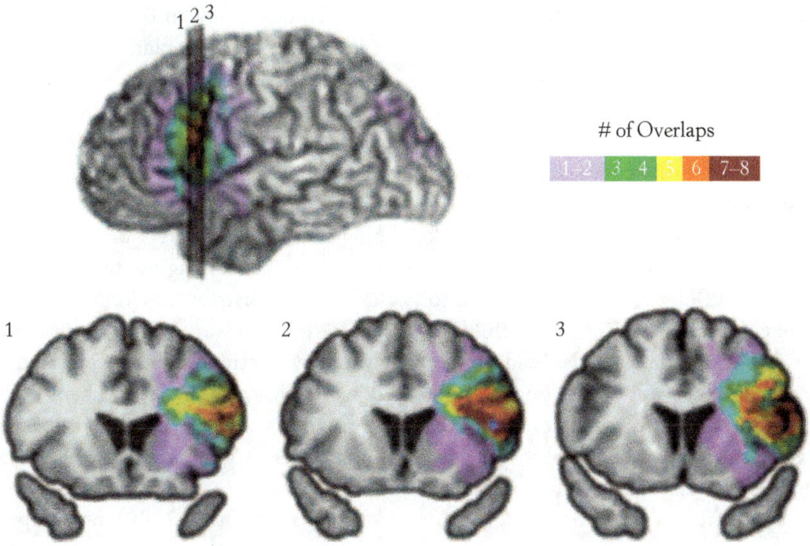

FIGURE 4.9: Lesion overlap map for 11 subjects with damage to the left posterior inferior frontal gyrus associated with a phonological deficit detected while reading aloud nonwords. Colors represent the number of subjects with overlap in the region.

Source: Fiez et al. (2006).

lexicons into articulatory sequences. Patient studies of individuals with lesions in approximately Broca's area demonstrated difficulties in reading aloud pronounceable nonwords (e.g., "trest") (Figure 4.9) (Fiez et al., 2006).

Disruption of conversion of phonological and orthographic lexical representations into intelligible articulations accounts for a subset of the symptoms of patients with Broca's aphasia, demonstrating the capability of the cognitive neuroscience approach to account for aphasic symptoms in the classical aphasic syndromes and aphasic symptoms in other patients with lesions including this brain region but not the other brain areas required for producing Broca's aphasia. Thus, although these patients do not necessarily present with a classical aphasic syndrome, most patients' deficits can be accounted for by the cognitive neuroscience approach of delineating the underlying cognitive units/processes that are disrupted, with disruptions of these units being the mechanisms producing the aphasic behavior.

Another aspect of localization that has developed with recent advances in modern neuroimaging is the ability to assess the structural integrity of white matter tracts in the brain. The fiber tracts of the proposed auditory dorsal stream system have been investigated using the white matter tracking technique of diffusion tensor imaging. Saur et al. (2008) found that word repetition was subserved via the arcuate and superior longitudinal fasciculi connecting the temporal and frontal lobes (Breier et al., 2008; Glasser & Rilling, 2008; Saur et al., 2008). Future studies using these techniques for white matter lesion mapping and correlating these with cognitive impairments will lead to a more detailed anatomic mapping of circuitry supporting cognitive functions, including phonology in language.

SYNTAX (SYSTEM OF GRAMMAR)

The term *syntax* refers to the rules governing word order by which sentences are constructed in a language. How the brain encodes these rules to form a system of grammar, even if such rules are overtly encoded, and whether these are encoded in circumscribed regions are controversial. Compared to the other language components of the brain, syntax does not have theoretical cognitive constructs based on a lexicon (storage of words) but, in general, consists of the process of ordering words in a grammatical manner to form sentences and interpreting the meaning of sentences based on word order during comprehension of other's sentences spoken to you.

The other language components with a lexical system organization allowed for development of cognitive units and processes more readily than syntax and are thus further ahead in delineating how these cognitive units are neutrally encoded. This lack of delineation of cognitive units may extend from syntactic cognitive processes not being intuitive or the fact that lesion studies have not resulted in disruption of syntax into recognizable cognitive subcomponents. This lack of delineation of cognitive aspects of syntax may also extend from a lack of knowledge of how syntax and syntactic operations are acquired developmentally. As opposed to the other language components, for which children are taught how to pronounce words, read words, and the meanings of those words, it is unclear how children first acquire the basic principles of syntactic order or even how later, more complex syntactic constructions are learned. This applies to both the production of syntactically correct sentences and the comprehension of sentences of varying syntactic complexity. Although grammar is taught in schools to some degree, it is relatively late in the language acquisition time frame, after proficiency in syntactic usage has developed to a large degree. It is proposed that syntactic knowledge is assimilated by children via the experience of using language in both production and comprehension, although how this occurs is not clearly understood. This lack of specification of the cognitive units of syntax or general anatomic regions previously associated with syntax has rendered developing fine-grained CAUs challenging.

The investigation of syntactical operations and performance includes examination of aspects of both syntactic production and comprehension. Typical assessment of syntactic production extends from evaluating spontaneous speech for grammatical complexity (Kaplan et al., 1983) and repetition of syntactically complex sentences or sentences with numerous function words (e.g., "no ifs, ands, or buts"). Syntactic comprehension is routinely assessed at a basic level in a picture–sentence matching task using semantically reversible (both the subject and the object can be reversed and the sentence would still be plausible) passive sentences ("Point to the correct picture describing this sentence, 'The car was hit by the truck'").

Anatomical localization of syntactic processes has been variable (see Caplan, 1999). One task-related activation study of syntactic comprehension processing showed involvement of a component of Broca's area, a right inferior frontal region, the left caudate nucleus, and the insula (Moro et al., 2001), whereas another studying sentences of increasing syntactic complexity noted only increased blood flow in Broca's area during syntactic judgment tasks (Caplan et al., 2000). Part of the variability in localizing syntactic processing may be attributable to different stimuli, testing paradigms, and investigative techniques, although some investigators have suggested that the variability is due to anatomical substrates of syntactic processes not being encoded as discrete brain regions detectable by current neuroimaging techniques (e.g., more anatomically distributed circuits).

Studies have suggested the existence of CAUs with the syntactic comprehension aspects of syntax. For example, syntactic comprehension of sentences for functions such as the relation between phrasal constituents (e.g., matching the sentence, "The cat that the dog is chasing is black," to the correct picture; Grodzinsky, 2000) or comprehension of spoken sentences that contain a syntactically ambiguous phrase (e.g., matching the sentence, "The boy is chased by the horse," to a picture of a boy chasing a horse; Tyler et al., 2011) have been localized to the left posterior inferior frontal gyrus (Broca's area). In addition, voxel-based lesion–symptom mapping in 50 Icelandic aphasics showed that impaired processing of syntactically complex sentences was associated with damage to the left anterior superior and middle temporal gyri and the temporal pole (Magnusdottir et al., 2013). As more of these types of studies across multiple individuals continue to provide converging evidence consistent with the previously discussed findings, these localizations can be considered consistent associations with syntactic cognitive units. Currently, there are enough inconsistencies between studies that clear localizations of syntactic functions are not reportable.

PROSODY

Prosody is defined as the melodic line of speech produced by variations of pitch, rhythm, and stress of pronunciation (Monrad-Krohn, 1963). The prosody of a sentence conveys considerable information, such as the type of sentence (statement, question, exclamatory, etc.) and its emotional content (spoken happily, angrily, etc.).

Studies of the localization of prosody-related functions have suggested some specific localizations of general aspects of prosody. Ross (1981) examined emotional expression and comprehension in right brain-damaged patients and suggested that the right hemisphere is organized for emotional expression and comprehension in a manner that is somewhat analogous to language in the left

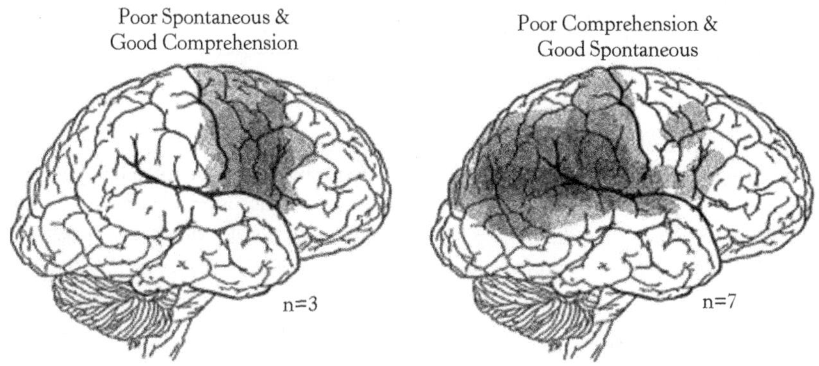

FIGURE 4.10: Lesion overlap designating regions associated with poor spontaneous affective prosody production and good affective prosody comprehension (left) and poor affective prosody comprehension and good spontaneous affective prosody production (right).

Source: Ross and Monnot (2008).

hemisphere. From those studies, Ross postulated an emotional prosody circuit in the right hemisphere, with that hemisphere mediating both expression and comprehension of emotional messages. This was further refined by Ross and Monnot (2008) in their study of 21 patients with right hemisphere lesions, 18 with left hemisphere lesions, and 42 controls tested with the aprosodia battery (Ross, Thompson, & Yenkosky, 1997). Overall, their findings showed that the right posterior inferior frontal region was essential for the production of affective prosody in speech and the right posterior superior temporal region was found to be essential for comprehension of affective prosody (Figure 4.10).

Other investigators have also implicated right perisylvian regions and other additional areas in prosody. Adolphs et al. (2002) studied 66 lesioned patients for impairments in recognizing emotions from prosody and then assessed for lesion overlap in those with impairments. Recognition of emotional prosody was associated with lesions of the right frontoparietal cortex (similar to Ross and colleagues), as well as bilateral frontal pole and left posterior inferior frontal regions (Adolphs et al., 2002). These latter two localizations have not received considerable corresponding support.

Subcortical regions have also been suggested to be essential for prosodic operations. Cancelliere and Kertesz (1990) studied 28 right hemisphere stroke patients, 18 left hemisphere strokes, and 20 controls using standardized tests of expression and comprehension of emotional prosody. Lesions of the basal ganglia were found to be most frequently associated with aprosodic deficits, followed by anterior temporal lobe and insula lesions (Cancelliere & Kertesz, 1990). Although it appears that the basal ganglia is involved in prosodic operations, basal ganglia lesions often do not result in prosodic deficits; thus, this localization does not appear to be a consistent one.

Overall, the cognitive neuroscience approach to language dysfunction is evolving as both functional imaging studies of normal and aphasic subjects continue to be conducted and linked to associated lesion studies. By describing patients' aphasic symptoms and linking them to anatomic correlates and underlying cognitive units disrupted, nearly all patients with aphasia can obtain an accurate account of their dysfunction (for CAUs, see Table 4.1). The success of this model will likely depend on several factors, including the combination of experimental paradigms with the evolving investigative techniques to explore, in both spatial and temporal domains, the multiple regions engaged in networks involved in the processing of these various linguistic components and what role each node in a network plays. As neuroimaging and analytic techniques evolve, the cognitive neuroscience framework will also need to incorporate in the model the neural mechanisms (e.g., electrophysiological coherence and neurotransmitter mediation) that subserve the cognitive operations involved in language. Finally, it will be essential to integrate in models not only the connections between the cognitive–linguistic components within language (e.g., the interface between orthography and phonology, and other units) but also other cognitive components outside the language system proper that contribute significantly

TABLE 4.1: LANGUAGE SUMMARY

Brain Region	Function
Lexical Semantics	
Left inferior parietal–posterior superior temporal region	Categorization, synonymity, and property judgment; sentence comprehension; multimodal integration
Left fusiform gyrus	Categorization, synonymity, and property judgment; multimodal integration
Orthography	
Left angular gyrus	Access to orthographic lexicon
Left ventromedial occipital region including underlying white matter to point of blocking/including posterior corpus callosum	Access to orthographic lexicon
Phonology	
Left posterior superior temporal gyrus	Access to phonology from speech input
Left supramarginal gyrus	Mapping sound structure to the phonological lexicon
Left posterior inferior frontal gyrus (within Broca's area)	Transform word representations into the corresponding articulatory sequences
Prosody	
Right posterior inferior frontal region	Affective prosody—production
Right posterior superior temporal region	Affective prosody—comprehension
Domain General for Lexical Processing	
Left pre-SMA	Cued generation; selection in retrieval
Left inferior frontal gyrus	Selection between multiple lexical stimuli

to successful task performance. For example, although not included directly in the previously discussed neural circuits, it has become increasing clear through a variety of functional imaging studies (D'Esposito et al., 1999) that the dorsal lateral prefrontal cortex is involved in aspects of working memory. As this region and its connections to other linguistic components are explored, it will be useful to integrate working memory and other cognitive control circuits (see Chapter 9) into the models proposed here for language processing.

APHASIA RECOVERY

A great deal could be gleaned about the cognitive neuroscience of language from recovery patterns of aphasic symptoms after acute lesions. Recovery from aphasia has traditionally been thought to depend on a complex interaction of lesion size and location, with patient characteristics such as age, gender, and handedness also playing a considerable role (Crosson et al., 2005). To date, large-scale prospective studies of aphasia recovery have not been conducted to confirm a significant predictive relationship between demographic variables and degree of recovery. Although methods for assessing initial severity have varied across studies, there is considerable agreement that the most important factor predicting recovery from aphasia after stroke is initial degree of severity of language symptoms (Pedersen et al., 1995). Few systematic studies have compared recovery from aphasia after etiologies other than stroke, but some have found that post-traumatic aphasia has a better prognosis than aphasia due to cerebral infarction (Kertesz & McCabe, 1977).

Although it is well-known that small lesions cause milder and shorter-lasting language impairments, only a few studies have examined the effect of lesion volume on aphasia recovery. Selnes and colleagues (1984) found that single word comprehension at 6 months after stroke was significantly related to lesion volume. Subsequent studies have also confirmed the importance of overall lesion volume for degree of recovery (Goldenberg & Spatt, 1994). Naeser and colleagues (1987) demonstrated that region-specific volume is also of importance, in that the degree of destruction within Wernicke's area was significantly related to levels of auditory comprehension recovery. Patients with less than 50% destruction of Wernicke's area had good recovery of auditory comprehension at 6 months, whereas patients with destruction of more than half of Wernicke's region had limited recovery even 1 year after onset. As with lesions of Broca's area, extension of a lesion beyond Wernicke's area was associated with a poorer outcome than lesions restricted to only that region (Naeser et al., 1987).

The time course of recovery after aphasia may also depend on the initial level of severity of the aphasic symptoms. Patients with mild initial symptoms of aphasia often recover within a few weeks after the onset of symptoms if from a stroke (Pedersen et al., 1995). Patients with severe global or Wernicke's aphasia may show some spontaneous recovery during the first 18 months after stroke, but the majority of the improvement takes place during the first 6 months (Nicholas et al., 1993). Findings from functional magnetic resonance imaging studies suggest that right hemisphere activation during language tasks early after stroke is also predictive of long-term aphasia outcome (Crinion & Price, 2005), and thus other neuroimaging markers may become useful as possible prognostic or treatment markers.

A number of studies have attempted to quantify the degree of improvement, over and beyond spontaneous recovery, offered by speech therapy. In a meta-analysis of the findings from 21 studies, better outcomes were obtained with treatment by a speech-language pathologist compared to treatment without a pathologist (Robey, 1994). Treatment initiated during the acute stages of recovery was found to be significantly more effective than treatment initiated at later stages. In addition to behavioral treatments, pharmacotherapy for the treatment of symptoms of aphasia has been explored. Some studies suggest that aphasic symptoms have significantly improved and/or improved recovery after treatment with medications such as piracetam (acetylcholine and glutamate effects) (Malykh & Sadaie, 2010), donepezil (acetylcholinesterase inhibitor) (Sarter et al., 2009), and dopamine agonists. These pharmacotherapies have not become prevalent in clinical practice at present. Constraint-induced therapy (CIT) (Pulvermüller et al., 2001) has been shown to be an effective training program for aphasia treatment. CIT requires a patient to use only an impaired function without compensatory help from other modalities to hasten recovery in that function. For example, a patient with a speech production problem would be required to use only his or her speech to communicate, with other communication methods not allowed to be used.

Other potential nonpharmacological treatments showing promise include repetitive transcranial magnetic stimulation (Martin et al., 2009), transcranial direct current stimulation (Baker et al., 2010), and more invasive techniques such as epidural stimulation (Cherney et al., 2010). Further studies are needed to assess their efficacy, dosages, and the optimal patient populations to be used for effective outcomes.

REFERENCES

Abdullaev, Y., & Posner, M. (1998). Event-related brain potential imaging of semantic encoding during processing single words. *Neuroimage, 7*, 1–13.

Adolphs, R., Damasio, H., & Tranel, D. (2002). Neuronal systems for recognition of emotional prosody: A 3-D lesion study. *Emotion, 2*, 23–51.

Alexander, M., & Benson, D. (1993). The aphasias and related disturbances. In R. Joynt (Ed.), *Clinical neurology* (pp. 1–58). Philadelphia, PA: Lippincott.

Baker, J., Rorden, C., & Fridriksson, J. (2010). Using transcranial direct current stimulation (tDCS) to treat stroke patients with aphasia. *Stroke, 41*(6), 1229–1236.

Basso, A., Lecours, A. R., Moraschini, S., & Vanier, M. (1985). Anatomo-clinical correlations of the aphasias as defined through computerized tomography: Exceptions. *Brain and Language, 26*, 201–229.

Berndt, R. S. (1988). Category-specific deficits in aphasia. *Aphasiology, 2*, 237–240.

Binder, J., & Desai, R. (2011). The neurobiology of semantic memory. *Trends in Cognitive Sciences, 15*(11), 527–536.

Binder, J., Desai, R., Graves, W., & Conant, L. (2009). Where is the semantic system? A critical review and meta-analysis of 120 functional neuroimaging studies. *Cerebral Cortex, 19*, 2767–2796.

Blumstein, S. (2009). Auditory word recognition: Evidence from aphasia and functional neuroimaging. *Language and Linguistics Compass, 3*(4), 824–838.

Boatman, D., Hall, C., Goldstein, M., Lesser, R., & Gordon, B. (1997). Neuroperceptual differences in consonant and vowel discrimination: As revealed by direct cortical electrical interference. *Cortex, 33*, 83–98.

Boatman, D., Lesser, R., & Gordon, B. (1995). Auditory speech processing in the left temporal lobe: An electrical interference study. *Brain and Language, 51*, 269–290.

Bowers, J., Bub, D., & Arguin, M. (1996). A characterization of the word superiority effect in a case of letter-by-letter surface alexia. *Cognitive Neuropsychology, 13*, 415–441.

Breier, J., Hasan, K., Zhang, W., Men, D., & Papanicolaou, A. (2008). Language dysfunction after stroke and damage to white matter tracts evaluated using diffusion tensor imaging. *American Journal of Neuroradiology, 29*(3), 483–487.

Bub, D., & Kertesz, A. (1982). Evidence for lexicographic processing in a patient with preserved written over oral single word naming. *Brain, 105*, 697–717.

Cancelliere, A., & Kertesz, A. (1990). Lesion localization in acquired deficits of emotional expression and comprehension. *Brain and Cognition, 13*, 133–147.

Caplan, D. (1999). Activating brain systems for syntax and semantics. *Neuron, 24*(2), 292–293.

Caplan, D., Alpert, N., Waters, G., & Olivieri, A. (2000). Activation of Broca's area by syntactic processing under conditions of concurrent articulation. *Human Brain Mapping, 9*, 65–71.

Cappa, S., Frugoni, M., Pasquali, P., Perani, D., & Zorat, F. (1998). Category-specific naming impairment for artefacts: A new case. *Neurocase, 4/5*, 391–398.

Caramazza, A. (1984). The logic of neuropsychological research and the problem of patient classification in aphasia. *Brain and Language, 21*, 9–20.

Caramazza, A., Berndt, R., & Basili, A. (1983). The selective impairment of phonological processing: A case study. *Brain and Language, 18*, 128–174.

Caramazza, A., & Shelton, J. (1998). Domain-specific knowledge systems in the brain the animate–inanimate distinction. *Journal of Cognitive Neuroscience, 10*, 1–34.

Cherney, L., Erickson, R., & Small, S. (2010). Epidural cortical stimulation as adjunctive treatment for non-fluent aphasia: Preliminary findings. *Journal of Neurology, Neurosurgery, and Psychiatry, 81*(9), 1014–1021.

Coltheart, M., Patterson, K., & Marshall, J. (1980). *Deep dyslexia*. Boston, MA: Routledge & Kegan Paul.

Coslett, H. B. (2000). Acquired dyslexia. *Seminars in Neurology, 20*, 419–426.

Crinion, J., & Price, C. (2005). Right anterior superior temporal activation predicts auditory sentence comprehension following aphasic stroke. *Brain, 128*(Pt. 12), 2858–2871.

Crosson, B., Moore, A., Gopinath, K., White, K., Wierenga, C., Gaiefsky, M., et al. (2005). Role of the right and left hemispheres in recovery of function during treatment of intention in aphasia. *Journal of Cognitive Neuroscience, 17*(3), 392–406.

Crosson, B., Sadek, J., Bobholz, J., Gökçay, D., Mohr, C., Leonard, C., et al. (1999). Activity in the paracingulate and cingulate sulci during word generation: An fMRI study of functional anatomy. *Cerebral Cortex, 9*(4), 307–316.

Damasio, A. (1990). Category-related recognition defects as a clue to the neural substrates of knowledge. *Trends in Neuroscience, 13*, 95–98.

Damasio, A., Damasio, H., Tranel, D., & Brandt, J. (1990). Neural regionalization of knowledge access: Preliminary evidence. *Cold Spring Harbor Symposia on Quantitative Biology, 55*, 1039–1047.

Damasio, H., Grabowski, T., Tranel, D., Hichwa, R., & Damasio, A. (1996). A neural basis for lexical retrieval. *Nature, 380*, 499–505.

Dejerine, J. (1892). Contribution a l'étude anatomo-pathologique et clinique des différentes variétés de cécité verbale.

Dejerine, J., & Thomas, A. (1891). Un cas de cécité verbale avec agraphie.

Demb, J., Desmond, J., Wagner, A., Vaidya, C., Glover, G., & Gabrieli, J. (1995). Semantic encoding and retrieval in the left inferior prefrontal cortex: A functional MRI study of task difficulty and process specificity. *Journal of Neuroscience, 15*, 5870–5878.

Demonet, J., Chollet, F., Ramsay, S., Cardebat, D., Nespoulous, J., Wise, R., et al. (1992). The anatomy of phonological and semantic processing in normal subjects. *Brain, 115*, 1753–1768.

D'Esposito, M., Postle, B., Jonides, J., & Smith, E. (1999). The neural substrate and temporal dynamics of interference effects in working memory as revealed by event-related functional MRI. *Proceedings of the National Academy of Sciences of the USA, 96*, 7514–7519.

Dronkers, N., Wilkins, D., Van Valin, R., Redfern, B., & Jaeger, J. (2004). Lesion analysis of the brain areas involved in language comprehension. *Cognition, 92*, 145–177.

Farah, M. (1989). The neuropsychology of mental imagery. In J. W. Brown (Ed.), *Neuropsychology of visual perception*. Hillsdale, NJ: Erlbaum.

Farah, M., McMullen, P., & Meyer, M. (1991). Can recognition of living things be selectively impaired? *Neuropsychologia, 29*, 85–193.

Farah, M., Meyer, M., & McMullen, P. (1996). The living/nonliving dissociation is not an artifact: Giving an a priori implausible hypothesis a strong test. *Cognitive Neuropsychology, 13*, 137–154.

Farah, M., & Wallace, M. (1992). Semantically-bounded anomia: Implications for the neural implementation of naming. *Neuropsychologia, 30*, 609–622.

Ferreira, C., Giusiano, B., & Poncet, M. (1997). Category-specific anomia: Implication of different neural networks in naming. *Neuroreport, 8*, 1595–1602.

Fiez, J., Tranel, D., Seager-Frerichs, D., & Damasio, H. (2006). Specific reading and phonological processing deficits are associated with damage to the left frontal operculum. *Cortex, 42*, 624–643.

Fox, P., Ingham, R., Ingham, J., Zamarripa, F., Xiong, J., & Lancaster, J. (2000). Brain correlates of stuttering and syllable production. A PET performance-correlation analysis. *Brain, 123*(Pt. 10), 1985–2004.

Friedman, R., & Hadley, J. (1992). Letter-by-letter surface alexia. *Cognitive Neuropsychology, 9*, 185–208.

Funnell, E., & Sheridan, J. (1992). Categories of knowledge? Unfamiliar aspects of living and nonliving things. *Cognitive Neuropsychology, 9*, 135–153.

Gainotti, G., Silveri, M., Daniele, A., & Giustolisi, L. (1995). Neuroanatomical correlates of category-specific semantic disorders: A critical survey. *Memory, 3/4*, 247–264.

Garrard, P., Patterson, K., Watson, P., & Hodges, J. (1998). Category-specific semantic loss in dementia of Alzheimer's type: Functional–anatomical correlations form cross-sectional analyses. *Brain, 121*, 633–646.

Glasser, M. F., & Rilling, J. K. (2008). DTI tractography of the human brain's language pathways. *Cerebral cortex, 18*(11), 2471–2482.

Goldenberg, G., & Spatt, J. (1994). Influence of size and site of cerebral lesions on spontaneous recovery of aphasia and on success of language therapy. *Brain and Language, 47*, 684–698.

Goodglass, H., Klein, B., Carey, P., & Jones, K. (1966). Specific semantic word categories in aphasia. *Cortex, 2*, 74–89.

Goodglass, H., Wingfield, A., Hyde, M., & Theurkauf, J. (1986). Category specific dissociations in naming and recognition by aphasic patients. *Cortex, 22*, 87–102.

Grodzinsky, Y. (2000). The neurology of syntax: Language use without Broca's area. *Behavioral and Brain Sciences, 23*, 1–71.

Grossman, M., Robinson, K., Biassou, N., White-Devine, T., & D'Esposito, M. (1998). Semantic memory in Alzheimer's disease: Representativeness, ontologic category, and material. *Neuropsychology, 12*, 34–42.

Hart, J., & Kraut, M. (2007). Neural Hybrid Model of semantic object memory (ver 1.1). In J. Hart & M. Kraut (Eds.), *Neural Basis of Semantic Memory*. Cambridge: Cambridge University Press.

Hart, J., Berndt, R., & Caramazza, A. (1985). Category-specific naming deficit following cerebral infarction. *Nature, 316*, 439–440.

Hart, J., Crone, N., Lesser, R., Sieracki, J., Miglioretti, D., Hall, C., et al. (1998). Temporal dynamics of verbal object comprehension. *Proceedings of the National Academy of Sciences of the USA, 95*, 6498–6503.

Hart, J., & Gordon, B. (1990). Delineation of single-word semantic comprehension deficits in aphasia, with anatomical correlation. *Annals of Neurology, 27*, 226–231.

Hart, J., & Gordon, B. (1992). Neural subsystems for object knowledge. *Nature, 359*, 60–64.

Hart, J., Kraut, M., Kremen, S., Soher, B., & Gordon, B. (2000). Neural substrates of orthographic lexical access as demonstrated by functional brain imaging. *Neuropsychiatry, Neuropsychology, and Behavioral Neurology, 13*, 1–7.

Hart, J., Maguire, M., Motes, M., Mudar, R., Chiang, H.-S., Womack, K., et al. (2013). Semantic memory retrieval circuit: Role of BA6 and thalamus. *Brain and Language, 126*(1), 89–98.

Hartwigsen, G., Baumgaertner, A., Price, C., Koehnke, M., Ulmer, S., & Siebner, H. (201). Phonological decisions require both the left and right supramarginal gyri. *Proceedings of the National Academy of Sciences of the USA, 107*(38), 16494–16499.

Hickok, G., Erhard, P., Kassubek, J., Helms-Tillery, S., Naeve-Velguth, S., Strupp, J., et al. (2000). A functional magnetic resonance imaging study of the role of left posterior superior temporal gyrus in speech production: Implications for the explanation of conduction aphasia. *Neuroscience Letters, 287*, 156–160.

Hickok, G., & Poeppel, D. (2004). Dorsal and ventral streams: A framework for understanding aspects of the functional anatomy of language. *Cognition, 92*, 67–99.

Hillis, A., & Caramazza, A. (1991). Category-specific naming and comprehension impairment: A double dissociation. *Brain, 114*, 2081–2094.

Hillis, A., Rapp, B., & Caramazza, A. (1999). When a rose is a rose in speech but a tulip in writing. *Cortex, 35*, 337–356.

Hinton, G. (1981). Implementing semantic networks in parallel hardware. In G. E. Hinton & J. A. Anderson (Eds.), *Parallel models of associative memory*. Hillsdale, NJ: Erlbaum.

Hodges, J., Patterson, K., Oxbury, S., & Funnell, E. (1992). Semantic dementia: Progressive fluent aphasia with temporal lobe atrophy. *Brain, 115*, 1783–1806.

Humphreys, G., & Riddoch, M. (1987). On telling your fruits from your vegetables: A consideration of category-specific deficits after brain damage. *Trends in Neuroscience, 10*, 145–148.

Kaplan, E., Goodglass, H., & Weintraub, S. (1983). *The Boston Naming Test* (2nd ed.). Philadelphia, PA: Lea & Febiger.

Kapur, S., Rose, R., Liddle, P., Zipursky, R., Brown, G., & Stuss, D. (1994). The role of the left prefrontal cortex in verbal processing: Semantic processing or willed action? *Neuroreport, 5*, 2193–2196.

Kertesz, A., & McCabe, P. (1977). Recovery patterns and prognosis in aphasia. *Brain, 1*, 1–18.

Kraut, M., Kremen, S., Segal, J., Calhoun, V., Moo, L., & Hart, J. (2002). Object activation from features in the semantic system. *Journal of Cognitive Neuroscience, 14*, 24–36.

Levy, D., Bayley, P., & Squire, L. (2004). The anatomy of semantic knowledge: medial vs. lateral temporal lobe. *Proceedings of the National Academy of Sciences U S A., 101*, 6710–6715.

Magnusdottir, S., Fillmore, P., den Ouden, D., Hjaltason, H., Rorden, C., Kjartansson, O., et al. (2013). Damage to left anterior temporal cortex predicts impairment of complex syntactic processing: A lesion–symptom mapping study. *Human Brain Mapping, 34*, 2715–2723.

Malykh, A., & Sadaie, M. (2010). Piracetam and piracetam-like drugs: From basic science to novel clinical applications to CNS disorders. *Drugs, 70*(3), 287–312.

Martin, A., Wiggs, C., Ungerleider, L., & Haxby, J. (1996). Neural correlates of category-specific knowledge. *Nature, 379,* 649–652.

Martin, P., Naeser, M., Ho, M., Treglia, E., Kaplan, E., Baker, E., et al. (2009). Research with transcranial magnetic stimulation in the treatment of aphasia. *Current Neurology and Neuroscience Reports, 9*(6), 451–458.

Mauri, A., Daum, I., Sartori, G., Riesch, G., & Birbaumer, N. (1994). Category-specific semantic impairment in Alzheimer's disease and temporal lobe dysfunction: A comparative study. *Journal of Clinical and Experimental Neuropsychology, 16,* 689–701.

McCarthy, R., & Warrington, E. (1988). Evidence for modality-specific meaning systems in the brain. *Nature, 334,* 428–430.

Monrad-Krohn, G. (1963). The third element of speech: Prosody and its disorders. In L. Halpem (Ed.), *Problems of dynamic neurology.* Jerusalem: Hebrew University Press.

Moore, C., & Price, C. (1999). A functional neuroimaging study of the variables that generate category-specific object processing differences. *Brain, 122,* 943–962.

Moro, A., Tettamanti, M., Perani, D., Donati, C., Cappa, S., & Fazio, F. (2001). Syntax and the brain: Disentangling grammar by selective anomalies. *Neuroimage, 13,* 110–118.

Naeser, M., Helm-Estabrooks, N., Haas, G., Auerbach, S., & Srinivasan, M. (1987). Relationship between lesion extent in "Wernicke's area" on computed tomographic scan and predicting recovery of comprehension in Wernicke's aphasia. *Archives of Neurology, 44,* 73–82.

Nicholas, M., Helm-Estabrooks, N., Ward-Lonergan, J., & Morgan, A. (1993). Evolution of severe aphasia in the first two years post onset. *Archives of Physical Medicine and Rehabilitation, 74,* 830–836.

Nielsen, J. (1946). *Agnosia, apraxia, aphasia: Their value in cerebral localization* (2nd ed.). New York, NY: Hoeber.

Nobre, A., Allison, T., & McCarthy, G. (1994). Word recognition in the human inferior temporal lobe. *Nature, 372,* 260–263.

Patterson, K., Marshall, J., & Coltheart, M. (1985). *Surface dyslexia: Neuropsychological and cognitive studies of phonological reading.* Hillsdale, NJ: Erlbaum.

Pedersen, P., Jorgensen, H., Nakayama, H., Raaschou, H., & Olsen, T. (1995). Aphasia in acute stroke: Incidence, determinants, and recovery. *Annals of Neurology, 38,* 659–666.

Pedersen, P., Vinter, K., & Olsen, T. (2004). Aphasia after stroke: type, severity and prognosis. The Copenhagen aphasia study. *Cerebrovascular Diseases, 17,* 35–43.

Petersen, S., Fox, P., Posner, M., Mintun, M., & Raichle, M. (1988). Positron emission tomographic studies of the cortical anatomy of single-word processing. *Nature, 331,* 585–589.

Petersen, S., Fox, P., Snyder, A., & Raichle, M. (1990). Specific extrastriate and frontal cortical areas are activated by visual words and word-like stimuli. *Science, 249,* 1041–1044.

Posner, M., Petersen, S., Fox, P., & Raichle, M. (1988). Localization of cognitive operations in the human brain. *Science, 240,* 1627–1631.

Price, C. (1998). The functional anatomy of word comprehension and production. *Trends in Cognitive Sciences, 2*(8), 281–288.

Pulvermüller, F., Neininger, B., Elbert, T., Mohr, B., Rockstroh, B., Koebbel, P., et al. (2001). Constraint-induced therapy of chronic aphasia following stroke. *Stroke, 32*(7), 1621–1626.

Race, D., Ochfeld, E., Leigh, R., & Hillis, A. (2012). Lesion analysis of cortical regions associated with the comprehension of nonreversible and reversible yes/no questions. *Neuropsychologia, 50,* 1946–1953.

Rapcsak, S., & Beeson, P. (2004). The role of the left posterior inferior temporal cortex in spelling. *Neurology, 62,* 2221–2229.

Rapcsak, S., Comer, J., & Rubens, A. (1993). Anomia for facial expressions: Neuropsychological mechanisms and anatomical correlates. *Brain and Language, 45,* 233–252.

Rapcsak, S., Kaszniak, A., & Rubens, A. (1989). Anomia for facial expressions: Evidence for a category-specific visual–verbal disconnection syndrome. *Neuropsychologia, 27,* 1031–1041.

Rapcsak, S., Rubens, A., & Laguna, J. (1990). From letters to words: Procedures for word recognition in letter-by-letter reading. *Brain and Language, 38,* 504–514.

Ricci, P., Zelkowicz, B., Nebes, R., Meltzer, C., Mintun, M., & Becker, J. (1999). Functional neuroanatomy of semantic memory: Recognition of semantic associations. *Neuroimage, 9,* 88–96.

Robey, R. (1994). The efficacy of treatment of aphasic persons: A meta-analysis. *Brain and Language, 47,* 582–608.

Robinson, K., Grossman, M., White-Devine, T., & D'Esposito, M. (1996). Category-specific difficulty naming with verbs in Alzheimer's disease. *Neurology, 47,* 178–182.

Ross, E. (1981). The aprosodias: Functional–anatomic organization of the affective components of language in the right hemispheric. *Archives of Neurology, 38,* 561–570.

Ross, E., & Monnot, M. (2008). Neurology of affective prosody and its functional–anatomic organization in right hemisphere. *Brain and Language, 104,* 51–74.

Ross, E., Thompson, R., & Yenkosky, J. (1997). Lateralization of affective prosody in brain and the callosal integration of hemispheric language functions. *Brain Lang, 56*(1), 27–54.

Sacchett, C., & Humphreys, G. (1992). Calling a squirrel a squirrel but a canoe a wigwam: A category-specific deficit for artefactual objects and body parts. *Cognitive Neuropsychology, 9*, 73–86.

Sarter, M., Parikh, V., & Howe, W. (2009). Phasic acetylcholine release and the volume transmission hypothesis: Time to move on. *Nature Reviews Neuroscience, 10*(5), 383–390.

Sartori, G., & Job, R. (1988). The oyster with four legs: A neuropsychological study on the interaction of visual and semantic information. *Cognitive Neuropsychology, 5*, 105–132.

Sartori, G., Job, R., Miozzo, M., Zago, S., & Marchiori, G. (1993). Category-specific form-knowledge deficit in a patient with herpes simplex virus encephalitis. *Journal of Clinical and Experimental Neuropsychology, 15*, 280–299.

Saur, D., Kreherb, W., Schnellb, S., Kummerer, D., Kellmeyer, P., Vrya, M.-S., et al. (2008). Ventral and dorsal pathways for language. *Proceedings of the National Academy of Sciences of the USA, 105*, 18035–18040.

Schwartz, M. (1984). What the classical aphasia categories can't do for us and why. *Brain and Language, 21*, 3–8.

Schwartz, M., Faseyitan, O., Kim, J., & Coslett, H. B. (2012). The dorsal stream contribution to phonological retrieval in naming. *Brain, 135*, 3799–3814.

Selnes, O., Niccum, N., Knopman, D., & Rubens, A. (1984). Recovery of single word comprehension: CT-scan correlates. *Brain and Language, 21*, 72–84.

Semenza, C., & Zettin, M. (1988). Generating proper names: A case of selective inability. *Cognitive Neuropsychology, 5*, 711–721.

Semenza, C., & Zettin, M. (1989). Evidence from aphasia for the role of proper names as pure referring expressions. *Nature, 342*, 678–679.

Shallice, T. (1994). Multiple semantics: Whose confusions? *Cognitive Neuropsychology, 10*, 251–261.

Silveri, M., Daniele, A., Giustolisi, L., & Gainotti, G. (1991). Dissociation between knowledge of living and nonliving things in dementia of the Alzheimer type. *Neurology, 41*, 545–546.

Silveri, M., & Gainotti, G. (1988). Interaction between vision and language in category-specific semantic impairment. *Cognitive Neuropsychology, 5*, 677–709.

Spitzer, M., Kwong, K., Kennedy, W., Rosen, B., & Bellivean, J. (1995). Category-specific brain activation in fMRI during picture naming. *Neuroreport, 6*, 2109–2112.

Temple, C. (1986). Anomia for animals in a child. *Brain, 109*, 1225–1242.

Thompson-Schill, S., D'Esposito, M., Aguirre, G. K., & Farah, M. J. (1997). Role of left inferior prefrontal cortex in retrieval of semantic knowledge: A reevaluation. *Proceedings of the National Academy of Sciences of the USA, 94*, 14792–14797.

Thothathiri, M., Kimberg, D., & Schwartz, M. (2012). The neural basis of reversible sentence comprehension: Evidence from voxel-based lesion–symptom mapping in aphasia. *Journal of Cognitive Neuroscience, 24*(1), 212–222.

Tippett, L., Glosser, G., & Farah, M. (1996). A category-specific naming impairment after temporal lobectomy. *Neuropsychologia, 34*, 139–146.

Tyler, L., Marslen-Wilson, W., Randall, B., Wright, P., Devereux, B., Zhuang, J., et al. (2011). Left inferior frontal cortex and syntax: Function, structure and behaviour in patients with left hemisphere damage. *Brain, 134*, 415–431.

Vandenberghe, R., Price, C., Wise, R., Josephs, O., & Frackowiak, R. (1996). Functional anatomy of a common semantic system for words and pictures. *Nature, 383*, 254–256.

Vignolo, L., Boccardi, E., & Caverni, L. (1986). Unexpected CT-scan findings in global aphasia. *Cortex, 22*, 55–69.

Warrington, E., & McCarthy, R. (1983). Category specific access dysphasia. *Brain, 106*, 859–878.

Warrington, E., & McCarthy, R. (1987). Categories of knowledge: Further fractionation and an attempted integration. *Brain, 110*, 1273–1296.

Warrington, E., & Shallice, T. (1984). Category specific semantic impairments. *Brain, 107*, 829–854.

Willmes, K., & Poeck, K. (1993). To what extent can aphasic syndromes be localized? *Brain, 116*, 1527–1540.

5

Praxis

The term *praxis* does not refer to a typical cognitive domain. Praxis refers to the process by which a skill is enacted or the performance of an action. It is predominantly a domain of complex motor skills. The skilled motor acts are assessed probing the integrity of this system from pantomime (visual imitation) or verbal command, thus having a direct link to the language system. It is this language-to-motor system interdependence that leads to its inclusion at this point.

In the early 1900s, Liepmann (1900, 1905) described the deficit of apraxia, which refers to an impairment in making skilled purposeful movements (Geschwind, 1965; Heilman & Rothi, 1993). This definition can be further refined and made more descriptive by saying that apraxia is characterized by a disruption of spatiotemporal properties of learned skilled movements, including improper translation of spatial plans into the correct angular motions at the joints (Poizner et al., 1990). By either of these descriptions, it is meant that an individual is unable to perform a previously known skilled movement (e.g., "Show me how you would comb your hair" and "Show me how you would brush your hair") to an external request (from an individual not performing the movement).

The optimal way to conceptualize apraxia is that an apraxic deficit in performing motor commands is not a pure motor deficit but, rather, a cognitive deficit of performing motor acts from a verbal or visual cue provided by a person testing the patient. As such, a patient cannot be called apractic if he or she is found on examination to have a sensory loss, weakness, tremors, dystonia, chorea, ballismus, athetosis, myoclonus, ataxia, or seizures.

The motor acts that are typically tested on patients center on the use of objects ("Show me how you use a hammer," "Show me how you use a toothbrush," etc.). One can speculate as to why the manipulation of objects plays such a central role in testing patients and in brain representational systems. In the semantic system, tools are one of the categories that are associated with a specific blood oxygenation level-dependent signal on functional magnetic resonance imaging (fMRI), and lesions have occurred that result in a selective impairment for tool information. It is suggested that this and other categories of items are uniquely organized in the brain due to their evolutionary significance (Caramazza & Shelton, 1998) or their importance for survival (Hart & Kraut, 2007). In either the evolution or the survival formulation of the organization of knowledge in the brain, tools and the representations associated with them have a distinctive neural organization. Thus, one must be careful in the examination of praxis to not assume a generalized praxis deficit when the patient may have a deficit that is more selective to one category of items.

Typically, testing for praxis begins by asking a patient verbally to perform a specific motor act. Examples include commands such as "Show me how you would comb your hair," "Show me how you would brush your teeth," "Show me how to use a hammer," or "Show me how you would throw a dart." The patient is not allowed to have the object in his or her hand while performing these acts. Other examples include asking a patient to show how to salute, throw a ball, wave goodbye, etc. No physical props are allowed to assist the patient in performing the action. If the patient fails, then the clinician performs the action and the patient is required to pantomime the action. A thorough set of commands for apraxia assessment, with normative data, is the Florida Apraxia Battery (Power et al., 2010).

IDEOMOTOR AND CONCEPTUAL APRAXIAS

From these assessments, a patient who has apraxia can be impaired in several ways (for a clinical summary, see Heilman, 2010; see Video 5). First, a patient can be impaired in performing a motor action from a verbal command but is better able to pantomime the action. This pattern is characteristic of the clinical condition referred to as *ideomotor apraxia*. When assessing patients with ideomotor apraxia, three types of errors are typical of their performance when performing the motor action from command. The patients make postural errors in which they hold the tool in an incorrect orientation due to improper positioning of the arm, hand, and/or fingers. They can also make two other types of movement errors referred to as egocentric and allocentric. Egocentric movement errors result from the subject using incorrect joints or poor coordination of the joints to perform the desired movement. Allocentric movement errors are an improper action demonstrated by the patient in applying the action of the item toward its target. For example, if a patient is asked to show how to use a hammer, an example of an allocentric error would be sliding a hammer backward and forward like one would do using a knife to slice a piece of meat. Another interesting type of error that patients with ideomotor apraxia can make is that they will often use their hand and fingers to represent the actual tool if they are requested to show an examiner how to use a tool. This type of error is referred to as a body part tool error.

Patients with ideomotor apraxia improve when imitating the examiner's pantomimes of actions, while still being somewhat impaired. They also improve their performance on showing how to use an item to command when given the actual item to use (e.g., placing a hammer in the patient's hand and asking him to demonstrate how he would use it). It has been speculated that this improvement occurs because of the visual input received and the ability to touch the item, both leading to the activation of multiple representational systems in the brain for that object, which are then able to access the motor system to allow for performance of the desired motor act. For example, by watching the examiner pantomime the intended movement of an item, the patient gains movement knowledge that may not have been readily accessible to her motor system internally in her brain (Poizner et al., 1990; this is explained further later). The general underlying cognitive dysfunction in ideomotor apraxia is inadequate or incomplete access of the motor system to intact movement representations, leading to poor production of the motor act.

Another type of disruption is to the conceptual system, termed *conceptual apraxia*, in which the patient cannot mimic the function of an object with or without a physical prop (e.g., if given a screwdriver and told to use it, the patient might hold it like a pen and try to write with it; De Renzi & Lucchelli, 1988). Patients with conceptual apraxia show impairment of the actual object or action knowledge representations in the brain. They may misuse objects, are unable to match objects and their actions, or cannot correctly judge whether a gesture refers to a specific object. As such, patients with conceptual apraxia tend to be severely impaired functionally by their condition in everyday life.

Thus, there are two key broad components to the praxis system: a production system (action plan and production) and a conceptual system (action knowledge). If a lesion occurs in the production system, the typical result will be ideomotor apraxia (e.g., difficulty showing how to use scissors to command but can to pantomime and functionally in real life), with a disruption to the conceptual system leading to conceptual apraxia (e.g., inability to perform or recognize the correct movement for scissors resulting in an error that may be showing the action for a completely different item).

Not discussed extensively in this chapter is *ideational apraxia*. Ideational apraxia, which has been confused as a term for conceptual apraxia, actually denotes an inability to *sequence correctly* a series of acts leading to an action goal (e.g., making a cup of coffee). It is more a deficit of linking together a series of acts to complete a complex action as opposed to a single, previously learned skilled movement (e.g., brushing teeth). This type of apraxia is associated with large left hemisphere lesions, dementia, or delirium without make correct object movements to command and cannot specific associated anatomic localizations.

GENERAL COGNITIVE–ANATOMIC FRAMEWORK AND COGNITIVE NEUROSCIENCE OF PRAXIS

Several cognitive units have been proposed to account for the previously described praxis behaviors. The general approach to conceptualize the stages involved in praxis is a three-stage approach:

1. "Memory" or knowledge of the skilled movement to be performed (e.g., the general idea of using a hammer). This is sometimes referred to as the representational system for these skilled movements. It is not a motor program of how to carry out the actual movements but, rather, an encoding of the

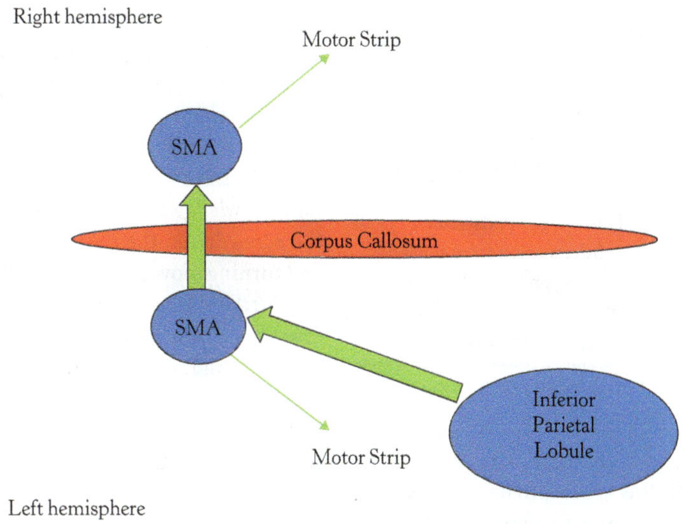

FIGURE 5.1: Schematic model of the brain regions involved in praxis. Movement representations are purported to be stored in the left inferior parietal lobule. Left supplementary motor area (SMA)/dorsal premotor area translates spatial–temporal representations into motor programs. This information from the left SMA is purported to be transferred across the anterior two-thirds region of the corpus callosum from the left to the right hemisphere. The SMA regions send the motor plan to the motor cortices for the movements to be performed.

representation of the concept of the act (e.g., what it means to hammer a nail). Consider the scenario of a loose screw that needs to be screwed in with several tools at one's disposal. A nonimpaired individual would recognize that the screwdriver is the correct tool for the job.

2. Translation of the movement representation into a motor code. This entails converting a single concept of a complex movement into a neural code for a series of muscle movements necessary to perform the coordinated act.
3. Motor system carries out the act. (See Figure 5.1 for a schematic of these concepts and general localization.)

The general anatomic framework associated with these cognitive units encompasses several distinct brain regions. The memory of or access to stored movement representations is generally associated with the left inferior parietal lobule region. The translation of these stored representations into motor programs is supported by each hemisphere's respective supplementary motor area (SMA) and/or premotor regions. For example, if the motor act is to be performed by the right hand, then left hemisphere structures are sufficient to perform the act. If the left hand is to be used to perform the motor act, information will have to be transferred from the left hemisphere to the right. The movement representation proceeds from the left inferior parietal lobe to the left SMA. There is then a transfer between the left SMA to the right SMA that is mediated by the anterior two-thirds of the corpus callosum. Then, the right hemisphere motor system carries out the motor acts transferred to the right SMA. Also, essential throughout this entire system are the white matter pathways connecting these regions together because effective execution of praxis acts requires efficient transferring of signals between these different regions. The following discussion describes details about the cognitive–anatomic units (CAUs) that are engaged in the praxis system (see Table 5.1 for CAUs).

Inferior Parietal Lobe

Damage to the left inferior parietal lobe (IPL) can induce apraxia, and it was proposed to disrupt the representations of skilled motor movements (Heilman et al., 1982). Heilman et al. referred to these movement representations as "visuo-motor engrams," using the term engram as it is used in descriptions of memory systems meaning the "store of a memory trace."

This role of the inferior parietal lobule was further modified by Halsband et al. (2001) after they examined patients with parietal lesions to find the presence of severe impairments in the recognition and imitation

TABLE 5.1: LIMB PRAXIS SUMMARY

Brain Region	Function
Supplementary motor area (SMA)/dorsal premotor area	Translating spatial–temporal representations into motor programs
Corpus callosum (anterior two-thirds)	Transfer of praxis-related information from the left hemisphere to the right
Left inferior parietal lobule	Spatial–temporal movement representations

of pantomimed actions in those with left parietal lesions (Figure 5.2). This appears to be the most consistent disruption to the praxis system: Inferior parietal lobe disruption, particularly left-sided lesions, is associated with an inability to follow verbal commands to perform acts, as well as impaired recognition and imitation of pantomimed actions.

Buxbaum et al. (2007) studied 16 ideomotor apraxia patients with left IPL lesions in great detail on tests of praxis and object manipulation, and they concluded that this region was essential in mediating representations of skilled hand–object interactions. They proposed that the representations contain pertinent information about both movement and posture representations as related to target actions with respect to specific objects. For example, the act of using a screwdriver should contain knowledge about the hand posture on grabbing the screwdriver, the position of the shoulder joint, and turning movements of the elbow joint.

Further detailed assessment of the movement mistakes made by apractic patients by Jax et al. (2006) found that apractic patients showed impairments not only in movements related to an object action but also in movements related to the patient's body (e.g., "Point to your left eye"). Lesion analysis suggests that damage to the left IPL (Brodmann's areas 39 and 40) may play a key role both in these apractic movement abnormalities and in body representation errors. This is consistent with the findings from Schwoebel and Coslett (2005), who showed that the left IPL region is also important for body representation encoding so that the apractic deficit with both incorrect movements related to the object and the patient's body is possibly associated with this location.

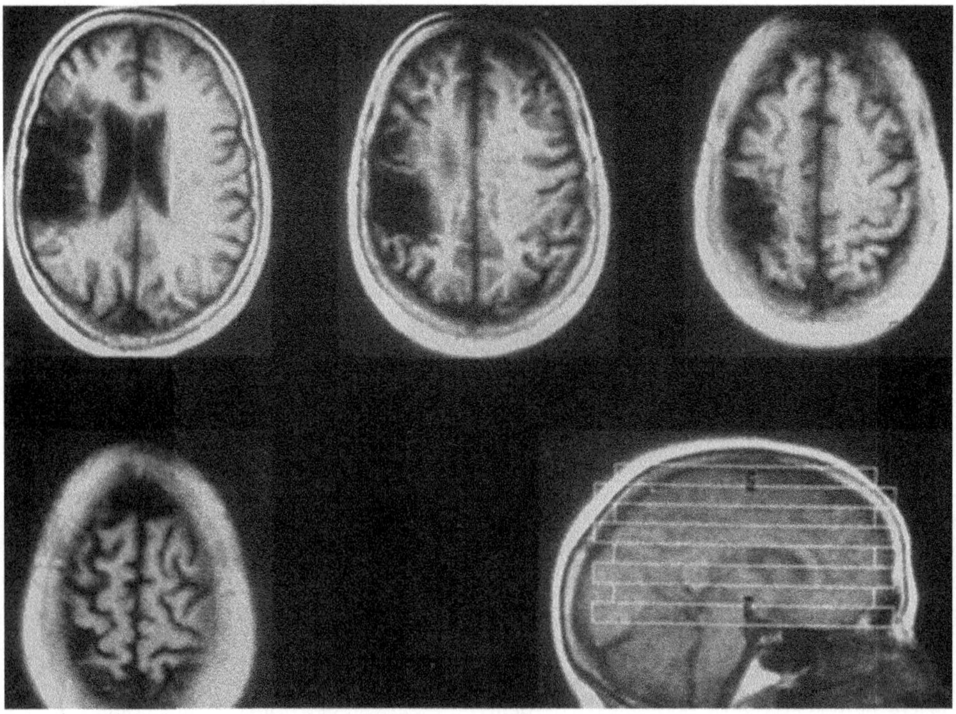

FIGURE 5.2: Patient with limb apraxia with lesion affecting her left inferior parietal lobule in addition to other regions. The blue arrows demonstrate the lesion that is affecting the left inferior parietal lobule and resulting in disruption of complex movement representation systems.

Manuel et al. (2013) studied 150 stroke and tumor patients to assess the role of the IPL and inferior frontal lobe in praxis. They conducted a large-scale voxel-based lesion–symptom mapping (VBLSM) analyses of pantomime errors of 150 left and right brain-damaged patients. Their findings support the notion that the left IPL is involved in pantomime and is involved in, the storage or access to storage of knowledge about previously learned manipulation of familiar objects (although Halsband et al. (2001) proposed that lesions to this region represent a motor production disorder from a dissociation between conceptual and production components of praxis). The analyses also revealed a key role for the white matter underlying the parietal lobe in addition to the parietal lobe cortex in these deficits, suggesting that a disruption of the functional interactions between the frontoparietal network can also impact the ability to pantomime (Peigneux et al., 2001).

Lesions disrupting white matter connections can separate an intact IPL with its movement representations from premotor regions that translate those representations. This would typically result from a lesion to aspects of the superior longitudinal fasciculus (SLF), the long white matter tract that connects the IPL to frontal lobe regions (for anatomical reference, see Figure 5.7). A study of 82 apractic patients with subcortical lesions showed that many had white matter disruption, particularly in aspects of the SLF (Pramstaller & Marsden, 1996). In general, these patients could not make skilled motor movements but could discriminate correct and incorrect pantomimes, supporting the notion that representations are supported by the IPL. This is due to the knowledge of movement representations for skilled motor acts stored in the IPL being intact so that patients are able to correctly access these representations for correct recognition of a pantomime presented to them. However, the white matter disconnection in these patients between the IPL and frontal lobe prohibits them from performing the action.

Overall, the data suggest that spatial–temporal movement representations (Heilman & Watson, 2008) or representations of skilled hand–object interactions (Buxbaum et al., 2007) are stored in the left IPL (aspects of the supramarginal and angular gyri). This is best exemplified by patients with lesions of this region resulting in an inability to perform skilled movements and not able to discriminate correctly versus incorrectly performed pantomimes of those movements. Studies also raise the issue that damage to the underlying white matter in this region can lead to significant deficits from an inability of the parietal and frontal lobe regions to communicate.

Supplementary Motor Area/Dorsal Premotor Area

Watson et al. (1986) reported that damage to the superior medial left frontal lobe leads to ideomotor apraxia of both hands, proposing that this premotor region is responsible for translating spatial–temporal representations stored in the left parietal lobe into motor programs (Heilman et al., 2008) (Figure 5.3). Support for this CAU claim also comes from activation studies that show the SMA involved with bimanual actions (Koski et al., 2002) and in planning and implementing skilled movements (Babiloni et al., 2003; Halsband et al., 2001). In addition, intraoperative electrical stimulation studies have shown that stimulation of this region results in the production of complex motor movements (Penfield & Welch, 1951). That this function is more lateralized to left than right superior medial frontal lobe is also supported to some degree by studies showing the left region to be dominant for action selection, including for those of the left hand (Schluter et al., 1998).

In support of this CAU localization, a VBLSM study was performed to investigate the lesion correlates of deficits in learning and retrieving sequential motor knowledge (Dovern et al., 2011). Apractic patients showed reduced ability to accurately retrieve previously learned motor sequences, with the correlation of this deficit being lesions to the dorsal premotor cortex.

Further studies are being conducted that more finely delineate finer-grained cognitive units involved in converting movement representations into motor sequence knowledge, including internally selecting appropriate actions, converting a learned motor sequence into an explicit motor plan, and predicting forthcoming actions (Dovern et al., 2011). Currently, there are no clear further anatomic subdivisions of the dorsal medial frontal premotor area to correlate with these proposed cognitive units. As additional studies are performed that provide anatomic correlates to these functions, the praxis model will develop further.

There are indications that other frontal lobe regions may be involved in aspects of praxis performance. A lesion analysis was performed in 21 left

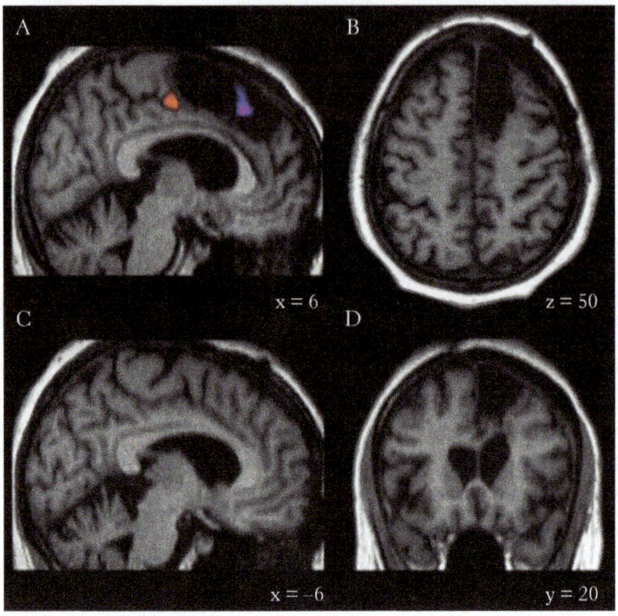

FIGURE 5.3: Left SMA lesion (dark area) resulting in apraxia of both limbs (radiological orientation). (The red and blue regions are part of an fMRI activation study in the patient.)

brain-damaged patients using a gesture comprehension task in which an actor performed correct or incorrect limb gestures. The left inferior frontal gyrus was found to also be involved in complex aspects of action-related processing (Pazzaglia et al., 2008). Further studies are needed to verify that this location consistently results in apractic-related deficits.

Corpus Callosum

Disconnection of the hemispheres via lesions of the corpus callosum has provided major insight into the important role that the anterior two-thirds of that structure plays in the hemispheric transfer of information between the bilateral SMAs. Because movement representations appear to be stored in the left IPL, it has been shown that if a patient is asked to perform a motor act with his or her left hand, information needs to be passed from the left IPL to the left SMA, across the corpus callosum, and to the right SMA for the motor act to be performed (see Figure 5.1).

Patients with Marchiafava–Bignami disease, a rare condition consisting of demyelination of the corpus callosum (Figure 5.4), often exhibit impaired praxis performance on commands using the left hand but intact praxis performance with the right hand (Berek et al., 1994). Apraxia of the left hand with intact praxis performance in the right hand is explained by the inability of the right hemisphere (to move the left hand properly and) to access complex movement knowledge representations localized to the left IPL. Whereas the left parietal lobe can transfer the movement information to the left SMA for the motor act to be carried out by the right hand, when there is a lesion to the corpus callosum, the movement information cannot transfer over to the right SMA for the motor act to be carried out by the left hand. As such, the right side of the brain does not have the complex motor act information to perform the act correctly with the left hand without instruction from the left IPL (Watson & Heilman, 1983).

Almost all cases of callosal disconnection (Figure 5.5) demonstrate apraxic errors when patients are asked to carry out verbal commands with the left hand (Graff-Radford et al., 1987; Watson & Heilman, 1983).

Subcortical Regions

Apraxia is common in basal ganglia diseases—Parkinson's disease, progressive supranuclear palsy, and most notably corticobasal degeneration, in which the presence of apraxia is a defining feature of the disease (Leiguarda, 2001). The striatum and globus pallidus have been proposed to be engaged in the cognitive operation of selection of individual

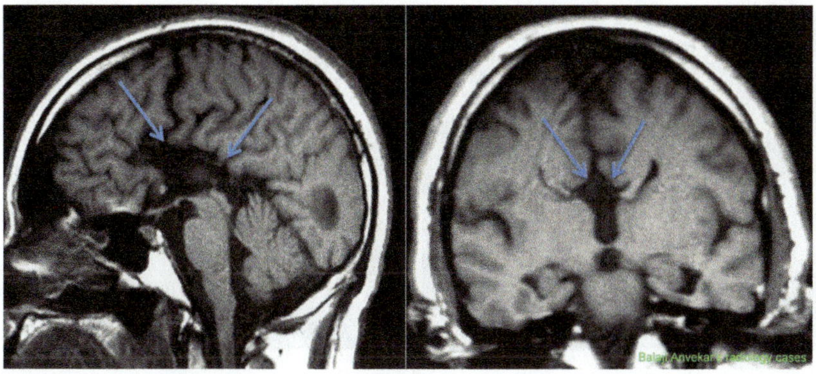

FIGURE 5.4: Patient with agenesis of the corpus callosum. The figure on the left is a sagittal image, and that on the right is a coronal image. The blue arrows designate where the corpus callosum should be located. This lack of a corpus callosum can lead to left limb apraxia.

Source: http://www.neuroradiologycases.com.

object-oriented responses (Hanna-Pladdy et al., 2001; Rushworth et al., 1998). As a consequence of dysfunction in this operation, the incorrect object for a motor act or the incorrect motor act for an object may be chosen, thus leading to apractic errors.

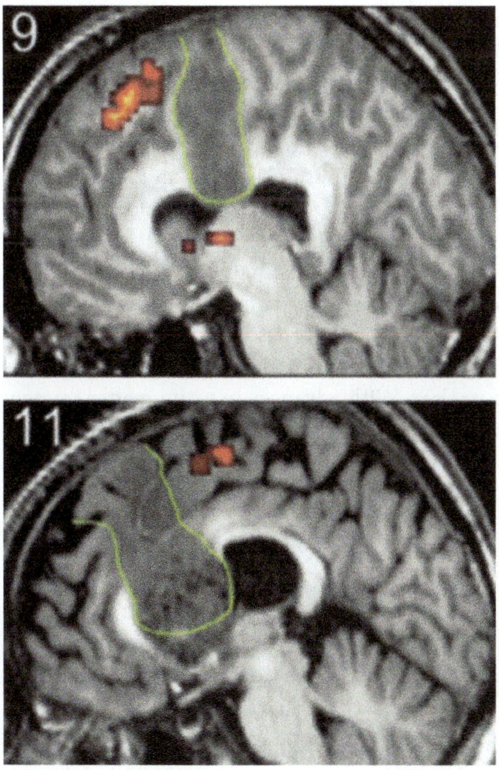

FIGURE 5.5: Region circled in yellow represents a tumor invading the corpus callosum resulting in disconnecting the two hemispheres and apraxia in the left hand.

Other studies, however, have not always found that basal ganglia lesions contribute significantly to specification of movement direction (Georgopoulos et al., 1983). Limb apraxia was assessed in 14 patients with strokes in the left basal ganglia, thalamus, or both, without cortical or white matter involvement. Only 3 patients in that study were impaired at pantomiming and imitating movements, and these patients had lesions of the lenticular nucleus of the basal ganglia and posterior limb of the internal capsule (De Renzi et al., 1986). Based on a meta-analysis of 82 cases of "deep apraxias" (apraxia with subcortical lesions), Pramstaller and Marsden (1996) concluded that lesions confined to the basal ganglia alone (caudate, putamen, and globus pallidus) rarely cause apraxia. Reassessment of cases that report apraxia from isolated damage to the lenticular nucleus of the basal ganglia were deemed to be likely secondary to disruption of the adjacent white matter in that region, likely the superior longitudinal fasciculus, which had been previously associated in multiple cases with apraxia (Figure 5.6).

Several studies further support the notion that basal ganglia pathology alone may not cause overt apraxia. For example, when basal ganglia lesions are combined with dysfunction in cortically based components of the praxis system (motor sequencing, response selection, etc.), different types of errors can occur that are similar to the types produced in ideomotor apraxia. This is supported by findings that Parkinson's disease (basal ganglia pathology) patients who also have evidence of frontal and parietal lobe dysfunction based on neuropsychological

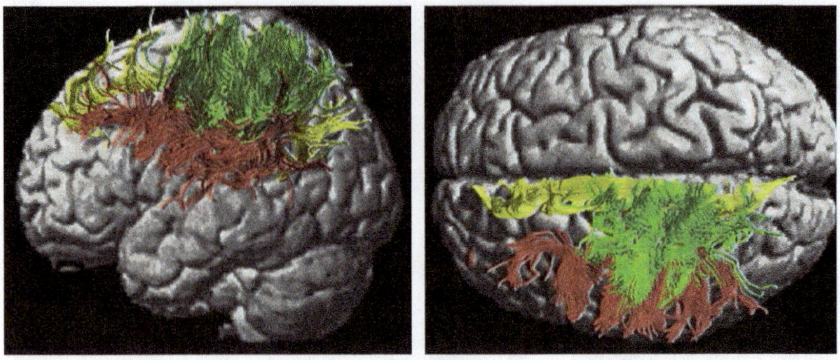

FIGURE 5.6: Apraxia from subcortical lesions may also occur by a disconnection of parietal lobe structures to the frontal lobe, typically occurring by lesioning of the superior longitudinal fasciculus. White matter connections between the parietal and frontal lobe are depicted in red, green, and yellow. The connections in red attach the left inferior parietal lobule to the premotor region in the superior frontal lobe, a key pathway in the praxis circuit that, if lesioned, leads to a disconnection-related apraxia.

Source: From Catani and ffytche (2005).

testing can exhibit apractic errors (Leiguarda et al., 1997).

Thus, it appears that basal ganglia pathology, on its own, does not consistently result in overt apraxia. However, when this pathology is combined with dysfunction of the cortical components of the neural circuits devoted to frontal and/or parietal functions, apraxia may then develop. The clearest example of this is the ideomotor apraxia in patients with corticobasal degeneration, in whom fronto-parietal cortical and basal ganglia damage coexists (Leiguarda, 2001).

DISSOCIATION APRAXIA

Several less common apractic disorders are also associated with the key regions noted, including dissociative apraxia. Patients who have intact complex movement knowledge representations but are impaired at activating these representations from stimuli in one modality (but not other modalities) have dissociation apraxia. This term is used because the movement representations have been dissociated from selective modalities of sensory input.

De Renzi and colleagues (1982) described patients who did not have a visual recognition deficit or difficulties with visual confrontation naming but could not perform correctly when seeing tools or taking cues to show the use of tools from visual input. These patients did demonstrate correct praxis movements to verbal command, however (Merians et al., 1997). Merians et al. (1997) also described three patients with dissociation apraxia associated with the verbal system.

Both the verbal and visual dissociation apraxia patients described had dissociation apraxia of both hands. This is likely due to dissociation apraxia being a "disconnection" phenomenon, in which there is an intact praxis system but a disconnection in accessing the system from a particular modality. This was likely secondary to a lesion in a left hemisphere gray matter relay station or a white matter connecting pathway from the verbal or visual system, respectively, to the praxis system to form the disconnection. Thus, depending on the location of the lesion, stimuli from one of these modalities (e.g., verbal) were not capable of activating the movement representations, but stimuli in other modalities (e.g., visual) were able to activate these representations. At this point, these conditions are not very common, and the anatomic location of these lesions is unclear. With advances in white matter tractography, more white matter disconnection lesions may well be detected to describe these dissociation apraxias.

LIMB KINETIC APRAXIA

Most daily acts performed by humans involve coordinated movements of both of their hands and fingers. Simple acts such as opening a can of soda, tying one's shoes, and buckling a belt utilize these movements regularly. Patients with a lack of "touch" and deftness to perform these actions that require a number of sequenced movements have limb kinetic apraxia.

Tests of dexterity are simple to devise at the bedside and can include tasks such as continuously flipping a coin, buttoning and unbuttoning all of the buttons on a shirt, or continually screwing and unscrewing the cap off of a bottle.

The brain regions that have been associated with limb kinetic apraxia in both lesion and activation studies are the premotor cortices, which are likely secondary to the representation and coordination of the fingers being encoded in these regions. Studies of right-handed individuals with left hemisphere premotor lesions involving the hand and finger areas showed that these individuals presented with limb kinetic apraxia of both the right and the left hand. A lesion of the right premotor hand/finger region resulted typically in just left limb kinetic apraxia. This suggested that the dominant hemisphere in right-handers exhibits some bilateral control over fine motor dexterity, whereas the right hemisphere controlled only left limb dexterity. Other studies have shown that lesions of the corticospinal tract can induce limb kinetic apraxia (Lawrence & Kuypers, 1968). Thus, disconnection of the primary motor cortex from the anterior horn cells of the spinal cord can lead not only to a loss of function of the affected hand but also to lack of dexterity in the intact hand and fingers. The lesion of the corticospinal tract resulting in limb kinetic apraxia can occur as high up in the central nervous system as the internal capsule and as far down as the brain stem.

With the syndrome resulting from lesions in either the gray matter of the primary motor cortex or the white matter corticospinal tract, it remains unclear how the clinically noted lack of dexterity occurs, which may be borne out with further investigations. In addition, further studies are needed on the role that the left premotor cortex plays in both limbs in terms of hand and finger dexterity compared to the right hemisphere's role in only left limb dexterity.

APRAXIA OF SPEECH

Apraxia is not limited to limb movements but can also be present when other body parts cannot perform skilled acts to command. An example is apraxia of speech (AOS), a condition in which the patient cannot perform oral movements when asked to do so verbally (e.g., "Touch your tongue to the roof of your mouth"). Dronkers (1996) studied stroke patients identified as having apraxia of speech and found them to have associated damage in the left superior precentral gyrus of the insula (Figure 5.7). Ogar et al. (2006) sought to characterize the performance of patients with AOS on motor speech

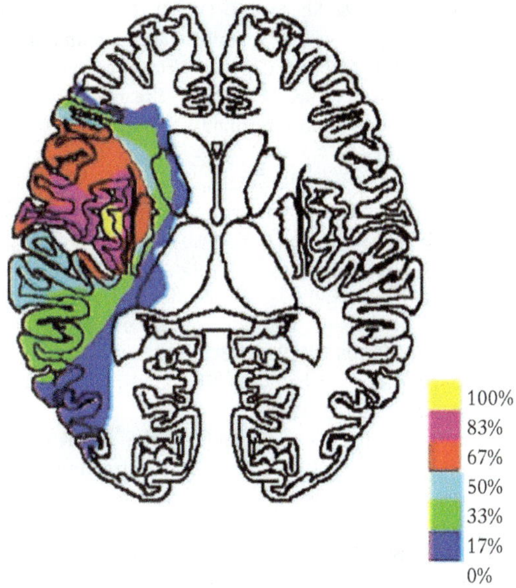

FIGURE 5.7: Overlap of lesions of 18 patients with apraxia of speech. The common area of infarction in bright yellow (100%) and is in the insula.

Source: Ogar et al. (2006).

evaluation and found that these patients made the most errors on tasks requiring the coordination of complex, but not simple, articulatory movements. These AOS patients also had lesions in the superior precentral gyrus of the insula, whereas patients without apraxia of speech did not. Others have suggested that the inferior aspect of the left precentral gyrus (Fox et al., 2001) or the left posterior inferior frontal gyrus (Hillis et al., 2004) could be responsible for AOS. Further consensus will be needed to establish a consistent localization for AOS.

REFERENCES

Babiloni, C., Del Percio, C., Babiloni, F., Carducci, F., Cincotti, F., Moretti, D., et al. (2003). Transient human cortical responses during the observation of simple finger movements: A high-resolution EEG study. *Human Brain Mapping, 20,* 148–157.

Berek, K., Wagner, M., Chemelli, A., & Aichner, F. (1994). Hemispheric disconnection in Marchiafava–Bignami disease: Clinical, neuropsychological and MRI findings. *Journal of the Neurological Sciences, 123,* 2–5.

Buxbaum, L., Kyle, K., Grossman, M., & Coslett, H. B. (2007). Left inferior parietal representations for skilled hand object interactions: Evidence from stroke and corticobasal degeneration. *Cortex, 43,* 411–423.

Caramazza, A., & Shelton, J. (1998). Domain-specific knowledgesystemsinthebraintheanimate–inanimate distinction. *Journal of Cognitive Neuroscience, 10,* 1–34.

Catani, M., & ffytche, D. (2005). The rises and falls of disconnection syndromes. *Brain, 128*(Pt. 10), 2224–2239.

De Renzi, E., Faglioni, P., Scarpa, M., & Crisi, G. (1986). Limb apraxia in patients with damage confined to the left basal ganglia and thalamus. *Journal of Neurology, Neurosurgery, and Psychiatry, 49,* 1030–1038.

De Renzi, E., Faglioni, P., & Sorgato, P. (1982). Modality-specific and supramodal mechanisms of apraxia. *Brain, 105*(Pt. 2), 301–312.

De Renzi, E., & Lucchelli, F. (1988). Ideational apraxia. *Brain, 113,* 1173–1188.

Dovern, A., Fink, G., Saliger, J., Karbe, H., Koch, I., & Weiss, P. (2011). Apraxia impairs intentional retrieval of incidentally acquired motor knowledge. *Journal of Neuroscience, 31,* 8102–8108.

Dronkers, N. (1996). A new brain region for coordinating speech articulation. *Nature, 384,* 159–161.

Fox, R., Kasner, S., Chatterjee, A., & Chalela, J. (2001). Aphemia: An isolated disorder of articulation. *Clinical Neurology and Neurosurgery, 103,* 123–126.

Georgopoulos, A., DeLong, M., & Crutcher, M. (1983). Relations between parameters of step-tracking movements and single cell discharge in the globus pallidus and subthalamic nucleus of the behaving monkey. *Journal of Neuroscience, 3,* 1586–1598.

Geschwind, N. (1965). Disconnexion syndromes in animals and man. *Brain, 88,* 237–294, 585–644.

Graff-Radford, N., Welsh, K., & Godersky, J. (1987). Callosal apraxia. *Neurology, 37,* 100–105.

Halsband, U., Schmitt, J., Weyers, M., et al. (2001). Recognition and imitation of pantomized motor acts after unilateral parietal and premotor lesions: A perspective on apraxia. *Neuropsychologia, 39,* 200–216.

Hanna-Pladdy, H., Heilman, K., & Foundas, A. (2001). Cortical and subcortical contributions to ideomotor apraxia: Analysis of task demands and error types. *Brain, 124,* 2513–2527.

Hart, J., & Kraut, M. (2007). Neural hybrid model of semantic object memory (ver 1.1). In J. Hart & M. Kraut (Eds.), *Neural basis of semantic memory.* Cambridge, England: Cambridge University Press.

Heilman, K. (2010). Apraxia. *Continuum, 16*(4), 86–98.

Heilman, K., & Rothi, L. (1993). Apraxia. In K. M. Heilman & E. Valenstein (Eds.), *Clinical neuropsychology.* New York, NY: Oxford University Press.

Heilman, K., & Watson, R. (2008). The disconnection apraxias. *Cortex, 44*(8), 975–982.

Heilman, K., Rothi, L., & Valenstein, E. (1982). Two forms of ideomotor apraxia. *Neurology, 32*(4), 342–346.

Heilman, K., & Watson, R. (2008). The disconnection apraxias. *Cortex, 44,* 975–982.

Hillis, A., Work, M., Barker, P., Jacobs, M., Breese, E., & Maurer, K. (2004). Re-examining the brain regions crucial for orchestrating speech articulation. *Brain, 127,* 1479–1487.

Jax, S., Buxbaum, L., & Moll, A. (2006). Deficits in movement planning and intrinsic coordinate control in ideomotor apraxia. *Journal of Cognitive Neuroscience, 18,* 2063–2076.

Koski, L., Iacoboni, M., & Mazziotta, J. (2002). Deconstructing apraxia: Understanding disorders of intentional movement after stroke. *Current Opinion in Neurology, 15,* 71–77.

Lawrence, D., & Kuypers, H. (1968). The functional organization of the motor system in the monkey: II. The effects of lesions of the descending brain-stem pathways. *Brain, 91*(1), 15–36.

Leiguarda, R. (2001). Limb apraxia: Cortical or subcortical. *Neuroimage, 14,* S137–S141.

Leiguarda, R., Pramstaller, P., Merello, M., Starkstein, S., Lees, A., & Marsden, C. (1997). Apraxia in Parkinson's disease, progressive supranuclear palsy, multiple system atrophy, and neuroleptic-induced parkinsonism. *Brain, 120,* 75–90.

Liepmann, H. (1900). Das Krankheitsbild der Apraxie (motorischen Asymbolie) auf Grundeines Falles von einseitiger Apraxie. *Monatsschrift fur Psychiatrie und Neurologie, 8,* 15–44.

Liepmann, H. (1905). Die linke Hemisphäre und das Handeln. *Muenchner Medizinische Wochenschrift, 52*(2), 2322–2326.

Manuel, A., Radman, N., Mesot, D., Chouiter, L., Clarke, S., Annoni, J., et al. (2013). Inter- and intrahemispheric dissociations in ideomotor apraxia: A large-scale lesion–symptom mapping study in subacute brain-damaged patients. *Cerebral Cortex, 23*(12), 2781–2789.

Merians, A., Clark, M., Poizner, H., Macauley, B., Gonzalez Rothi, L., & Heilman, K. (1997). Visual-imitative dissociation apraxia. *Neuropsychologia, 35*(11), 1483–1490.

Ogar, J., Willock, S., Baldo, J., Wilkins, D., Ludy, C., & Dronkers, N. (2006). Clinical and anatomical correlates of apraxia of speech. *Brain and Language, 97,* 343–350.

Pazzaglia, M., Smania, N., Corato, E., & Aglioti, M. (2008). Neural underpinnings of gesture discrimination in patients with limb apraxia. *Journal of Neuroscience, 28,* 3030–3041.

Peigneux, P., Salmon, E., Garraux, G., et al. (2001). Neural and cognitive bases of upper limb apraxia in corticobasal degeneration. *Neurology, 57,* 1259–1268.

Penfield, W., & Welch, K. (1951). The supplementary motor area of the cerebral cortex; A clinical and experimental study. *AMA Archives of Neurology and Psychiatry, 66,* 289–317.

Poizner, H., Mack, L., Verfaellie, M., Gonzales Rothi, L., & Heilman, K. (1990). Three-dimensional computer graphic analysis of apraxia. *Brain, 113,* 85–101.

Power, E., Code, C., Croot, K., Sheard, C., & Gonzalez-Rothi, L. (2010). Florida Apraxia Battery-Extended and Revised Sydney (FABERS): Design, description, and a healthy control sample.

Journal of Clinical and Experimental Neuropsychology, 32, 1–18.

Pramstaller, P., & Marsden, C. (1996). The basal ganglia and apraxia. *Brain, 119*, 319–340.

Rushworth, M., Nixon, P., Wade, D., Renowden, S., & Passingham, R. (1998). The left hemisphere and the selection of learned actions. *Neuropsychologia, 36*, 11–24.

Schluter, N., Rushworth, M., Passingham, R., & Mills, K. (1998). Temporary interference in human lateral premotor cortex suggests dominance for the selection of movements: A study using transcranial magnetic stimulation. *Brain, 121*, 785–799.

Schwoebel, J., & Coslett, H. (2005). Evidence for multiple, distinct representations of the human body. *Journal of Cognitive Neuroscience, 17*, 543–553.

Watson, R., Fleet, W., Gonzalez-Rothi, L., & Heilman, K. (1986). Apraxia and the supplementary motor area. *Archives of Neurology, 43*, 787–792.

Watson, R., & Heilman, K. (1983). Callosal apraxia. *Brain, 106*, 391–403.

6

Episodic Memory and Amnesia

There is a great deal of confusion regarding what is meant when the term "memory" is used by individuals as opposed to when it is used by researchers and clinicians. When older individuals and patients complain of memory difficulties, they typically say they have a "short-term memory problem." In fact, short-term memory, which is also referred to by investigators as working memory, is rarely impaired in these individuals. Working memory (which is discussed further in Chapter 10) most often refers to the system that holds information for a short, transient period (e.g., on the order of seconds to minutes with an average of 7 units) to keep it available for information processing. Working/short-term memory requires monitoring, allows for manipulating information (repeating a string of numbers backwards as in the reverse digit span test), and the information is either eventually stored in another, longer term memory system or is forgotten. The best example is calling information for a phone number and keeping it in your head and rehearsing it until you can dial it. Do you remember the number 1 minute later if you were not continually rehearsing it and trying to remember it? The short period of time during which you have that number available to you is what constitutes working or short-term memory.

The type of memory potentially disrupted as individuals age, experience dementia, or have symptoms of amnesia is referred to as episodic memory. *Episodic memory* is defined as recollecting things or events that have happened in the recent past in particular spatial and temporal contexts (Tulving, 1972). A real-life example is being given a list of items to remember to buy at the grocery store in 20 minutes. The types of errors that occur in individuals with an episodic memory impairment for this example are forgetting to purchase items on the list or purchasing the wrong or extra items when at the grocery store.

Another type of memory that is commonly misunderstood is semantic memory. *Semantic memory* refers to remembering facts and general knowledge about the world that are constant and not time dependent (e.g., "knowing what a cup is"). Episodic memory and semantic memory are two different types of declarative memory (Squire, 1987; Tulving, 1983) (Figure 6.1). Although it is clear that there is an interdependence between these two memory systems (e.g., one has to access semantic memory of the concept "corn" to store it on a list of items in episodic memory to be bought at the grocery store 20 minutes from now), we view these as clearly separable entities.

The studies of Vargha-Khadem et al. (1997) described patients with amnesia in whom there had been hippocampal damage early in life. They experienced impaired episodic memory throughout their lives; however, these individuals successfully acquired general fact knowledge (semantic memory) throughout schooling and life, even with hippocampal damage. These findings demonstrate that at some level, there are processes/mechanisms that are distinctly dedicated to semantic memory systems and others to episodic memory systems.

This chapter focuses on cognitive and anatomic units associated with episodic memory. When episodic memory is impaired to a severe degree, it is referred to as *amnesia*. There are two types of amnesia: anterograde and retrograde. After a lesion to the brain occurs and an individual develops an anterograde memory loss, he or she develops an inability to create new episodic memories from the time after the lesion occurred. A retrograde memory loss refers to a loss of or inability to access memories created prior to the event. When a retrograde amnesia occurs, there are noted patterns in terms of the characteristics of the material that cannot be remembered. A temporal gradient to which types of memories are lost can be noted in retrograde amnesia (Ribot's law) and refers to the observation that items that were encoded and remembered far in the past (e.g., 10 years prior to the lesion) are relatively

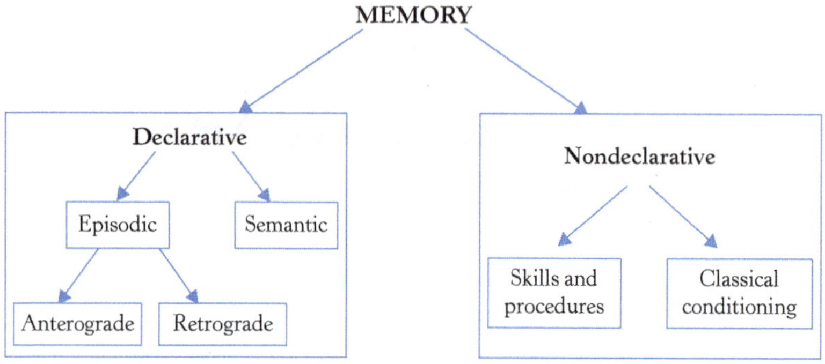

FIGURE 6.1: Components of memory. In declarative (explicit) memory (red box), there are two types—episodic and semantic memory. Episodic memory consists of anterograde and retrograde components.

preserved, whereas items that were encoded and remembered more recently (e.g., 10 days prior to the lesion) are the most at risk of being lost. The occurrence (or co-occurrence) of these amnesias and the severity, types of materials, and length are discussed in this chapter with the specific etiologies that cause them.

To best understand these cognitive–anatomic units (CAUs) in relation to the different types of memory loss associated with episodic memory, an understanding of the cognitive models of episodic memory is useful. Two major functional neural-based models of episodic memory are described: cognitive map theory and multiple trace theory (Moscovitch et al., 2006). *Cognitive map theory* proposes that the hippocampus is essential in creating a memory by creating internal maps of the spatial representations of items and their external surroundings (Burgess et al., 2002; O'Keefe & Nadel, 1978). Within this framework, the hippocampus forms spatial maps, which are representations encoding the relationship between objects in a spatial setting, one that is independent of the observer's position in viewing the scene (e.g., remembering that you placed your keys on the kitchen table). The hippocampus is essential for retaining and retrieving both recent and remote spatial memories and purportedly does not distinguish between cognitive maps acquired recently and those acquired long ago. Consequently, hippocampal damage should lead to impaired spatial memory no matter how long ago it was previously acquired the same as a more recently constructed spatial memory. Thus, in cognitive map theory, there would be no proposed "gradient effect" if a retrograde amnesia were to develop.

In some researchers' view, the cognitive map theory has morphed into the multiple trace theory, whereas others view these as two separate models. In *multiple trace theory,* the ability to re-experience the past is mediated by the hippocampus (Squire & Zola-Morgan, 1991; Teyler & DiScenna, 1986; Teyler & Rudy, 2007; Yonelinas, 2002). Memories are first formed by the hippocampus creating the spatial encoding maps noted previously. Recalling an event requires the hippocampus accessing the trace of the initial memory by re-encoding and re-forming the memory again along with the cortical regions that encoded those parts of the memory. In such a scheme, the hippocampus basically stores an index of cortical regions that were activated when the memory was first experienced. Thus, each time a memory is retrieved, it becomes re-encoded, resulting in "multiple traces" of the memory. Older episodic memories are distributed more widely in the hippocampal–cortical networks than newer ones (Moscovitch et al., 2005). Thus, the theory proposes that damage to the hippocampus would lead to a temporally graded retrograde amnesia.

Both of these theories of episodic memory support the three major cognitive units that are necessary for the formation and recollection of an episodic memory: encoding, storage, and retrieval (Figure 6.2). The encoding stage entails attending to and registering the information that is to be remembered. It also includes the process of transforming this information into a stored representation of the information in the brain. Using the example of being told items to remember to buy at the grocery store ("Don't forget to pick up a gallon of milk and a loaf of rye bread when you go to the store this afternoon"), it is necessary to attend to and hear the items to be remembered, call up from semantic memory the representation of the items to remember, and place them in episodic memory as part of the list to

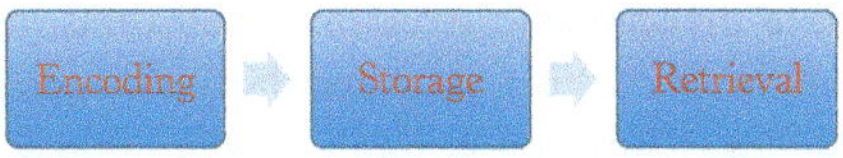

FIGURE 6.2: The three general stages of episodic memory.

be remembered. The storage stage requires that the specific items on the list be retained and maintained in some capacity over time in the absence of active rehearsal/retrieval. This storing of a specific group of items for a designated time frame differs from semantic memory, in which the representations are not dependent on some temporal relationship (e.g., bread is always bread and not just one type, such as rye bread, to be bought at the store today). This storage of a group of items (previously encoded in semantic memory; Vargha-Khadem et al., 1997) at a specific period of time in episodic memory requires a process of storing this list of items as a group to be remembered.

This storage stage has been proposed across models to best be accounted for by what is referred to as the consolidation process. Up to this point, the stages described have been from a cognitive perspective. To best account for the storage stage and the consolidation mechanism, anatomical considerations are helpful to explain the storage stage. The identification of the existence of "place cells" in the hippocampus had a great deal to do with development of both the cognitive map and multiple trace theories' accounts of the storage stage. These cells have been found in animals to become active when an animal enters a particular place in the environment, with that place in the environment referred to as its place field. The place cells function as a spatial frame that links to other neurons throughout the cortices that encode for specific items that would be located in a given location in space that the place cell has in its field. Forming a new memory then requires the complex interaction between the cortical neurons encoding for aspects of an object and the environment in which the object is found and the connections to the hippocampal place cells that stamp that object into a memory for storage. When first experiencing the item during encoding, incoming sensory information (color, shape, smell, etc.) activates various sensory and association cortical regions simultaneously at the time of encoding. For example, for encoding the memory of your wet dog coming out of the rain and into your kitchen, you activate the cortical areas in the brain that encode for the perceptual characteristics of that item (dog) and place (kitchen). The activity of neurons in these sensory/association regions in the cortex then projects those signals to the hippocampus. The synapses between the cortex and the hippocampus are then purportedly strengthened. Thus, the encoded instance is represented as a set of strengthened synapses between the hippocampus and the cortex. This strengthening of the synapses, referred to as "cellular consolidation," consists of the synthesis of new proteins after the experience (Squire & Kandel, 2009). The newly stabilized synapses in the hippocampus support the memory for just a short period of time, and if not further reinforced, it will decay away. The reinforcement (consolidation) process is again proposed to occur by further changes in the cortical–hippocampal synapses that yield to a more permanent connection for a stored memory that can be retrieved at a later time (Squire & Kandel, 2009).

The retrieval stage refers to the processes engaged in searching and finding the specific items to be recalled and producing them in some representational manner for retrieval (e.g., "Can you tell me the list of items you are supposed to pick up at the store?"). There is a "dual-process" framework by which to conceptualize retrieval: A retrieval cue (item presented for recognition) activates two signals—a *recollection* signal entailing qualitative aspects of the event to be remembered and a *familiarity* signal that is a quantitative measure of the event that is adequate for simple judgments (Rugg & Vilberg, 2013; Rugg & Yonelinas, 2003; Wixted, 2007; Wixted & Mickes, 2010; Yonelinas, 2002). A successful recollection judgment consists of confidence from past exposure of an item along with additional information from the original presentation of the stimulus (spatial location of the stimulus, color of the stimulus, etc.). Familiarity is the degree of confidence in memory strength for a particular event, which is a continuous rather than an absolute measure, without necessarily accounting for detailed information about the setting of the given stimuli (Rugg & Yonelinas, 2003).

These two retrieval processes have been accounted for either as conjoined or distinct processes within two models (Wixted, 2007). The signal-detection model describes familiarity and recollection as one entity, with recollection representing the ceiling threshold for confidence in a memory judgment. Proponents of this model propose the hippocampus as the only structure involved in these types of judgments, with damage impacting both processes equally (Wais et al., 2006; Wixted & Squire, 2004). The dual-process detection model (Yonelinas, 1994) treats familiarity and recollection as functionally independent and that correspond to different anatomical regions. Functional neuroimaging studies report that different regions are engaged for both aspects of recognition (Yonelinas et al., 2005), with further studies showing the hippocampus and parahippocampal cortex to be activated in recollection, whereas the perirhinal cortex is more involved in familiarity (Diana et al., 2007).

To reiterate, the two major cognitive theories presented to account for episodic memory are cognitive map and multiple trace theory. Both theories support and account for three cognitive units: encoding, storage, and retrieval. The goal of this chapter is not to distinguish between the previously delineated models but, rather, to determine if there are CAUs that can be identified that account for aspects of these models.

Other stimulus types need to be included in any cognitive formulation of episodic memory, including, but not limited to, memory for objects that are not associated with a particular place, nonspatial memory (e.g., verbal memory/words to remember), auditory nonverbal sound memory (e.g., the sound of a bat hitting a ball), and face memory. These issues are addressed throughout the chapter as they arise.

Irrespective of the underlying cognitive neuroscience theories, a majority of the lesion-deficit findings in episodic memory have greatly aided in generating these theories. Episodic memory difficulties due to lesions occur in a variety of brain regions, including the medial temporal lobes, midline diencephalic structures (thalamus, mammillary bodies, fornix, etc.), and the frontal and parietal lobes (Knowlton & Squire, 1995; Shimamura & Squire, 1987; Squire, 1987). The case of amnestic patient H. M., who years ago had a bilateral medial temporal lobectomy and is one of the most well-studied cases in the history of cognitive neuroscience, has led to considerable insight into the neuroanatomical regions associated with subcomponents of episodic memory (Scoville & Milner, 1957). To best understand how episodic memory is supported in the brain and how lesions result in impairment of episodic memory, the following sections are organized by anatomic structures and roles that they play in amnestic syndromes. First, the neural circuit that has been most often associated with episodic memory and amnestic disorders—the Papez circuit—is discussed.

PAPEZ CIRCUIT

The Papez circuit is a neural pathway in the brain first described in 1937 by James Papez. It begins and ends with the hippocampus (or the hippocampal formation). Fiber dissection indicates that the average size of the circuit is 350 mm. The Papez circuit goes through the following neural pathway: hippocampal formation (including hippocampus, dentate gyrus, and rhinal sulcus) → fornix → mammillary bodies → mammillothalamic tract → anterior nucleus of the thalamus → cingulum and prefrontal regions → entorhinal cortex → hippocampal formation (for schematics of the circuit, see Figure 6.3; for anatomic visualization, see Figures 6.4, 6.5, and

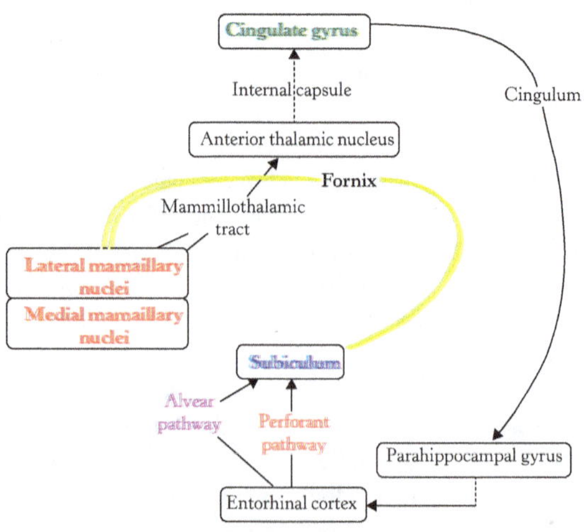

FIGURE 6.3: Schematic of connections in the Papez circuit.

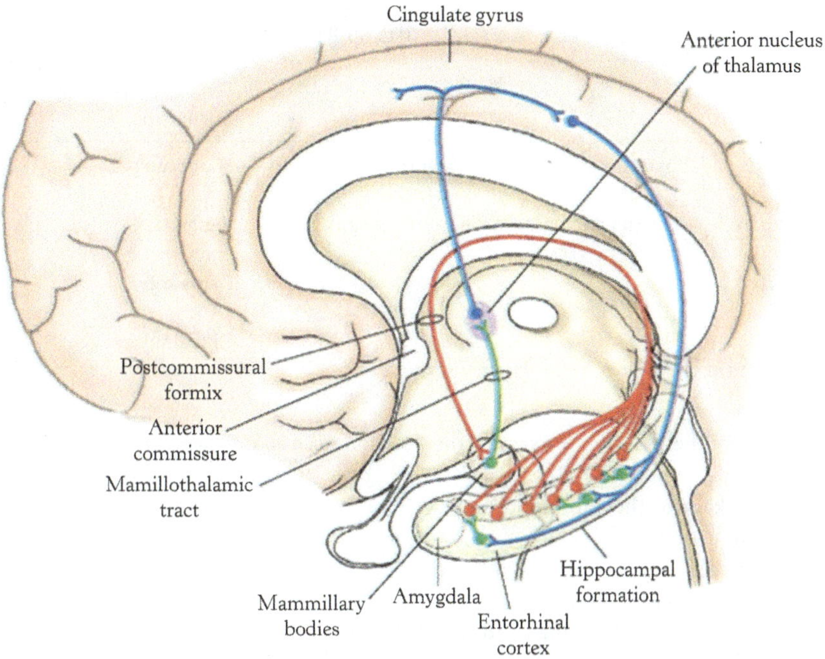

FIGURE 6.4: Schematic of Papez circuit showing some key neuronal connections.

6.10; and for subdivisions of aspects of this circuit, see Table 6.1).

To aid in further visualizing the extent and connections of the Papez circuit, follow the structures in the figures as follows: The parahippocampal gyrus extends medially and inferiorly along the temporal lobe, with its most anterior portion curving inward to join the hippocampus. The anterior aspects of the parahippocampal region consist of the perirhinal (Brodmann areas (BAs) 35 and 36) and entorhinal cortex (ventral and medial to the perirhinal cortex). The portion of the parahippocampal gyrus at the edge of the hippocampal fissure is called the subiculum. The axons from the subiculum and the projections of cells of the hippocampus form the fornix. The fornices on each side curve superiorly, curve over the thalamus, and then proceed anteriorly and join at the midline to form the body of the fornix. This is how information can transfer between hemispheres within the Papez system. The body of the fornix proceeds anteriorly until it reaches the anterior end of the thalamus, where it splits apart again into two branches. These branches of the fornix terminate primarily in the mammillary bodies, although fibers also terminate in lateral and anterior nuclei of the thalamus, the anterior commissure (white matter pathway connecting the two hemispheres), and septal nuclei (nuclei in the medial inferior frontal lobe that play a role in reinforcement and rewards). Fibers from the mammillary bodies, known as the mamillothalamic tract, connect to the anterior nucleus of the thalamus. The anterior nucleus of the thalamus also receives direct input from the hippocampus via the fornix. Fibers from

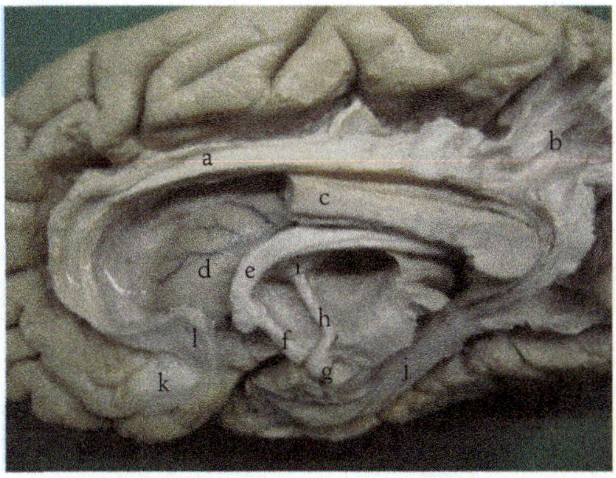

FIGURE 6.5: Photo of the cingulum and surrounding structures: a, cingulum; b, fibers of cingulum going to parietal lobe; c, corpus callosum; d, caudate head; e, fornix body; f, fornix columns; g, mammillary body; h, mamillothalamic tract; i, anterior nucleus of thalamus; j, radiation of the cingulum; k, paraolfactory gyrus; l, paraterminal gyrus.

Source: Shah et al. (2012).

TABLE 6.1: LIMBIC STRUCTURES

Parahippocampal Gyrus		Cingulate Cortex/ Gyrus	Hippocampal Formation	Uncus
Anterior	**Posterior**	Anterior cingulate (BA 24, 32, 33)	Hippocampal sulcus	
Entorhinal cortex	Posterior parahippocampal gyrus	Posterior cingulate (BA 23, 31)	Fimbria of hippocampus	
Perirhinal cortex		Retrosplenial cortex (BA 26, 29, 30)	Dentate gyrus	
			Rhinal sulcus	

the anterior nucleus of the thalamus project to the cingulate gyrus and prefrontal lobe. The cingulate gyrus then connects back to the parahippocampal gyrus to complete the circuit.

Connections between the anterior thalamus and frontal lobe, reciprocal connections between the frontal lobe and medial temporal cortices, and connections between the dorsomedial nucleus of the thalamus and medial temporal cortices all provide modulatory influences on memory functions in the Papez circuit. The hippocampus, parahippocampus, fornix, mammillary bodies, mamillothalamic tract, anterior nucleus of the thalamus, and frontal lobe play key roles in the primary cognitive processes of episodic memory—encoding, storage, and retrieval. The role that these regions play in these cognitive processes in episodic memory is detailed next. This is best organized by the memory deficits associated with regions in the Papez circuit and corresponding cognitive operations that are disrupted.

MEMORY DEFICITS FROM BRAIN LESIONS

Lesions affecting memory performance provide the opportunity to delineate CAUs associated with aspects of episodic memory. In describing memory deficits, it is worth repeating that there are two distinct types of memory loss: anterograde and retrograde. The anterograde deficit refers to the inability to lay down new memories after the point when the lesion occurred, whereas retrograde amnesia refers to a loss of memories created prior to the event. The description of the time period that the retrograde amnesia covers (months/years after illness, lifetime, etc.) and whether it is "temporally graded" (greater loss of memory for events that are closer in time to when the lesion occurs and less loss for events that happened farther in time from when the lesion occurs) or "flat" (loss of memories is equivalent across all time points of the retrograde amnesia) are key features in characterizing a retrograde memory loss with respect to the time point that a lesion occurred.

Several other factors are important in describing the memory deficits from a cognitive perspective. A key factor is the type of testing performed on the patient. Neuropsychological tests used to assess anterograde memory include paragraph memory, list learning, and drawing from memory. Retrograde memory assessments include tasks assessing memories from the patient's past, such as memory for famous faces, personally familiar faces, personal events, and public events. The types of responses required from any kind of test, for anterograde or retrograde amnesia, are important. For example, free recall requires the subject to actively search his or her memory to find and access the exact items that were to be remembered and report them to the examiner (i.e., placing considerable demands on retrieval processes). These demands are diminished when the subject is provided multiple choices and asked to recognize the correct item to be remembered.

There is little disagreement on the types of tasks to use to determine the presence of anterograde amnesia from a clinical assessment. The patient's previous history and knowledge are removed as confounding factors because they are presented a list to remember of common items or a story in which all the elements in the story should be easily recognizable to the average person. However, there is no clear consensus as to which tasks to use for assessing retrograde amnesia, and there is less consensus as to which brain regions are dedicated to cognitive aspects of retrograde amnesia. In addition, the length of time of retrograde memory loss or whether the loss is temporally graded vary by the type of memory disrupted (e.g., memory for famous faces, personally familiar faces, personal events, and public events) across patients. In addition, it appears that retrograde amnesia can vary considerably *within an individual patient* for the length of time of memory loss for each stimulus group type (including memory for public events, autobiographical memory for personal events, famous faces, and/or familiar faces). Thus, brain regions associated with retrograde memory loss are described, but note that the description of the specific roles for these regions in retrograde memory is still evolving.

The CAUs for episodic memory, with the majority of the anatomic units being part of the Papez circuit, have several unique features compared to the other cognitive domains discussed. First, the dissociable anatomic units are associated with multiple cognitive units of encoding, storage, and retrieval, which are documented in the text and summary table. This is due to the multiple roles these regions play, lack of specification of the cognitive units, and/or lack of clear dissociation of the anatomic regions that clearly support specific cognitive operations. The second characteristic is that based on studies of the Papez circuit, there are clear anatomic units associated with cognitive units that are connections between neural regions that, if lesioned consistently, yield a disruption of the Papez circuit via disconnection of brain regions. These are delineated clearly in the following sections. The other characteristic concerning the roles of these CAUs in episodic memory is that they perform operations that, when disrupted, can result in both the clinical syndromes of anterograde and retrograde amnesia, which are noted with each CAU.

Diencephalic Amnesia

The diencephalon is a region of nuclei located at the top of the brain stem. The regions of importance to memory functioning include portions of the thalamus and its connections located in the diencephalon. In particular, patients who have injuries involving the midline structures of these regions demonstrate severe anterograde amnesia and often demonstrate a temporally graded retrograde amnesia. The structures most often implicated in diencephalic amnesia include the dorsomedial and anterior nuclei of the thalamus, the mammillary bodies (parts of the hypothalamus), and the white matter (mamillothalamic) tract connecting these two structures. Common etiologies of diencephalic amnesia are presented in the following two sections.

Wernicke–Korsakoff's Encephalopathy and Amnesia

Wernicke–Korsakoff's amnestic syndrome (Wernicke–Korsakoff's encephalopathy (WKE)) is caused by damage to medial diencephalic structures, including the dorsomedial nucleus of the thalamus and mammillary bodies, resulting from severe thiamine deficiency, most often related to excessive alcohol consumption and its associated malnutrition. Patients who have amnesic WKE demonstrate clinically normal intelligence and working memory ability, but their ability to place new information into recent or remote memory (anterograde amnesia) is severely impaired (Butters & Cermak, 1980; see Video 6); they also develop a retrograde amnesia. The severe anterograde amnesia appears to affect all of the cognitive units of episodic memory (encoding, storage, and retrieval) (Pitel et al., 2008). Patients demonstrate equally poor recall and recognition for both anterograde and retrograde components (Butters et al., 1988; Cermak, 1984), and occasionally "recall" information that was never presented—a phenomenon known as confabulation (Butters & Stuss, 1989).

A review of studies suggested that isolated limbic diencephalic lesions generally produce a relatively brief period of retrograde amnesia, 3 years or less, including autobiographical memory (Race et al., 2012). Those with WKE showed a striking temporal gradient to the retrograde amnesia with relative sparing of early memories, and the length of retrograde amnesia varied depending on the type of stimulus material assessed (e.g., personal events, world events, and familiar faces).

The neuropathology of WKE brains has routinely demonstrated shrinkage and brown discoloration of the mammillary bodies consistent with previous hemorrhage (Figures 6.6 and 6.7). In the majority of patients, there is the occasional appearance of gray discoloration indicative of necrosis of the tissue in the mammillary bodies (Kril & Harper, 2012). Cohort studies of WKE patients suggest that the mammillary bodies and dorsomedial nucleus of the thalamus are the key regions in the diencephalon to be lesioned to result in impairment of successful episodic memory. Other studies suggest that the additional involvement of damage to the anterior thalamus is also required to develop the memory impairment of WKE. Rare cases support the role of only the anterior thalamus and mammillary bodies

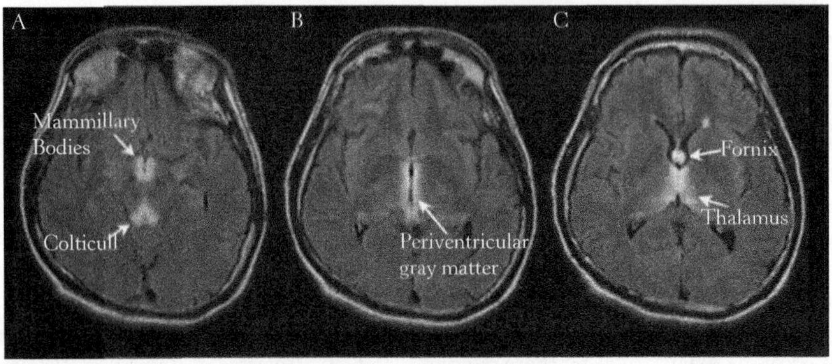

FIGURE 6.6: MRI findings of acute Wernicke's encephalopathy. FLAIR images demonstrating symmetric high signal in the mammillary bodies and colliculi (A), periventricular gray matter (B), and fornix and thalamus (C).

Source: Jung et al. (2012).

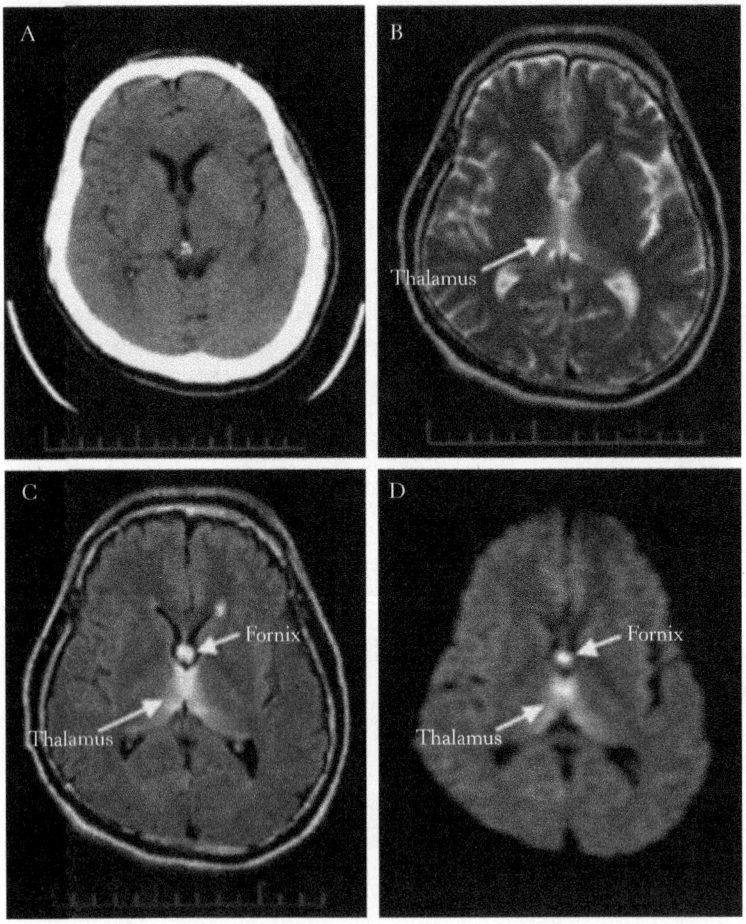

FIGURE 6.7: Computed tomography (CT) and MRI images of acute Wernicke's encephalopathy: (A) CT, (B) T2 fast spin echo image, (C) FLAIR image, and (D) diffusion-weighted image.

Source: Jung et al. (2012).

in WKE. Because these nuclei form part of wider memory circuits, damage to the interconnecting white matter tracts (fornix and mamillothalamic tracts) can also result in a deficit similar to that of direct damage to these nuclei (Kril & Harper, 2012). Although Victor et al. (1989) concluded that damage to the mammillary bodies and dorsomedial nuclei is necessary to result in the amnesia of WKE, taken together, the evidence to date suggests that damage to the thalamus (anterior thalamic and dorsomedial nuclei) and mammillary bodies (medial mammillary nucleus of the hypothalamus) appears to be required to have the clinical syndrome of WKE. It is also of note that acute lesions to these same regions by pathologies other than WKE (e.g., cerebrovascular accident (CVA)) can result in the same memory impairments as the behavioral description for WKE (Schmahmann, 2003).

The incidence of WKE appeared to be on a steady decline; however, there has been a recent increase in the incidence of patients who present with thiamine deficiency. The current cases are now secondary to elective abdominal procedures for bariatric surgery (Ba & Siddiqui, 2010).

Diencephalic Connections

Van der Werf et al. (2003) studied a group of patients with infarctions in the thalamic region, with 10 cases demonstrating a pure amnestic syndrome with sparing of other cognitive functions (including working memory, semantic memory, and intellectual capacity). These symptoms occurred with lesions disrupting the mammillothalamic tract connecting the mammillary bodies to the thalamus (Figure 6.8). These patients showed an anterograde memory deficit characterized by a failure to encode both verbal and visual information, but it appears that retrograde memory was not tested in this study, so the extent of its involvement is unknown.

Fornix lesions typically occur as part of surgical removal of colloid cysts located in the third ventricle and can result in anterograde amnesia and a pronounced retrograde amnesia for autobiographical memory, including extending back to cover the entire life of the patient (Poreh et al., 2006). Because the fornix is a major afferent and efferent pathway of the hippocampus, a severe disconnection to the hippocampus results from a fornix lesion. In the reported case, there was a lifelong retrograde amnesia for all autobiographical memory but a limited retrograde amnesia for memory of public events (Poreh et al., 2006) (Figure 6.9). These findings were most consistent with theories in which a hippocampal system is essential for recovering autobiographical memories no matter how old they are (i.e., more consistent with multiple trace theory) but is not as essential for retrieving public events. Further studies with comprehensive testing of multiple types of retrograde memory will help clarify if this is a consistent association with the fornix.

In addition, patients with isolated damage to the fornix and mammillary bodies demonstrate impaired recollection-based recognition and spared familiarity-based recognition. These findings supported the claim that retrieval was a distinct dual process that was functionally and anatomically

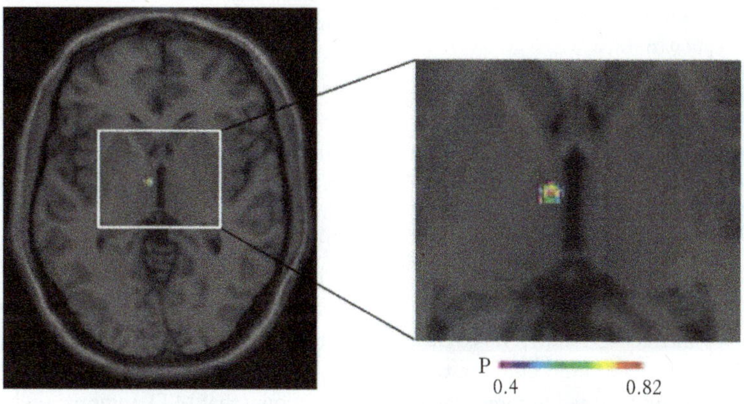

FIGURE 6.8: Amnesic syndrome with lesion in mamillothalamic tract. The colored voxels show the degree of overlap of lesions of patients with amnesic syndromes compared to those without. Ten patients with pure amnesic deficits represent the overlap.

Source: Van der Werf et al. (2003).

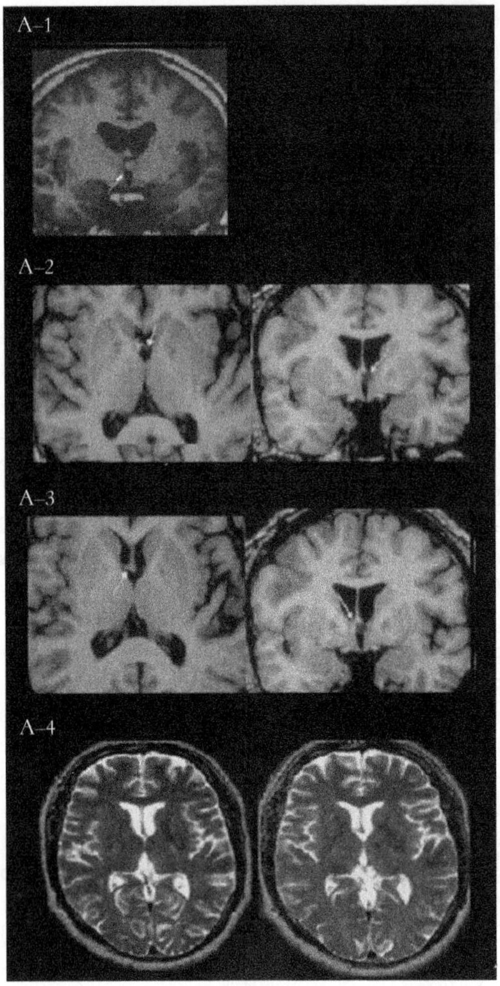

FIGURE 6.9: Presurgical MRI shows third ventricle colloid cyst (A-1). Post-surgical fornix lesions seen in axial and coronal views on T1 images for the left fornix transection (A-2) and right fornix disruption (A-3). T2 scan showing fornix disruption (A-4).

Source: Poreh et al. (2006).

isolatable, demonstrating separate recognition and familiarity units in the retrieval mechanism (Vann et al., 2009).

Medial Temporal Lobe Amnesia

Some of the most intriguing studies in cognitive neuroscience have centered around amnesia that is associated with lesions of the medial temporal lobe (MTL) and its relationship with episodic memory. It is still an ongoing debate as to the extent of the MTL lesion and whether there are subdivisions of the region that may correspond to specific cognitive units or stimulus types in episodic memory (related to either anterograde or retrograde processes). It is clear, however, that the midline (medial) aspects of the temporal lobes are essential neural substrates for some of the cognitive units responsible for anterograde and retrograde episodic memory (for anatomy, see Figure 6.10).

In 1957, Scoville and Milner described patient H. M., who had a profound amnesia following bilateral medial temporal lobectomies to surgically remove the anterior two-thirds of his hippocampi, parahippocampi, and amygdalae to treat his epilepsy. Following his surgery, H. M. demonstrated a dense anterograde and retrograde amnesia, and he allowed himself to be widely studied from 1957 until his death. His amnestic disorder persisted following his surgery, allowing for extensive testing as well as neuroimaging (Figure 6.11) (Corkin et al., 1997).

Since the studies of H. M., numerous studies of patients with MTL lesions have been conducted. In terms of the MTL lesion localization with the three major stages of episodic memory, there has been no clear association of MTL with a specific, single stage. The most prominent role the MTL appears to play as a CAU is in the storage stage via the process of consolidation. Based on extensive investigation of this circuit, the CAU is specified for not only its anatomic substrate but also its neural mechanism because the neurophysiological contribution in the consolidation mechanism for MTL—indexing of posterior cortices to store/integrate information (e.g., spatial and object information)—appears most essential (Mayes & Roberts, 2001).

These MTL regions may also be engaged in the retrieval stage via reactivating associations between representations in the cortices that the hippocampus established previously, with the hippocampus being necessary for at least some critical time period for this memory recollection (Mayes & Roberts, 2001). An alternative but related account of the hippocampal role in retrieval is that the hippocampus "binds" contextual information from the parahippocampal cortex with object information from the perirhinal cortex to retrieve an integrated memory (Diana et al., 2007; Montaldi & Mayes, 2010). An integrated account of retrieval including the MTL has been proposed by Rugg and Vilberg (2013), who have shown that MTL regions, anchored by the hippocampus, are connected with a network of cortical regions, including the posterior cingulate gyrus, posterior parietal cortex, and medial prefrontal cortex, to form a retrieval network.

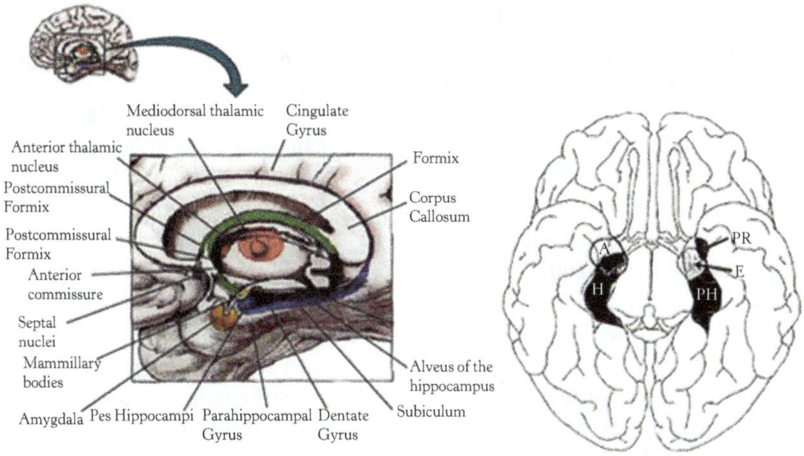

FIGURE 6.10: Graphic of medial temporal lobe structures and relationship to other structures in the Papez circuit.

Source: Moscovitch et al. (2005).

In addition to the prominent role that the MTL plays in storage, Daselaar et al. (2004) did not demonstrate a clear dissociation between encoding and retrieval processes in the MTL but did show that both are supported by the MTL. A region in the left MTL, including the parahippocampal cortex and hippocampal formation, appears on functional imaging studies to be engaged in both encoding and retrieval, whereas a small region in the left MTL, including the entorhinal cortex, was found to be

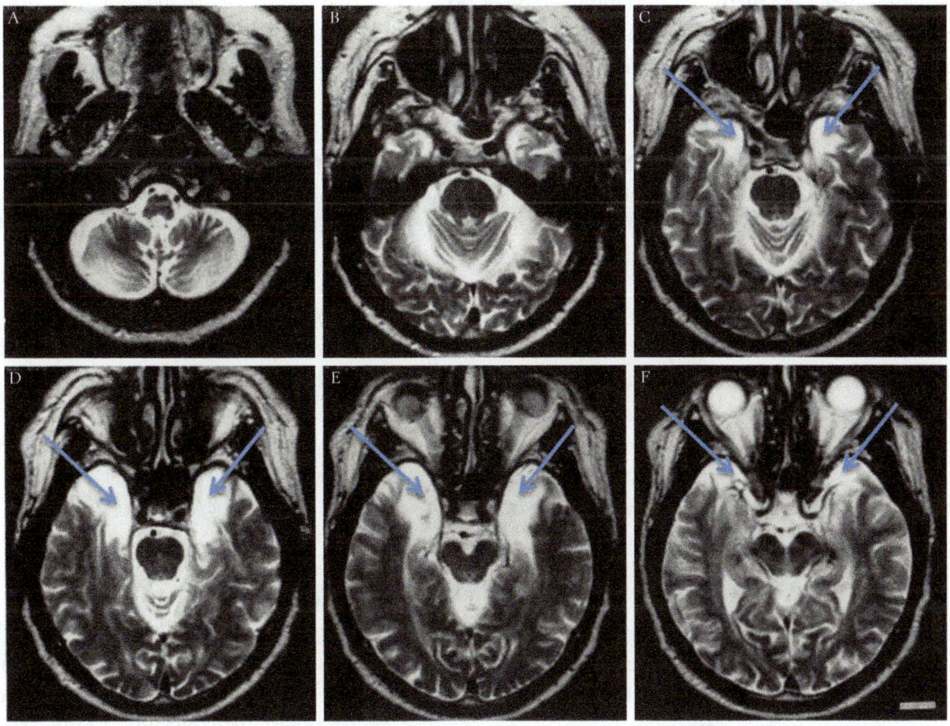

FIGURE 6.11: MR images (T2 weighted) of the patient H. M. with the bright signal (blue arrows) at the tip of the temporal lobes indicating the extent of the bilateral resections.

Source: Corkin et al. (1997).

activated exclusively during encoding. To date, the contributions of the specific regions in the MTL to encoding, storage, and retrieval have not been fully established, nor has it been determined if these can clearly be anatomically dissociated into independent regions supporting specific processes. Investigations are ongoing to determine if separate MTL regions for encoding and retrieval can be distinguished (Mayes & Roberts, 2001). However, it may well result in the general finding that MTL lesions are involved in disruption of all aspects of encoding, storage, and retrieval.

Retrograde amnesia attributed to MTL lesions has led to some localization findings. In general, when lesions are limited to the hippocampus alone, retrograde amnesia is limited to include a few years prior to the lesion. If the lesion extends to the entire hippocampal formation (or to other regions in the MTL adjacent to the hippocampus), retrograde amnesia becomes more severe, encompassing past memories ranging from several years prior to the injury to decades of one's life. The remote memory loss in these cases is temporally graded with preservation of the most remote memories. If the MTL damage extends out to include regions of the inferior temporal gyrus and further to the lateral temporal lobe, then retrograde amnesia can be extensive and ungraded. An example of this type of ungraded retrograde amnesia with MTL lesions extending laterally out to the parahippocampal and inferior temporal gyri resulted in severe impairments on free recall (anterograde amnesia) and ungraded retrograde deficits in autobiographical remote memory as well as personal semantic knowledge (Bright et al., 2006; Insausti et al., 2013).

In a summary of the inconsistent results from retrograde amnesia studies, Squire and Bayley (2007) summarized their interpretation of the data accumulated up to that time on retrograde amnesia for factual information in MTL lesions and determined that it can be either temporally limited, covering only a few years, or prolonged, depending on the locus and extent of damage. The findings on locus and extent of damage were as follows:

1. Damage only to hippocampus plus dentate gyrus and subiculum → retrograde amnesia for past news events is temporally graded and extends for only a few years.
2. Limited hippocampal lesions plus cell loss in the entorhinal cortex results in temporally limited, retrograde amnesia that covers one or two decades.
3. Large lesions of the medial temporal lobe and extending into the lateral temporal lobe produce extended retrograde amnesia that can cover many decades, with sparing only of memories from early life. Remote autobiographical memory is intact when damage is limited to the hippocampus or adjacent medial temporal lobe structures. The findings emphasize the importance of lateral temporal (and possibly other pathologies, including the frontal lobe) for understanding retrograde amnesia involving autobiographical memory.

An alternative account of this same literature comes from multiple trace theories' contention that complex memories involve the hippocampus for re-experiencing detailed episodic and spatial memories, no matter how old they are (Moscovitch et al., 2005). The model predicts that the temporal extent and severity of retrograde amnesia is related to the amount of hippocampal complex damage. Ranganath (2010) alternatively suggests that there is functional heterogeneity in the medial temporal lobes, and that there exist subregions that differ in terms of the kind of information they process and represent. However, these subregions have yet to be identified.

Overall, it has yet to be clarified how MTL lesions account for the varying stimulus types (personal events, famous faces, etc.), temporal gradient or not, and extent of time of the retrograde amnesia. There are several key reasons for this, one of which has to do with the lack of realization that the different stimulus group types have different degrees of length of retrograde amnesia within the same individual who develops it. The fact that this has only become evident during approximately the past decade has led to many instances of retrograde amnestics who had incomplete data acquisition sets. Based on the data collected thus far, there appear to be different degrees and characteristics of retrograde amnesia for at least the following stimulus group types: autobiographical memory for personally familiar faces, personal events, public events, and famous faces. It is clear that to best clarify possible subdivisions of anatomic structures that may contribute to specific episodic memory functions or specific stimulus types, consistent evaluation of amnestic patients with relatively similar testing batteries would be helpful. This is quite difficult in retrograde memory assessments

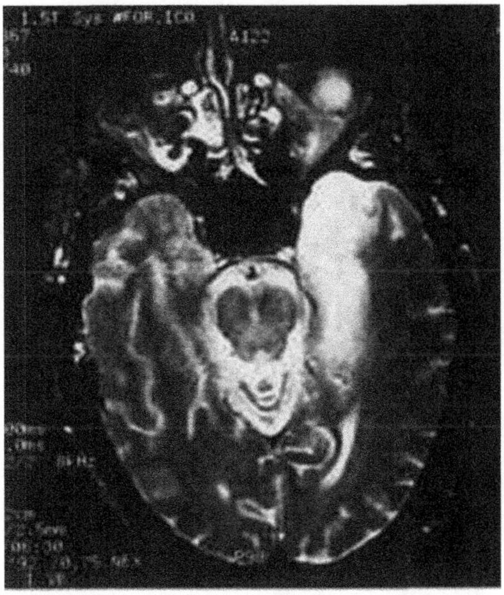

FIGURE 6.12: MRI scan of a patient with herpes simplex encephalitis with an extensive lesion (increased signal) in the left medial temporal lobe extending to the temporal pole.

because there is a lack of norms for these tests and the personal autobiographical memories are unique to each individual patient. This latter point makes each test battery unique for each patient and thus difficult to compare across patients. Another factor making it difficult to perform adequate assessments is that without premorbid testing, it is unclear how well any patient remembered his or her unique information prior to developing the lesion.

The type of pathology that typically results in MTL lesions includes herpes simplex encephalitis (O'Connor et al., 1992) (Figure 6.12), post-irradiation, and neurodegenerative diseases such as frontotemporal lobar degeneration (Knibb et al., 2006) and Alzheimer's disease (Weintraub et al., 2012). However, the same symptoms have developed from similar lesions resulting from CVA (Szabo et al., 2009). These unilateral stroke lesions in MTL do help to solidify the association of lesions to the left MTL with verbal episodic memory loss (anterograde amnesia) (Szabo et al., 2009). (There is a suggestion that right MTL damage leads to nonverbal episodic memory loss; however, this has not been a consistent finding.)

Aggleton (2008) described episodic memory functions associated with specific regions of the Papez circuit but noted that additional brain areas external to the circuit are engaged in episodic memory, such as the medial prefrontal cortex and retrosplenial cortex. The following section describes these other brain regions and the correlations with amnestic behavior.

Frontal Lobe Amnesia

It has been proposed that the interaction between frontal and medial temporal systems is essential for normal memory function, with the frontal lobes subsuming cognitive control functions in such varied roles as organization, search, selection, monitoring, or decision-making in episodic memory (Moscovitch & Winocur, 2002; Shallice, 2002; Shimamura, 2002).

Studies have shown the frontal lobes to be directly involved in the retrieval processes of episodic memory by engaging in organizing information in episodic memory (contributing to encoding and retrieval aspects) and in directed search for episodic memories supporting a significant aspect of episodic retrieval (Rugg & Wilding, 2000). On the other hand, MTL structures are not necessary for recognition of familiar items; thus, an MTL lesion may leave some sparing of recognition episodic memory (mediated by the frontal lobes to some extent) but strongly affects recall of episodic memories (Aggleton, 2008).

In terms of specific frontal lobe regions engaged in episodic memory, the basal forebrain is most often implicated. The basal forebrain is located superior to the optic chiasm and includes the medial septal nuclei, nucleus basalis of Meynert, nucleus accumbens, diagonal band of Broca, anterior hypothalamus, and part of the prefrontal cortex (Figure 6.13). The septal nuclei function as a relay station from the hippocampus to the hypothalamus (the nuclei receive their input from the hippocampus via the fornix). The nucleus basalis of Meynert lies inferior to the basal ganglia and lateral to the hypothalamus. The nucleus basalis provides the acetylcholine input to extensive cortical regions, particularly the MTL, and thus affects episodic memory storage via regulation of the medial temporal lobes neurochemically (Johnston et al., 1979). These basal forebrain structures also have extensive structural connections to and from the hippocampus and cortex essential to episodic memory functioning (Mesulam et al., 1983; Zola-Morgan & Squire, 1993).

Key cases in which this area was disrupted and resulted in the development of primarily anterograde amnesia occurred after clipping of an unruptured anterior communicating artery (ACA) aneurysm with a lesion in the basal forebrain area

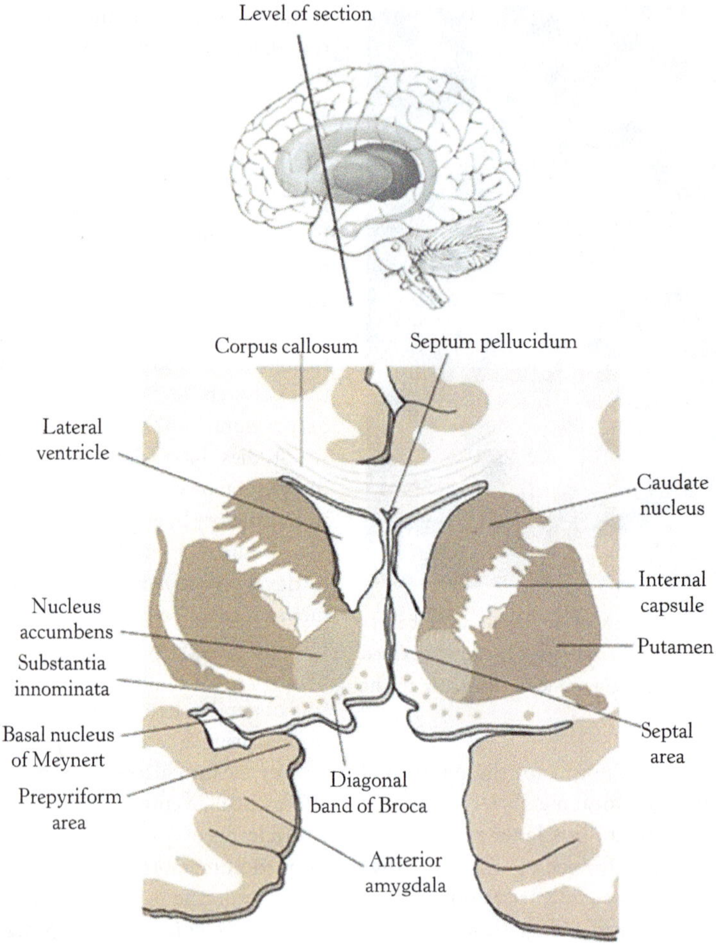

FIGURE 6.13: Cross section taken through the forebrain (top figure shows plane of the section). Key nuclei related to episodic memory include the nucleus basalis of Meynert, septal nuclei, and the diagonal band of Broca.

Source: http://what-when-how.com.

centered in the diagonal band of Broca including the anterior hypothalamus, septal nucleus, lamina terminalis, and paraterminal gyrus. The nucleus basalis of Meynert was minimally affected, and the diencephalon was not damaged. It was assumed that disconnection of the pathway between the diagonal band of Broca and the hippocampus contributed to the memory impairment (Abe et al., 1998).

Group studies of patients with lesions in the previously mentioned regions demonstrate some general patterns of performance. Bilateral frontal lesions result in more retrograde memory impairment on news events than do unilateral frontal lesions, and in patients with unilateral lesions, those with right frontal pathology performed worse on these memory measures than those with left frontal pathology (Kopelman et al., 1999).

Overall, it is clear from multiple lesion studies, particularly those of midline lesions resulting from ACA aneurysm rupture, that the medial frontal lobes play an integral role in episodic memory, with corresponding lesions resulting in notable impairment. However, it is unclear what specific regions of the medial frontal structures correlate with specific episodic memory cognitive operations (encoding, retrieval, etc.).

PARIETAL LOBE CONTRIBUTIONS TO EPISODIC MEMORY

Medial parietal (precuneus) and caudomedial limbic (e.g., posterior cingulate) regions have been implicated in lesion studies as being engaged in retrieval aspects of episodic memory (Davidson et al., 2008). Several case studies have reported memory impairment after damage to these regions, although the specific contributions of precuneus and posterior cingulate to episodic memory operations are still unclear (for reviews, see Aguirre & D'Esposito, 1999; Maguire, 2001). Patients with damage to this broad set of regions may either show a full-blown amnesia similar to that following medial temporal damage (Rudge & Warrington, 1991; Valenstein et al., 1987; Von Cramon & Schuri, 1992) or show a more selective topographical disorientation, in which they can recognize familiar landmarks but get lost when asked to go from one place to another (Takahashi et al., 1997). Further studies concerning these regions are warranted because these areas appear to play a role in episodic memory functions as implicated by functional connectivity magnetic resonance imaging (fcMRI) rest state and plaque deposition in Alzheimer's disease.

PSYCHOGENIC AMNESIA

It is common for anterograde deficits to occur in the absence of retrograde amnesia. The reverse pattern, however, is rare. Isolated retrograde impairments, including loss of past memories, personal history, and personal identity, typically are psychological rather than neurologic in origin (Kopelman, 1987).

SUMMARY

Lesions of the diencephalon including the mammillary bodies and dorsomedial and anterior nuclei of the thalamus produce anterograde and retrograde episodic memory amnesia while appearing to affect encoding, storage, and retrieval stages. Disruption of the fornix connecting the MTL to these areas yields a similar deficit. MTL structures (including the parahippocampal gyri and hippocampus) produce an anterograde amnesia (all three stages affected) and a retrograde amnesia, with the extent and quality depending on the stimulus type and regions affected. Although the hippocampus is involved in all three stages of episodic memory, it is essential for the storage stage due to its key role in the consolidation process of stamping and storing a memory. If MTL damage extends to the lateral temporal cortices, then an extensive retrograde amnesia can occur that covers up to many decades of life, with the type of material most affected involving autobiographical memory. Lesions affecting midline frontal lobe structures (e.g., septal nuclei, diagonal band of Broca, and nucleus basalis of Meynert) can result in an anterograde amnesia assumed to arise from impaired retrieval processes and retrograde amnesia that is greater in temporal extent for bilateral > right > left frontal involvement.

Compared to those discussed in other chapters, the CAUs in this chapter do not always have a clear correspondence to the defined units of encoding, storage, and retrieval, but in multiple instances there is overlap (a lesion affects multiple cognitive units). It is clear, however, that the lesions disrupt cognitive units in episodic memory, and thus in Table 6.2, the CAUs of episodic memory that can be attributed to

TABLE 6.2: EPISODIC MEMORY SUMMARY

Brain Region	Functions
Diencephalic	
Mammillary bodies; dorsomedial and anterior nuclei of thalamus (WKE)	Anterograde—encoding, storage, retrieval Retrograde—temporal gradient, varying length
Fornix (connection)	Anterograde; retrograde for autobiographical memory even for the entire life of the patient
Mammillothalamic tract (connection)	Anterograde (encoding) for verbal and visual information
Temporal lobe	
Hippocampal formation (hippocampus, hippocampal sulcus, fimbria of hippocampus, dentate gyrus, rhinal sulcus)	Anterograde (if on left, predominantly verbal anterograde) Retrograde—limited to several years—temporally graded
Parahippocampal gyrus (entorhinal cortex, perirhinal cortex, posterior parahippocampal gyrus)	Anterograde; hippocampus plus this region gives 10–20 year retrograde—not considerable autobiographical memory effect
Lateral temporal cortex (including inferior temporal gyrus)	If MTL + this region → retrograde, especially for autobiographical and personal semantic memory—extensive and ungraded
Frontal lobe	
Midline frontal structures (septal nuclei, diagonal band of Broca, nucleus basalis of Meynert)	Anterograde—retrieval (search) and indirectly storage via ACh effect on MTL from nucleus basalis Retrograde—greater temporal length if bilateral

these regions are listed as best as currently can be discerned.

This lack of finer specification may be due to the fact that the lesion and activation studies that were used to form these localizations do not have the resolution to distinguish the anatomic units that correspond to the defined cognitive units (encoding, storage, and retrieval), the lesions that have occurred are too large to isolate the size of anatomic unit to correspond to the cognitive units described, the cognitive units need to be better delineated, or that these cognitive units are not organized by discrete anatomic units but a more anatomically distributed schema. It is also clear that lesions of the white matter tracts (fornix) can result in a disconnection in the circuit and affect cognitive units.

Utilizing the network models can also provide an account of the anatomic localizations and cognitive units described. When a lesion in a region is involved in disrupting multiple cognitive units, then one can ascribe that the region is engaged in multiple cognitive operations and consequently the anatomic support for that operation is distributed across several anatomic regions.

Studies of both retrograde and anterograde amnesia must specify the type of stimuli studied for memory performance (e.g., autobiographical memory for personally familiar faces, personal events, public events, and famous faces for retrograde amnesia; visual words, auditory words, pictures, faces, nonverbal shapes, and paragraphs/stories for anterograde amnesia). In addition, it is important to note when these materials are used in testing and if the stimuli and tests have been standardized with appropriate norms. Using these types of approaches can lead to finer localizations and clearer cognitive–brain associations, even with the variability in what individuals know about remote world knowledge and the variability inherent in each individual's personal history.

REFERENCES

Abe, K., Inokawa, M., Kashiwagi, A., & Yanagihara, T. (1998). Amnesia after a discrete basal forebrain lesion. *Journal of Neurology, Neurosurgery, and Psychiatry, 65*, 126–130.

Aggleton, J. (2008). Understanding anterograde amnesia: Disconnections and hidden lesions. *Quarterly Journal of Experimental Psychology, 61*(10), 1441–1471.

Aguirre, G., & D'Esposito, M. (1999). Topographical disorientation: A synthesis and taxonomy. *Brain, 122*, 1613–1628.

Ba, F., & Siddiqi, Z. (2010). Neurologic complications of bariatric surgery. *Reviews in Neurological Diseases*, 7(4), 119–124.

Bright, P., Buckman, J., Fradera, A., Yoshimasu, H., Colchester, A., & Kopelman, M. (2006). Retrograde amnesia in patients with hippocampal, medial temporal, temporal lobe, or frontal pathology. *Learning & Memory, 13*, 545–557.

Burgess, N., Maguire, E., & O'Keefe, J. (2002). The human hippocampus and spatial and episodic memory. *Neuron, 35*, 625–641.

Butters, N., & Cermak, L. (1980). *Alcoholic Korsakoff's syndrome*. New York, NY: Academic Press.

Butters, N., Salmon, D., Cullum, C., et al. (1988). Differentiation of amnesic and demented patients with the Wechsler Memory Scale–Revised. *Clinical Neuropsychology, 2*, 133–148.

Butters, N., & Stuss, D. (1989). Diencephalic amnesia. In F. Boller & J. Grafman (Eds.), *Handbook of neuropsychology* (Vol. 3, pp. 107–148). Amsterdam: Elsevier.

Cermak, L. (1984). The episodic–semantic distinction in amnesia. In L. R. Squire & N. Butters (Eds.), *Neuropsychology of memory* (pp. 55–62). New York, NY: Guilford.

Corkin, S., Amaral, D., Gonzalez, R., Johnson, K., & Hyman, B. (1997). H. M.'s medial temporal lobe lesion: Findings from magnetic resonance imaging. *Journal of Neuroscience, 17*(10), 3964–3979.

Daselaar, S., Veltman, D., & Witter, M. (2004). Common pathway in the medial temporal lobe for storage and recovery of words as revealed by event-related functional MRI. *Hippocampus, 14*, 163–169.

Davidson, P., Anaki, D., Ciaramelli, E., Cohn, M., Kim, A., Murphy, K., et al. (2008). Does lateral parietal cortex support episodic memory? Evidence from focal lesion patients. *Neuropsychologia, 46*(7), 1743–1755.

Diana, R., Yonelinas, A., & Ranganath, C. (2007). Imaging recollection and familiarity in the medial temporal lobe: A three-component model. *Trends in Cognitive Sciences, 11*, 379–386.

Insausti, R., Annesee, J., Amarala, D., & Squire, L. (2013). Human amnesia and the medial temporal lobe illuminated by neuropsychological and neurohistological findings for patient E.P. *Proceeding of the National Academy of Sciences of the USA,110*(21), E1953–E1962.

Johnston, M., McKinney, M., & Coyle, J. (1979). Evidence for a cholinergic projection to neocortex from neurons in basal forebrain. *Proceedings of the National Academy of Sciences of the USA, 76*(10), 5392–5396.

Jung, Y., Chanraud, S., & Sullivan, E. (2012). Neuroimaging of Wernicke's encephalopathy and Korsakoff's syndrome. *Neuropsychology Review, 22*, 170–180.

Knibb, J., Kipps, C., & Hodges, J. (2006). Frontotemporal dementia. *Current Opinion in Neurology, 19*(6), 565–571.

Knowlton, B., & Squire, L. (1995). Remembering and knowing: Two different expressions of declarative memory. *Journal of Experimental Psychology: Learning, Memory, and Cognition, 21*, 699–710.

Kopelman, M. (1987). Amnesia: Organic and psychogenic. *British Journal of Psychiatry, 150*, 428–442.

Kopelman, M., Stanhope, N., & Kingsley, D. (1999). Retrograde amnesia in patients with diencephalic, temporal lobe or frontal lesions. *Neuropsychologia, 37*, 939–958.

Kril, J., & Harper, C. (2012). Neuroanatomy and neuropathology associated with Korsakoff's syndrome. *Neuropsychology Review, 22*, 72–80.

Maguire, E. (2001). The retrosplenial contribution to human navigation: A review of lesion and neuroimaging findings. *Scandinavian Journal of Psychology, 42*, 225–238.

Mayes, A., & Roberts, N. (2001). Theories of episodic memory. *Philosophical Transactions of the Royal Society of London B, 456*, 1395–1408.

Mesulam, M., Mufson, E., Levey, A., & Wainer, B. (1983). Cholinergic innervation of cortex by the basal forebrain: Cytochemistry and cortical connections of the septal area, diagonal band nuclei, nucleus basalis (substantia innominata), and hypothalamus in the rhesus monkey. *Journal of Comparative Neurology, 214*, 170–197.

Montaldi, D., & Mayes, A. (2010). The role of recollection and familiarity in the functional differentiation of the medial temporal lobes. *Hippocampus, 20*, 1291–1314.

Moscovitch, M., Nadel, L., Winocur, G., Gilboa, A., & Rosenbaum, R. (2006). The cognitive neuroscience of remote episodic, semantic and spatial memory. *Current Opinion in Neurobiology, 16*, 179–190.

Moscovitch, M., Rosenbaum, R., Gilboa, A., Addis, D., Westmacott, R., Grady, C., et al. (2005). Functional neuroanatomy of remote episodic, semantic and spatial memory: A unified account based on multiple trace theory. *Journal of Anatomy, 207*, 35–66.

Moscovitch, M., & Winocur, G. (2002). The frontal cortex and working with memory. In D. Stuss & R. Knight (Eds.), *The frontal lobes* (pp. 188–209). Oxford, England: Oxford University Press.

O'Connor, M., Butters, N., Miliotis, P., Eslinger, P., & Cermak, L. (1992). The dissociation of anterograde and retrograde amnesia in a patient with herpes encephalitis. *Journal of Clinical and Experimental Neuropsychology, 14*(2), 159–178.

O'Keefe, J., & Nadel, L. (1978). *The hippocampus as a cognitive map*. Oxford, England: Oxford University Press.

Pitel, A., Beaunieux, H., Witkowski, T., Vabret, F., de la Sayette, V., Viader, F., et al. (2008). Episodic and working memory deficits in alcoholic Korsakoff patients: The continuity theory revisited. *Alcoholism: Clinical and Experimental Research, 32*(7), 1229–1241.

Poreh, A., Winocur, G., Moscovitch, M., Backon, M., Goshen, E., Ram, Z., et al. (2006). Anterograde and retrograde amnesia in a person with bilateral fornix lesions following removal of a colloid cyst. *Neuropsychologia, 44*, 2241–2248.

Race, E., & Verfaellie, M. (2012). Remote memory function and dysfunction in Korsakoff's syndrome. *Neuropsychology Review, 22*, 105–116.

Ranganath, C. (2010). A unified framework for the functional organization of the medial temporal lobes and the phenomenology of episodic memory. *Hippocampus, 20*, 1263–1290.

Rudge, P., & Warrington, E. (1991). Selective impairment of memory and visual perception in splenial tumors. *Brain, 114*, 349–360.

Rugg, M., & Vilberg, K. (2013). Brain networks underlying episodic memory retrieval. *Current Opinion in Neurobiology, 23*, 255–260.

Rugg, M., & Wilding, E. (2000). Retrieval processing and episodic memory. *Trends in Cognitive Science, 4*, 108–115.

Rugg, M., & Yonelinas, A. (2003). Human recognition memory: A cognitive neuroscience perspective. *Trends in Cognitive Sciences, 7*, 313–319.

Schmahmann, J. (2003). Vascular syndromes of the thalamus. *Stroke, 34*, 2264–2278.

Scoville, W., & Milner, B. (1957). Loss of recent memory after bilateral hippocampal lesions. *Journal of Neurology, Neurosurgery, and Psychiatry, 20*, 11–21.

Shah, A., Jhawar, S., & Goel, A. (2012). Analysis of the anatomy of the Papez circuit and adjoining limbic system by fiber dissection techniques. *Journal of Clinical Neuroscience, 19*, 289–298.

Shallice, T. (2002). Fractionation of the supervisory system. *Principles of frontal lobe function*, 261–277.

Shimamura, A. (2002). Relation between binding theory and the role of consolidation in memory retrieval. In L. R. Squire & D. L. Schacter (Eds.), *Neuropsychology of memory* (3rd ed., pp. 61–72). New York, NY: Guilford.

Shimamura, A., & Squire, L. (1987). A neuropsychological study of fact memory and source amnesia. *Journal of Experimental Psychology—Learning Memory and Cognition, 13*(3), 464–473.

Squire, L. (1987). *Memory and brain*. New York, NY: Oxford University Press.

Squire, L., & Bayley, P. (2007). The neuroscience of remote memory. *Current Opinion in Neurobiology, 17*(2), 185–196.

Squire, L., & Kandel, E. (2009). *Memory from mind to molecules* (2nd ed.). Grand Junction, CO: Roberts.

Squire, L., & Zola-Morgan, S. (1991). The medial temporal lobe memory system. *Science, 253*, 1380–1386.

Szabo, K., Förster, A., Jäger, T., Kern, R., Griebe, M., Hennerici, M., et al. (2009). Hippocampal lesion patterns in acute posterior cerebral artery stroke: Clinical and MRI findings. *Stroke, 40*, 2042–2045.

Takahashi, N., Kawamura, M., Shiota, J., Kasahata, N., & Hirayama, K. (1997). Pure topographic disorientation due to right retrosplenial lesion. *Neurology, 49,* 464–469.

Teyler, T., & DiScenna, P. (1986). The hippocampal memory indexing theory. *Behavioral Neuroscience, 100,* 147–154.

Teyler, T., & Rudy, J. (2007). The hippocampal indexing theory and episodic memory: Updating the index. *Hippocampus, 17,* 1158–1169.

Tulving, E. (1972). Episodic and semantic memory. In E. Tulving & W. Donaldson (Eds.), *Organization of memory* (pp. 381–403). New York, NY: Academic Press.

Tulving, E. (1983). *Elements of episodic memory.* Oxford, England: Clarendon.

Valenstein, E., Bowers, D., Verfaellie, M., Heilman, K., Day, A., & Watson, R. (1987). Retrosplenial amnesia. *Brain, 110,* 1631–1646.

Van der Werf, Y., Scheltens, P., Lindeboom, J., Witter, M., Uylings, H., & Jolles, J. (2003). Deficits of memory, executive functioning and attention following infarction in the thalamus: A study of 22 cases with localized lesions. *Neuropsychologia, 41,* 1330–1344.

Vann, S., Tsivilis, D., Denby, C., Quamme, J., Yonelinas, A., Aggleton, J., et al. (2009). Impaired recollection but spared familiarity in patients with extended hippocampal system damage revealed by 3 convergent methods. *Proceedings of the National Academy of Sciences of the USA, 106,* 5443–5447.

Vargha-Khadem, F., Gadian, D., Watkins, K., Connelly, A., Van Paesschen, W., & Mishkin, M. (1997). Differential effects of early hippocampal pathology on episodic and semantic memory. *Science, 277,* 376–380.

Victor, M., Adams, R., & Collins, G. (1989). *The Wernicke–Korsakoff syndrome and related neurological disorders of alcoholism and malnutrition.* Philadelphia, PA: Davis.

Von Cramon, D., & Schuri, U. (1992). The septo-hippocampal pathways and their relevance to human-memory—A case-report. *Cortex, 28,* 411–422.

Wais, P., Wixted, J., Hopkins, R., & Squire, L. (2006). The hippocampus supports both the recollection and the familiarity components of recognition memory. *Neuron, 49,* 459–466.

Weintraub, S., Wicklund, A., & Salmon, D. (2012). The neuropsychological profile of Alzheimer disease. *Cold Spring Harbor Perspectives in Medicine, 2*(4), a006171.

Wixted, J. (2007). Dual-process theory and signal-detection theory of recognition memory. *Psychological Review, 114,* 152–176.

Wixted, J., & Mickes, L. (2010). A continuous dual-process model of remember/know judgments. *Psychological Review, 117,* 1025–1054.

Wixted, J., & Squire, L. (2004). Recall and recognition are equally impaired in patients with selective hippocampal damage. *Cognitive Affective & Behavior Neuroscience, 4*(1), 58–66.

Yonelinas, A. (1994). Receiver-operating characteristics in recognition memory: Evidence for a dual-process model. *Journal of Experimental Psychology—Learning Memory and Cognition, 20,* 1341–1354.

Yonelinas, A. (2002). The nature of recollection and familiarity: A review of 30 years of research. *Journal of Memory and Language, 46,* 441–517.

Yonelinas, A., Otten, L., Shaw, K., & Rugg, M. (2005). Separating the brain regions involved in recollection and familiarity in recognition memory. *Journal of Neuroscience, 25,* 3002–3008.

Zola-Morgan, S., & Squire, L. (1993). Neuroanatomy of memory. *Annual Review of Neuroscience, 16,* 547–63.

7

Higher-Order Visual Processing

The term "disorders of higher-order visual processing" generates confusion as to what represents a "higher-order" function. This is distinguished in two ways for the purposes of this text, both functionally and anatomically. *Higher-order visual processing* is defined as visual processing that is beyond the circuitry from the eye to the primary visual cortices and also more complex than simple visual perception processing performed cortically in the primary visual cortices.

One of the first higher-order visual components to be addressed after visual perception is visual object processing and recognition, which is also dependent on visual object memory. The visual memory storage system has been the subject of extensive study in terms of both the cognitive and the anatomic organization of visual object memory. It has been possible to study this system in a different manner than the language system because the visual object memory system can be investigated in multiple animal species in addition to humans, most notably nonhuman primates. Mishkin and colleagues (1983) have shown through lesion studies of nonhuman primates that there are bilateral "strips" extending from the primary visual cortex inferiorly and then anteriorly along the base of the brain from the occipital to the inferior temporal lobes that encode for visual object memory (Mishkin et al., 1983; Ungerleider & Mishkin, 1982) (Figure 7.1). These bilateral pathways then extend superiorly to the posterior aspect of the Sylvian fissure in nonhuman primates. This is possible in nonhuman primates because they do not have to encode for language in the brain, which is occupying these regions in humans. Also, nonhuman primate brains dedicate extensive regions to visual processing because it is their primary sensory system engaged in functions necessary for survival (defense against large predators, finding food, etc.) In humans, the two visual strips encompassing the "what" system remain inferior on the base of the temporal lobes and do not extend superiorly from the base of the temporal lobe nor do they extend as far forward anteriorly. These limitations in the size of the region are deemed to be due to the language system occupying large portions of the temporal lobes.

Considerable attention has also been paid to possible subdivisions—both cognitively and anatomically—within the visual "what" object memory system. Whereas some researchers have suggested that there are regions selective to particular categories of knowledge, such as houses and places (Spiridon & Kanwisher, 2002), others have proposed that *object memory* is encoded as distributed representations of parts of the objects throughout both the right and left sides of the "what" system (Haxby et al., 2001). Disruptions of the "what" system has led to further insights into some aspects of its cognitive–anatomic organization, which are detailed in this chapter with the disorders associated with impaired recognition of objects presented visually—termed *visual agnosia*.

VISUAL AGNOSIA

Apperceptive Visual Agnosia

Visual agnosia was first described by Lissauer (1890) and Freud (1891) as a disorder of visual recognition, which could not be attributed to a pure peripheral visual deficit (see Video 7). The hallmark feature of the agnosias is a failure of item/object recognition. Agnosias can occur in any sensory modality, where an item cannot be recognized if presented to an individual in that modality. These patients can recognize the item if presented in another modality; for example, visual agnosics cannot recognize an item when it is presented to them visually but can recognize it tactilely if placed in their hand. To designate that an individual has an agnosia, he or she must be intact in terms of the peripheral nervous system for the modality proposed to be involved with the agnosia (e.g., in tactile agnosia, no loss of peripheral

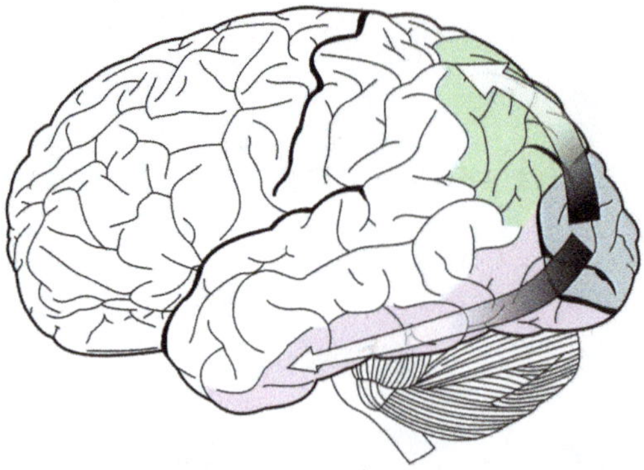

FIGURE 7.1: Schematic of the "what" system in nonhuman primates. Without a language system, the visual object recognition "what" system (purple region) extends more anteriorly into the inferior temporal lobe (Mishkin et al., 1983). This visual object memory system extends ventrally from the primary and secondary association visual cortices (blue) forward to the inferior temporal region. (The "where" system, shown in green, extends dorsally from the visual cortices into the parietal lobes.)

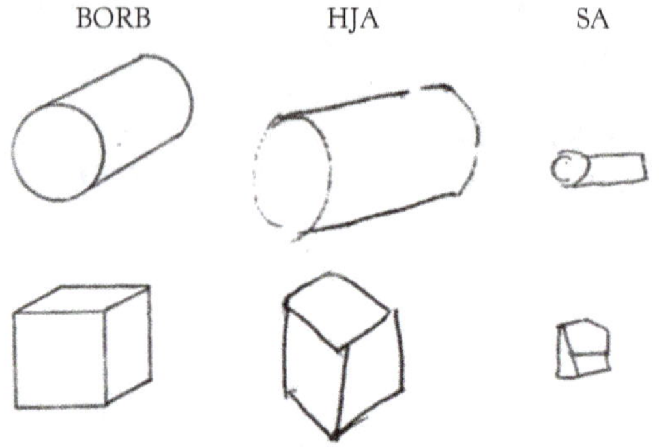

FIGURE 7.2: Copying of objects from the BORB battery, with the original to be copied under the heading BORB; the copy from patient HJA, who has integrative visual agnosia; and the copy from patient SA, who has visual form agnosia.

Source: Riddoch et al. (2008).

sensation; in auditory agnosia, no loss of hearing acuity). Lissauer first described two major types of visual agnosia—apperceptive agnosia, which was described as a disorder in higher-order visual perceptual processing impeding recognition, and associative agnosia, which is a deficit in accessing stored memories of visual concepts or a disruption of the concepts themselves.

Apperceptive agnosias have been further divided (Riddoch et al., 2008) into *form* and *integrative* apperceptive agnosia. Although object recognition is impaired in both types of these apperceptive agnosias, form agnosia is distinguished as being defined as an inability to recognize familiar items; in addition, the subject cannot perform shape matching or even trace the contours of items (e.g., patient SA in Figure 7.2) (Benson & Greenberg, 1969; Riddoch et al., 2008).

On further examination, individuals with form apperceptive agnosia have intact primary peripheral (eye up to primary visual cortex) visual function but an inability to recognize objects presented to them visually. Also, they are unable to recognize or match simple stimuli (e.g., showing subjects two pictures of stimuli and asking them if the stimuli are identical in each picture), including simple geometric shapes. They are also unable to copy or trace visually presented stimuli. Notably, these patients demonstrate poor performance on discriminating overlapping shapes (e.g., see Figure 7.3), with an inability to identify the outlines of various items (Benson & Greenberg, 1969; Riddoch et al., 2008). These patients have intact semantic knowledge of the items and can describe the items and their features if asked verbally to describe items from memory. Taking these abilities and deficits into account, it has been proposed that the cognitive unit that appears to be disrupted, resulting in this dysfunction, is the ability to shift between focusing on local features and focusing on global features of an item.

Integrative apperceptive agnosia is defined as an inability to integrate local parts with more

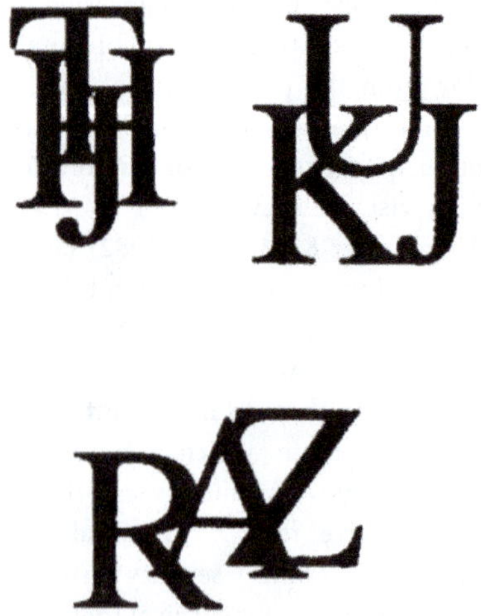

FIGURE 7.3: Overlapping letters test. Subjects are required to identify the three letters in each overlapping triad of letters.

holistic properties of an object. Patients demonstrate poor part–whole integration (when looking at an item, they cannot easily put the parts together to make a whole item), have difficulty decomposing scenes in terms of telling objects from the background (referred to as dissecting figure–ground relationships), and cannot group parts of objects correctly. This is proposed to be secondary to an inability to integrate perceptual information into a coherent whole item or loss of stored perceptual knowledge as related to integrated, whole items.

On testing, these patients still have difficulty matching objects to a sample target if the matching is strongly dependent on the perceptual information of the objects to match. Impaired performance on this test distinguishes the integrative agnosics (impaired on test for perceptually based matches) from individuals with associative visual agnosias. In copying figures, those with integrative agnosia are only mildly impaired; they have the general shape and size outlines intact but details incorrect, which differs from form agnosics, who are inaccurate in details and general outline of an item (see Figure 7.2, form agnosic SA). Thus, disruption of the cognitive unit of integrating complex perceptual information is the hallmark feature of integrative agnosics.

Anatomic Correlates of the Apperceptive Agnosias

Patients with apperceptive agnosias, in general, were thought to have associated lesions in the bilateral dorsal occipital–parietal (OP) regions (Riddoch & Humphreys, 1987). Using the divisions of form and integrative agnosia as subtypes of apperceptive agnosia, form agnosia has been previously found to be associated with lesions involving bilateral frontal and right PO lesions including the underlying white matter (Charnallet et al., 1996), patient DF with a lesion of the lateral occipital cortex plus posterior parietal involvement (Milner et al., 1991), and a patient with bilateral occipital plus right parietal lobe involvement (Vecera & Behrmann, 1997). This has led to the proposition that bilateral dorsal PO damage is important to developing form agnosia (Figure 7.4) (Riddoch et al., 2008). However, there are so few cases and notable anatomic exceptions that more evidence is required for this localization to be considered consistent (Riddoch et al., 2008). In addition, many of the cases of form agnosia resulted from carbon monoxide poisoning, which

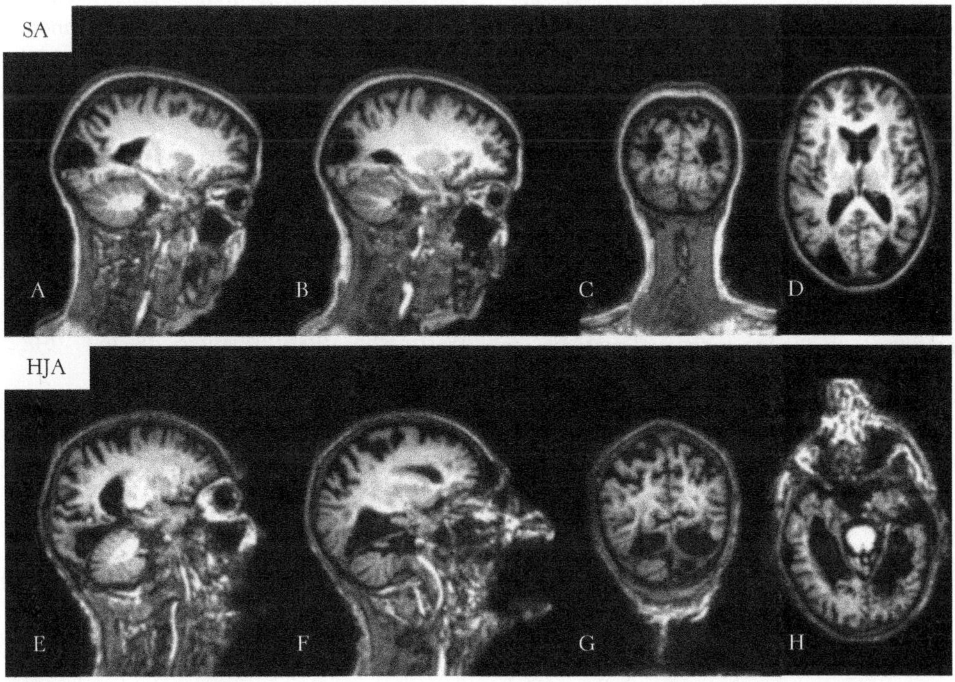

FIGURE 7.4: Lesions in patient SA, who has form agnosia, and patient HJA, who has integrative visual agnosia.

Source: Riddoch et al. (2008).

can manifest with neuronal death in regions that are not always detected by structural imaging methods.

Integrative agnosia, on the other hand, is associated with bilateral lesions of the lateral temporo-occipital region at the most posterior extent, sparing Brodmann area 17, medial extrastriate regions, and the parietal lobes (Figure 7.4) (James et al., 2003; Riddoch et al., 2008). However, the anatomic correlations initially were inconsistent in that there were additional regions disrupted in these patients, rendering this localization unreliable.

In addition to the lack of a clear anatomic localization for the apperceptive agnosias, the localization of one of the more finer-grained visual cognitive units underlying apperceptive agnosias is also not consistently localizable. The dorsal OP region has been linked to local/global perceptual processing and where these local parts are located in space (e.g., the "where" system). Although there has been disruption to this cognitive unit with lesions in the dorsal OP area, there have also been cases of impaired local feature processing in global figures after inferior medial occipital lesions (Fink et al., 1999).

Associative Visual Agnosia

An inability to connect the mental representation of a visually acquired item with its associated semantic knowledge (including name, use, description, etc.) is referred to as *associative visual agnosia*. Patients still do not recognize, nor can they name, visually presented items as a result of the loss of object meaning from the disconnection of visual processing areas from regions encoding semantic object meaning (Riddoch & Humphreys, 2003). Associative visual agnosia is distinguished from apperceptive agnosias in that patients with the apperceptive form have an inability to produce a complete percept of the item presented to them, due to a lack of feature integration, even though individual features can be identified. Associative agnosics can recognize the integrated whole of the item presented because they can copy or draw it. While being able to determine that the item presented to them is a "whole," single item, they still do not recognize what it is. Associative agnosics can draw a copy, not necessarily a "whole object" version, but will copy it in a piecewise, slow manner, typically drawing each "part" or "piece" of the figure separately. Thus, the copied object looks like pieces put together without a sense of the "whole" object, which can easily be detected from a normal subject's copying.

On examination, these patients cannot describe or mimic functions of items. When asked to say what the item is, their typical response is, "I don't know what it is." Individuals can access intact semantic knowledge (e.g., semantic knowledge stored in other modalities, such as sound, gesture, and lexical semantics) when the objects are presented through an unaffected modality (e.g., touch and sound). These patients again have intact primary peripheral visual functions as well as intact language functions.

This lack of information exchange between visual processing and visual semantic knowledge can potentially occur from two types of cognitive impairment: (1) inability to access stored representations of objects and (2) disruption of the stored representations of the objects (Barton, 2011; Ramon & Rossion, 2010). One proposed method to distinguish these two subtypes of associative visual agnosia is that those with impaired access have intact visual imagery when asked to visualize internally an object from a verbal cue, whereas those with impaired representations have disrupted imagery.

The lesions associated with associative visual agnosia have commonly been bilateral lesions of the inferior temporo-occipital junction and subjacent white matter (De Renzi, 2000; McCarthy & Warrington, 1986) (Figures 7.5 and 7.6). It is

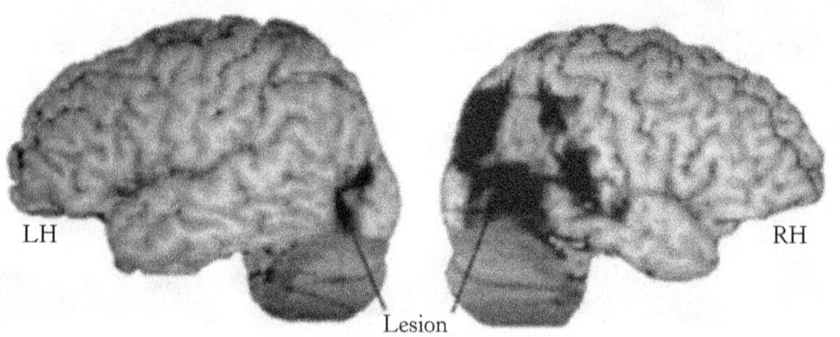

FIGURE 7.5: Sagittal view of both the right hemisphere (RH) and the left hemisphere (LH) in a patient with associative visual agnosia demonstrating bilateral lesions involving the inferior temporo-occipital regions.

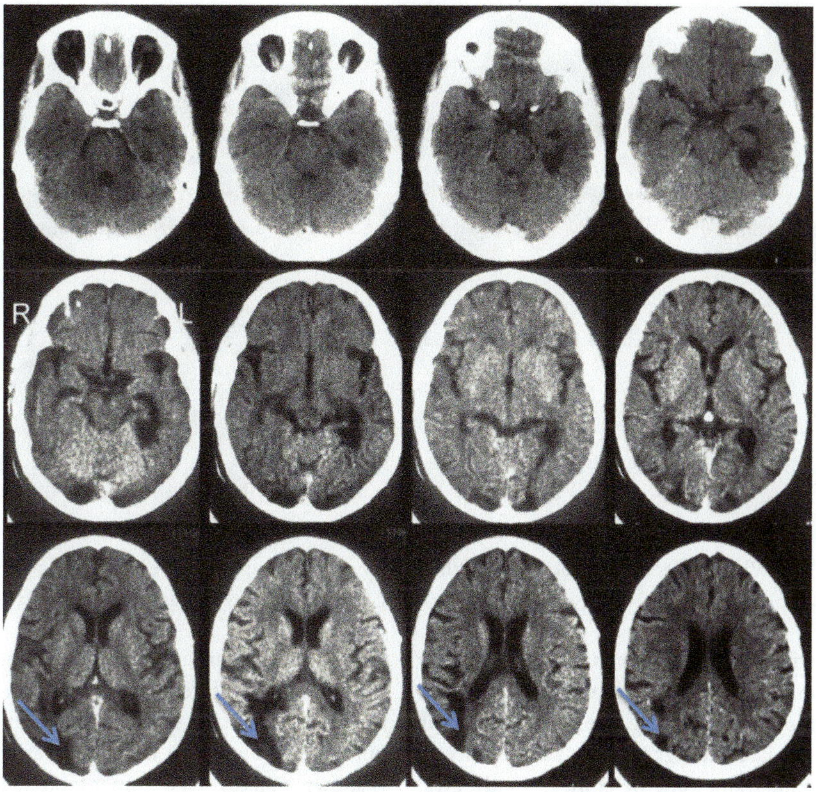

FIGURE 7.6: Axial images of a patient with associative visual agnosia resulting from a lesion in the right inferior temporo-occipital region. (Radiological convention on the scans, where the right side of the image is the left side of the brain.) Blue arrows designate the lesioned area.

important to note, however, that one can have associative visual agnosia with unilateral damage to the left or right temporo-occipital region (Farah, 1994). White matter disconnections between visual and temporal semantic regions (e.g., lesions affecting the inferior longitudinal fasciculus) that occur bilaterally can also result in visual associative agnosia (Damasio et al., 2000) (Figure 7.7).

These deficits have been incorporated in a model of visual object recognition by Marr (1980). The proposed cognitive stages begin with peripheral visual processing starting from the retina and ending in primary visual cortex. Initial higher-order visual perception then proceeds to extracting an initial visual representation. This occurs by extracting features and shapes from the visual peripheral input. Then, these features are integrated into a visual representation of a whole object. In Marr's model, a proposed internal 2½-dimensional representation is first formed, which is referred to as a viewer-centered representation, meaning that this first integrated object representation is just for the object in the perspective of the viewer. Next, a three-dimensional object-centered object representation is generated that is independent of the view in which the object is seen when encountered on presentation from the experimenter to the patient. This fully integrated internal visual representation of the object can then access semantic object knowledge. The apperceptive agnosias appear to have difficulty in the cognitive stages prior to generating an integrated representation. Impaired visual semantic representations or access to these representations are the characteristic deficit types in associative agnosia. The specificity of the cognitive unit and a consistent lesion location to the bilateral inferior temporo-occipital junction led to this one cognitive–anatomic unit (CAU) associated with associative agnosia. Due to the lack of specification of apperceptive agnosia subtypes to specific cognitive operations and the lack of an adequate number of patients with a consistent deficit, the identification of CAUs, if present, in the visual perceptual processing domain is a continually evolving area of investigation. With this in mind, several

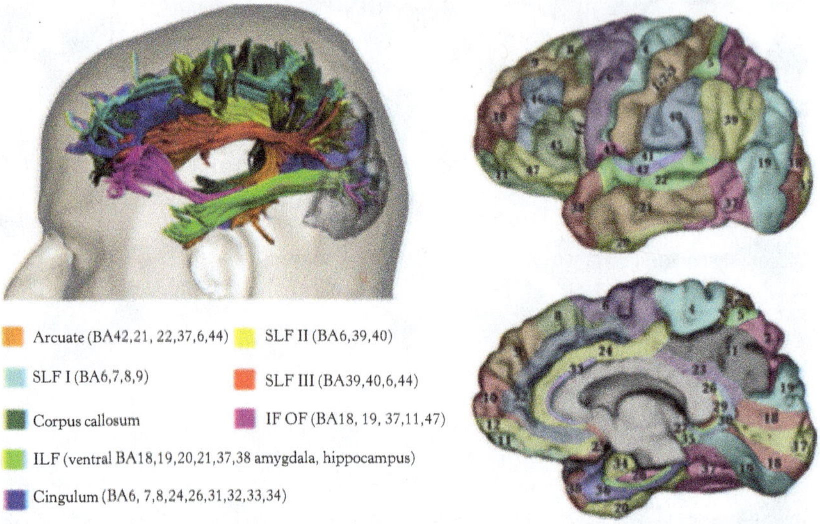

FIGURE 7.7: White matter tracts associated with the visual system. Disruption of the inferior longitudinal fasciculus (light green tract) can disconnect visual areas from semantic regions resulting in visual associative agnosia.

of the following sections (e.g., those on simultanagnosia, achromatopsia, and prosopagnosia) describe more circumscribed cognitive operations and their anatomic correlates in higher-order visual processing within the framework of clinical syndromes. Throughout this chapter, the basic organization of cognitive and behavioral functions is delineated using the approach outlined via normal functioning, disease states, and/or both. In this chapter, the optimal mapping of CAUs (see Table 7.1 for CAUs) proceeds best from this point forward with insights gained from the disease states.

SIMULTANAGNOSIA

Simultanagnosia refers to difficulty in detecting or perceiving multiple items in a scene, even though perception of each of the single items is preserved. These subjects can best see one item at a time. The more items that are present in one's visual field, the more confusing it is for these patients to pick out a single object. In a typical scenario, a patient is shown a picture of a dinner table with plates and bowls of food (a bowl of corn, a plate with turkey on it, a bowl with mashed potatoes, and a bowl of peas). The patient will report only seeing in front of them a bowl of corn. The patient can be told that there are multiple items on the table and will still only report seeing the bowl of corn. The amount of time given to the patient makes no difference in his or her performance; the patient will still report seeing only the bowl of corn. If all the items, including the bowl of corn, are removed except for the plate of turkey, the patient will then report correctly that he or she sees a plate of turkey. Typically, a reduction in the number

TABLE 7.1: HIGHER-ORDER VISUAL PROCESSING SUMMARY

Brain Region	Function
Bilateral inferior temporo-occipital junction (rarely unilateral)	Visual semantic representations or access to these representations → associative visual agnosia
Bilateral posterior superior parietal lobes	Ability to shift attention to multiple items → simultanagnosia (dorsal subtype)
Either right or left fusiform face area in the lingual/fusiform gyri *and* right occipital face area (region in the lingual and fusiform gyri)	Face recognition → prosopagnosia
Middle third of the lingual gyrus	Color perception → achromatopsia
Right inferior parietal lobule (and superior longitudinal fasciculus)	Neglect

of items in front of the patient leads to improving performance. These patients have normal vision and full visual fields, so this is not a result of a peripheral visual problem.

This cognitive dysfunction has been explained with several plausible accounts. One is that the subjects are impaired at shifting visual attention (Pavese et al., 2002) or in the allocation of attention. An alternative account is that there is a failure to bind information of where an object is ("where" system) with what an object's identity is ("what" system) (Coslett & Lie, 2008a). Based on these two differing descriptions of the dysfunction associated with simultanagnosia, there have been two proposed subtypes of simultanagnosia—a dorsal and ventral subtype. Dorsal simultanagnosia patients have as their major dysfunction restricted attention to one object when multiple objects are present in view or an inability to shift attention to other objects (perseveration of attention). This attentional focus is so narrow that patients can only "see" parts of objects to the point of not being able to correctly identify a whole object. Ventral simultanagnosia patients can see and recognize whole objects and do not misidentify them, but they can only see one object at a time.

Regarding anatomic correlates, one voxel-based lesion–symptom mapping (VBLSM) study of simultanagnosia (subtypes were not specified) lesion analysis of five patients suggested that the key damage involved the medial occipitoparietal junction, cuneus, and inferior intraparietal sulcus (Riddoch et al., 2010). Lesion overlap and VBLSM measures were then conducted with seven patients with simultagnosia (again subtypes were not specified and likely including some of the five subjects noted previously) and indicated that bilateral parieto-occipital white matter disconnections are needed to result in the symptoms of simultanagnosia. White matter tractography revealed that the pathway damage was to bilateral pathways within the visuospatial attention network, including the superior longitudinal fasciculus, the inferior fronto-occipital fasciculus, and the inferior longitudinal fasciculus. The authors concluded that damage to the parieto-occipital regions together with bilateral white matter disconnections were the lesions that contributed to poor visual processing of multiple objects of simultanagnosia (Chechlacz et al., 2012).

It was clear from these studies that determining anatomic correlates for simultanagnosia would require analyses of the cognitive subtypes (dorsal and ventral), even if few cases were available for

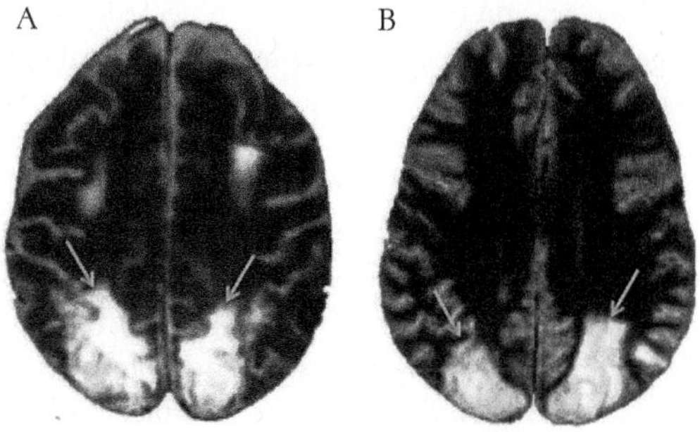

FIGURE 7.8: Lesion sites associated with simultanagnosia. Bilateral superior parietal lesions (blue arrows) in two MRI axial cuts.

Source: http://www.cell.com.

study. When accounting for the two types of simultanagnosia, dorsal simultanagnosia is associated with bilateral superior parietal–occipital lesions (Figure 7.8) (Coslett & Lie, 2008b; Jackson et al., 2006; Kase et al., 1977; Rizzo & Hurtig, 1987). The etiologies of these types of lesions are strokes typically "watershed" infarctions. In these types of strokes, there is a decrease in blood pressure so that the farthest branches of brain arteries start to receive decreased flow. In brain regions that receive their blood supply from the far ends of two arteries, these regions become infarcted if the blood flow is reduced for an extended period of time (e.g., during a myocardial infarction). These are referred to as watershed infarctions. When these occur at the junction of branches of the posterior cerebral and middle cerebral arteries that supply the superior parietal lobes, bilateral infarctions can occur in these regions and result in isolated dorsal simultanagnosia. Watershed infarcts have also been associated with visual associative agnosia from bilateral temporo-occipital infarcts resulting from watersheds at posterior cerebral and middle cerebral arteries that feed inferior temporo-occipital regions.

Ventral simultanagnosia was attributable to the bilateral posterior inferior parietal lesions involving the angular gyrus. Other lesions associated with ventral simultanagnosia have been reported in the left posterior temporal or temporo-occipital cortex (Kinsbourne & Warrington, 1963), bilateral fusiform, right calcarine sulcus, V4, and lingual gyrus (Leek et al., 2012). Due to this inconsistent localization, it has not been possible to make a consistent cognitive anatomic association with ventral simultanagnosia. This is similar to other non-disease-based investigations showing that binding location information with object identity is in general associated with the inferior parietal cortex, but no consistent locations within this region have been identified with this cognitive function.

OPTIC ATAXIA

Optic ataxia is characterized by the key symptom of misreaching for visual targets, without the co-occurrence of weakness, incoordination, or clumsiness. Patients can describe the object in front of them that they are to pick up, but they are unable to grasp it while reaching for it. Paradoxically, they can correctly reach for the object if (1) their eyes are closed after first visualizing where the object is located or (2) they have their eyes closed and reach for the object by its sound. This is best explained by dysfunction in the cognitive operation that maps retinal coordinates from where an object is seen into spatial coordinates that can be used by the motor system (Buxbaum & Coslett, 1998).

The anatomic correlate for optic ataxia has typically been extensive bilateral posterior parietal lobe lesions. The localization of this operation has not become any finer due to the limited number of cases identified. It often forms part of Balint's syndrome, along with the symptoms of simultagnosia and paralysis of gaze. As more cases of optic ataxia or Balint's syndrome are identified, this localization may become more clearly consistent.

PROSOPAGNOSIA

Prosopagnosia is an inability to recognize familiar faces, despite intact intellectual and cognitive functioning and intact visual acuity. These patients typically try to compensate by identifying individuals through other mechanisms. For example, prosopagnosics will compensate for this face recognition problem by identifying individuals by their gait, the smell of the perfume they wear, the smell of the soap or shampoo they use, and, most commonly, by recognizing their voice when they speak. These types of compensatory mechanisms are necessary because in severe cases, prosopagnosic patients may not be able to recognize their spouse or immediate family members by their faces alone. Prosopagnosics can identify the parts of the face (mouth, eyes, nose, etc.) so that the notion of what constitutes a "face concept" is not disrupted. Many cases of prosopagnosia are accompanied by an inability to recognize objects (visual object agnosia) so that its development in isolation is not common.

Interestingly, prosopagnosics patients can show intact "implicit" recognition of faces, as demonstrated by studies in which these patients have preservation of the galvanic skin response to familiar faces that they report not being able to recognize. By implicit recognition of faces, it is meant that while consciously the patient does not recognize the face, there is still evidence—such as pulse, heart rate, blood pressure, pupillary response, or sweat on the skin as measured by the galvanic skin response—that at least at some unconscious level, the individual shows physiological signs from his or her autonomic nervous system that he or she recognizes the face. This finding in prosopagnosics has been used to suggest that the disruption in prosopagnosia is not an impairment of internal representation of known faces but, in fact, an inability to purposefully access these intact representations.

The lesions resulting in prosopagnosia are located in bilateral inferomesial visual association cortices (lingual and fusiform gyri) and subjacent white matter—territories that are similar to that occupied by lesions causing visual object agnosia (Rapcsak et al., 2003). (The lesions resulting in visual object agnosia are typically more extensive than those in prosopagnosia.) Rarely, isolated right mesial occipito-temporal lobe lesions (Figure 7.9) can produce permanent prosopagnosia (Nachson, 1995). The fact that prosopagnosia has never been reported following unilateral left hemisphere lingual and fusiform gyri lesions suggested initially that right ventromedial occipito-temporal damage is both necessary and sufficient to produce prosopagnosia.

Subsequent studies have revealed a region, the right occipital face area (OFA), whose integrity is believed to be essential for normal face perception. This was proposed because in some cases of prosopagnosia, the right OFA (located in the lateral occipital cortex) was the only area that was critical or required to be involved in a lesions to produce prosopagnosia (Busigny et al., 2010; Rossion, Schiltz, & Crommelinck, 2003).

By reviewing jointly the lesion and functional neuroimaging findings, it has been proposed that both the fusiform face area (FFA) in the lingual/fusiform gyri (right or left) and the OFA in the right hemisphere are required to be intact for normal face recognition to be accomplished (Rossion, Schiltz, & Crommelinck, 2003) (for anatomical localizations, see Figure 7.10). Lesion evidence has now shown that acquired prosopagnosia can result

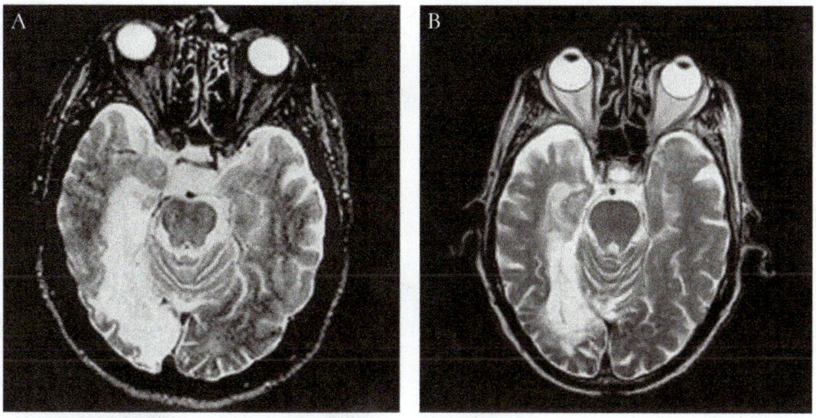

FIGURE 7.9: Lesions associated with prosopagnosia involving the right ventromedial occipito-temporal region.
Source: Rapcsak et al. (2003).

from damage principally to the right fusiform in the region of FFA (Barton et al., 2002) or to the right OFA and left fusiform gyrus (Atkinson & Adolphs, 2011; Ramon & Rossion, 2010). This has led to an overall localization of lesions of either the right or the left FFA in the lingual/fusiform gyri and right OFA (region in the lingual and fusiform gyri) as being necessary to develop prosopagnosia. Disruption of this FFA–OFA network can also result in prosopagnosia with disruption of the white matter regions connecting these areas (Fox et al., 2008). The cases of prosopagnosia from lesions in any of these regions usually follow embolic infarction of the posterior cerebral artery distribution or butterfly gliomas crossing the splenium of the corpus callosum.

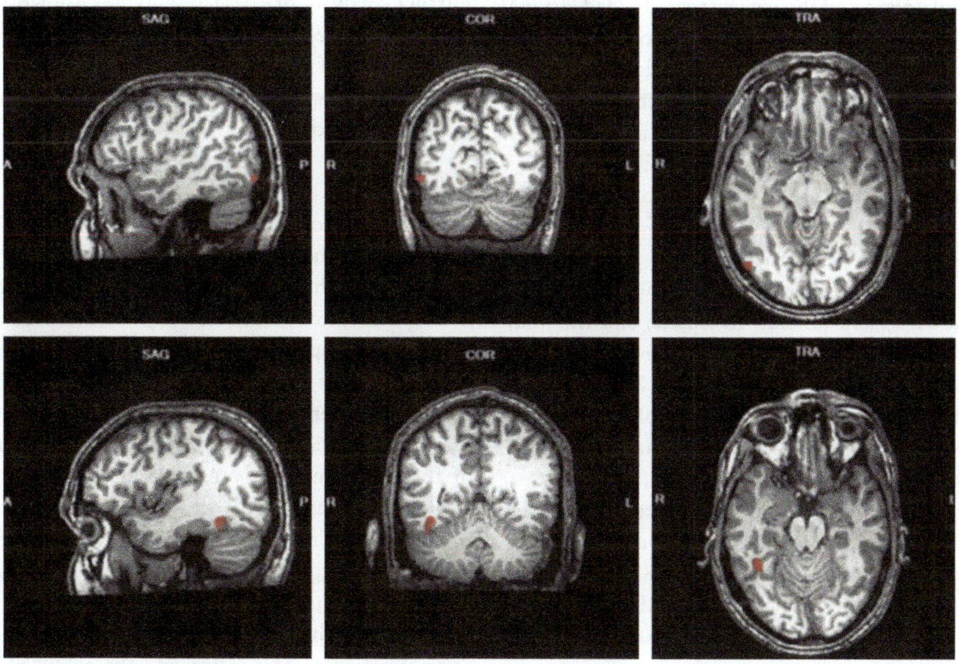

FIGURE 7.10: Key regions to face processing designated by red voxels. Top row designates occipital face area, and second row shows fusiform face area.
Source: Fox et al. (2008).

ACHROMATOPSIA

Cerebral achromatopsia is an isolated disorder of color perception, without other visual deficits (visual acuity, brightness, etc.) (Cowey & Heywood, 1997). When tested, many achromatopsics cannot name colors and, most important, cannot sort colors when tested for color hue perception with the Farnsworth–Munsell 100 color hue test. Achromatopsics are differentiated from color agnosics in that achromatopsics can tell an examiner the correct color that an object is supposed to be if asked verbally. In contrast, color agnosics perform normally on perceptual tests but have impaired knowledge of colors and in knowing the colors that items are supposed to be (e.g., that ketchup is red) (Barton, 2010). Patients with achromatopsia report that everything in their affected fields appears as shades of gray (similar to a black-and-white television). They have impaired color discrimination when viewing objects so that patients may pick up the wrong objects if they are similarly shaped and color is used to discriminate them from other objects.

Patients can have hemiachromatopsia, in which there is only disrupted color perception in either the right or the left visual field of view, with right-sided lesions (discussed later) resulting in left-sided achromatopsia and the reverse for left-sided lesions. Many subjects compensate if they have hemiachromatopsia by directing their visual field of view to the one intact for color processing when important color-related decisions are required. The best way to assess these patients is to move a colored object (a pin with a red ball at the top) from one visual field to the other and ask the patients if there are any changes in the color of the object.

Lesion localizations associated with achromatopsia have been difficult to isolate, and this may well be due to the fact that detecting these types of deficits is uncommon because a lesion extending to this region would likely involve the striate cortex and lead to a visual field cut that would obviate achromatopsia (Barton, 2010). Irrespective, achromatopsia has been most consistently reported to occur with lesions of the fusiform gyrus, the lingual gyrus, or both (Meadows, 1974; Verrey, 1888). Bilateral lesions of the lingual and fusiform gyri have been shown to result in achromatopsia, and unilateral lesions cause hemiachromatopsia (loss of color in half of the visual field) (Barton, 2010) (Figure 7.11). A meta-analysis of 92 cases with some deficit in color discrimination confirmed this localization using a voxel-based lesion analysis approach (Figure 7.12) (Bouvier & Engel, 2006). Further analysis of these lesions has shown that there is a more focal region within this area, the middle third of the lingual gyrus or its underlying white matter, that when damaged in isolation results in impaired color processing.

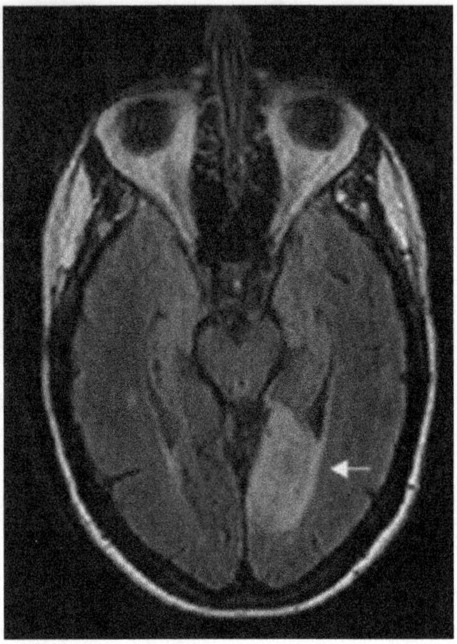

FIGURE 7.11: Lesion of left lingual gyrus resulting in hemiachromatopsia.

Source: Barton (2010).

NEGLECT

The syndrome of neglect refers to patients who are not aware of the space on the side opposite their brain lesion. These patients, typically with a right hemisphere stroke, will not pay attention to any objects in the space on the left side of the environment in front of them. They may even go so far as to deny the existence of that side of space in front of them. This denial and lack of attention to that side of the world remains present and adjusts/moves as they turn their heads or move throughout the world (Chatterjee & Coslett, 2010). It is important to note that neglect is different from a visual field cut. Patients with field cuts are blind and cannot see in the affected half of the space in front of them. In neglect patients, their vision and the extent of the visual field in front of them are normal; they just do not attend to the things that exist in the affected side of the space in front of them.

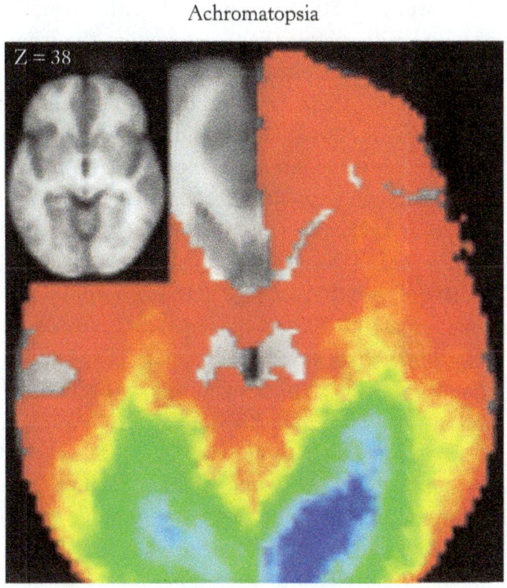

FIGURE 7.12: Lesion overlap for cases of achromatopsia. The intensity of blue is the highest region of overlap, and the intensity of red is the lowest region of overlap.

Source: Bouvier and Engel (2006).

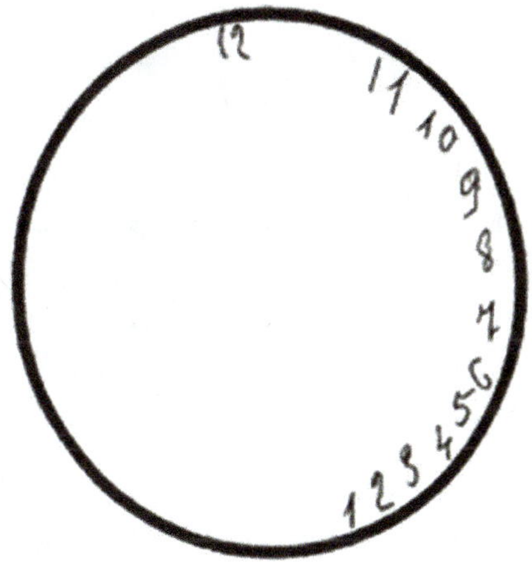

FIGURE 7.13: Example of clock face drawn by a neglect patient.

Neglect is typically tested for with several tasks, including the line bisection task, drawing to command, and the cancellation task. The line bisection task consists of giving patients a line and asking them to place a mark in the middle of the line when placed in front of them. Normal individuals will place their mark typically in the middle of the line. Neglect patients—for example, the most typical type, left-sided neglect—will place their mark to the right side of the actual middle of the line. Typically, the mark will be at the one-fourth point of the length of the line, as if they were bisecting the half of the line that they can attend to. When asked to draw an object from memory or copy an object or a scene in front of them, neglect patients will leave out the left side of what they are supposed to draw (Figure 7.13). On the cancellation task, subjects are presented with a sheet of paper with multiple copies of several shapes scattered throughout the page. They are instructed to cross out all of one particular shape on the page. A neglect patient will cross out the shapes only on one side of the page and will not cross out the ones on the side that he or she neglects.

There are several accounts for neglect or actually several cognitive units or combination of units that when disrupted account for the neglect syndrome. One account is that a major impairment in neglect is one of impaired spatial attention. Heilman et al. (1979) suggested that right hemisphere lesions disrupt both arousal and spatial attention (functions that had been proposed to be right hemisphere dominant). The combined disruption of both of these functions leads to a shift in attentional bias to stimuli only in the right side of space in front of the patient. Another account of neglect is that it results from impaired spatial intention. Spatial intention refers to the processes needed to select locations in space for actions to be performed. Disruption of spatial intention processes after a right hemisphere lesion results in a patient being unable to start or continue movements into the left side of space in front of him or her. The third account is that there is a disruption in the patient's internal spatial representations. Disruptions of internal spatial representations caused by a lesion in the right hemisphere can impair a patient's ability to form a normal representation of the left side of the world in front of him or her.

Lesions to the right hemisphere have long been associated with left-field neglect, particularly to the inferior parietal lobule (angular and supramarginal gyri), premotor cortex in the frontal lobe, subcortical regions (thalamus and basal ganglia), and white matter tracts (Figure 7.14) (Vallar, 2001). In a series of 19 patients, 8 of 9 patients with neglect had right posterior parietal lobe (particularly supramarginal gyrus) damage, whereas 8 of 10 without neglect did not have lesion involvement of this region (Vallar & Perani, 1987). In a study of right hemisphere lesion patients (n = 51) tested with a cancellation task,

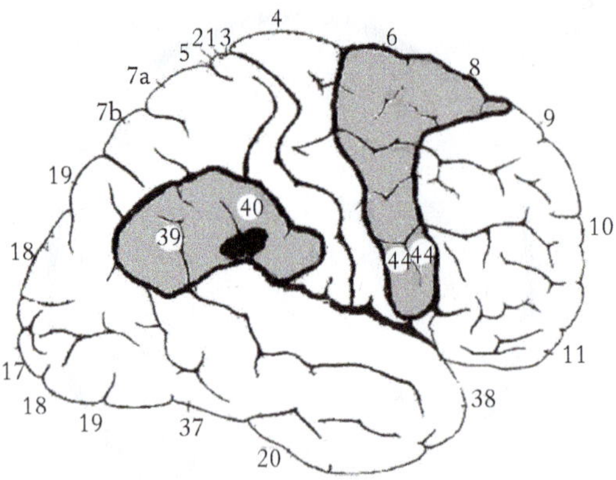

FIGURE 7.14: Cortical regions previously identified to be associated with neglect.

Source: Vallar (2001).

all cases of neglect had lesions including involvement of the thalamus, the basal ganglia, and the subcortical white matter, demonstrating the additional importance of these subcortical structures in neglect (Vallar & Perani, 1986).

A study of 80 stroke patients with disruption of long white matter tracts connecting the frontal and parietal lobe found a significant association of disruption of these tracts and neglect syndrome (Verdon et al., 2010). These findings were taken as support for the contention that a fronto-parietal disconnection may account for some forms of neglect and play a role in the severity of the disorder (Figure 7.15) (Doricchi et al., 2008). Further studies have shown that damage to the superior longitudinal fasciculus white matter tract and the network it supports in the right hemisphere is specifically associated with neglect syndromes (Bartolomeo, 2006; Chechlacz et al., 2012).

Given these anatomic correlates with neglect, the question can be posed whether further delineation of neglect into more fine-grained cognitive operations is possible and whether there are anatomic correlates to these operations. The best model that currently accounts for this approach involves the subsequent classification of spatial attention in neglect by some investigators in terms

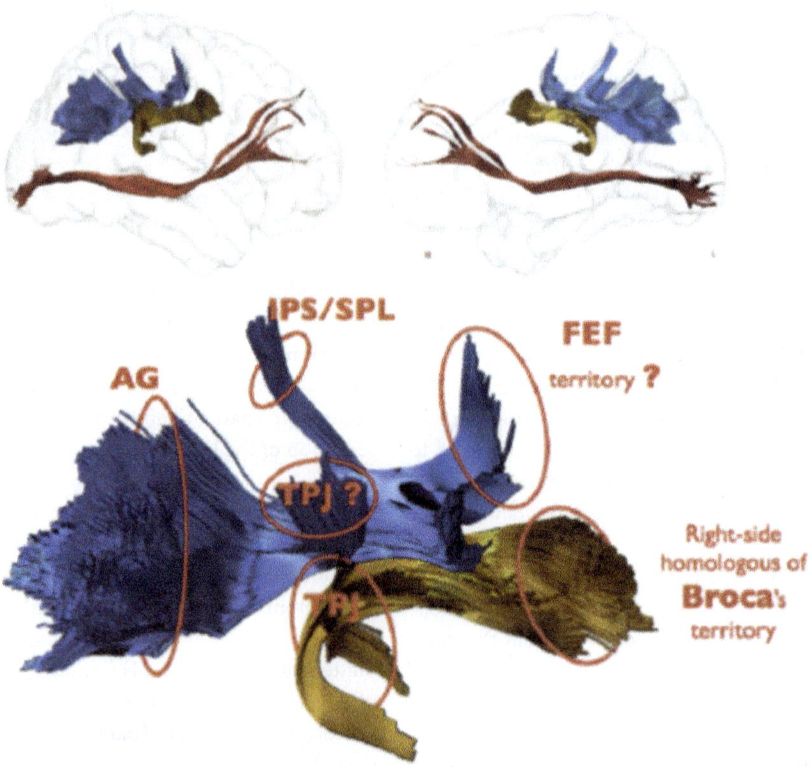

FIGURE 7.15: White matter pathway known as superior longitudinal fasciculus (SLF) with its branches. Damage to this frontoparietal connection (bottom figure) can result in neglect.

Source: Doricchi et al. (2008).

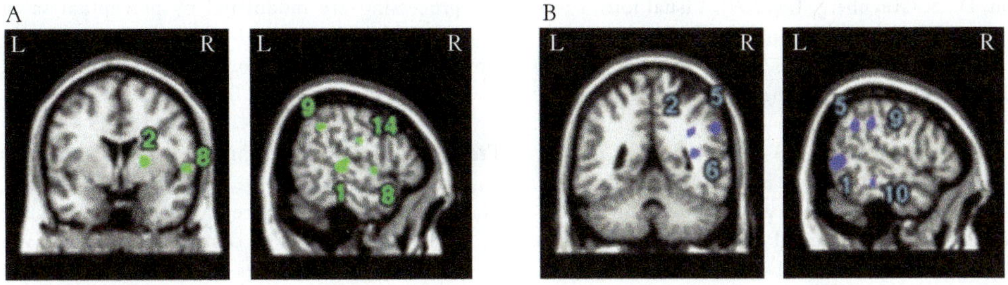

FIGURE 7.16: Concurrence of lesion sites with symptoms of allocentric neglect (blue) and egocentric neglect (green).
Source: Chechlacz et al. (2012).

of (1) interpreting errors from the perspective of the patient viewing the environment or (2) viewing the errors from the perspective of objects in space. In terms of interpreting errors from the perspective of the patient viewing the world, this is best assessed with tasks such as the line bisection task in which deficits can reflect problems in assessing where patients perceive the ends of the lines in relation to themselves (viewing things from the perspective of the patient is called an egocentric frame of reference). Taking the view of interpreting errors from the perspective of the object in space (referred to as the allocentric frame of reference) can be accounted for by looking at the line bisection task and assessing line bisection deficits as reflecting impaired perception of the line as a single, complete object.

Using this framework to interpret performance in spatial attention, it was proposed that egocentric symptoms are associated with damage within the perisylvian network (prefrontal, supramarginal, and superior temporal gyri) and subcortical structures; allocentric symptoms are associated with more posterior lesions, including the angular, middle temporal, and middle occipital gyri. These structures were further proposed to be highly linked by white matter tracts for exchanging information between the regions. When Chechlacz et al. (2012) applied this framework to a meta-analysis of neglect studies in the literature, "egocentric" neglect errors were associated with the right superior temporal gyrus, right insula, and subcortical structures including the right putamen and thalamus. "Allocentric" neglect errors were associated with lesions of the right angular gyrus, right temporo-parietal junction, right middle temporal gyrus, and the right superior longitudinal fasciculus (Figure 7.16).

Overall, lesions of the right inferior parietal lobule have appeared to continuously and consistently result in neglect syndromes in general, without further specification of finer delineated cognitive units associated with this location. The lesions in this region may also need to extend to a certain overall volume and/or involvement of the underlying white matter to lead to a clinically significant or long-lasting deficit. In addition, involvement of aspects of the white matter pathway—the right superior longitudinal fasciculus connecting the inferior parietal lobule to frontal lobe regions engaged in attentional processes—is emerging as another likely candidate for a consistent localization. As imaging and localization techniques develop, this region may become a consistent localization. A network-based model describing two attentional networks—dorsal and ventral—has been proposed, delineating the interaction of these networks and the cognitive operations that are associated with each (Corbetta & Shulman, 2002). Lesion models affecting these networks and the resultant neglect symptoms are being developed by Corbetta and colleagues as well as other investigators, and these show promise to eventually provide a functioning account for spatial attention cognitive units with fine-grained specification (see Chapter 13).

REFERENCES

Atkinson, A., & Adolphs, R. (2011). The neuropsychology of face perception: Beyond simple dissociations and functional selectivity. *Philosophical Transactions of the Royal Society of London Series B*, *366*, 1726–1738.

Bartolomeo P. (2006). A parietofrontal network for spatial awareness in the right hemisphere of the human brain. *Archives of Neurology*, *63*, 1238–1241.

Barton, J. (2010). Disorders of color and object recognition. *Continuum*, *16*(4), 111–127.

Barton, J. (2011). Disorder of higher visual function. *Current Opinion in Neurology*, *24*, 241–245.

Barton, J., Press, D., Keenan, J., & O'Connor M. (2002). Lesions of the fusiform face area impair perception of facial configuration in prosopagnosia. *Neurology*, *58*, 71–78.

Benson, D., & Greenberg, J. (1969). Visual form agnosia: A specific deficit in visual discrimination. *Archives of Neurology, 20*, 82–89.

Bouvier, S., & Engel, S. (2006). Behavioral deficits and cortical damage loci in cerebral achromatopsia. *Cerebral Cortex, 16*(2), 183–191.

Busigny, T., Graf, M., Mayer, E., & Rossion, B. (2010). Acquired prosopagnosia as a face-specific disorder: Ruling out the general visual similarity account. *Neuropsychologia, 48*, 2051–2067.

Buxbaum, L., & Coslett, H. (1998). Spatio-motor representations in reaching: Evidence for subtypes of optic ataxia. *Cognitive Neuropsychology, 15*(3), 279–412.

Charnallet, A., Rousset, S., Carbonnel, S., & Pellat, J. (1996). A case study of a strong perceptual deficit without agnosia: Evidence against sequential perception and memory? *Brain and Cognition, 32*, 115–117.

Chatterjee, A., & Coslett, H. B. (2010). Disorders of visuospatial processing. *Continuum, 16*, 99–110.

Chechlacz, M., Rotshtein, P., Hansen, P., Riddoch, J., Deb, S., Humphreys, G. (2012). The neural underpinnings of simultanagnosia: Disconnecting the visuospatial attention network. *Journal of Cognitive Neuroscience, 24*(3), 718–735.

Chechlacz, M., Rotshtein, P., & Humphreys, G. (2012). Neuroanatomical dissections of unilateral visual neglect symptoms: ALE meta-analysis of lesion–symptom mapping. *Frontiers in Human Neuroscience, 6*, article 230.

Corbetta, M., & Shulman, G. (2002). Control of goal-directed and stimulus-driven attention in the brain. *Nature Reviews Neuroscience, 3*, 201–215.

Coslett, H., & Lie, G. (2008a). Simultanagnosia: When a rose is not red. *Journal of Cognitive Neuroscience, 20*(1), 36–48.

Coslett, H., & Lie, G. (2008b). Simultanagnosia: Effects of semantic category and repetition blindness. *Neuropsychologia, 46*(7), 1853–1863.

Cowey, A., & Heywood, C. (1997). Cerebral achromatopsia: Colour blindness despite wavelength processing. *Trends in Cognitive Science, 1*(4), 133–139.

Damasio, A., Tranel, D., & Rizzo, M. (2000). Disorders of complex visual processing. In M. M. Mesulam (Ed.), *Principles of behavioral and cognitive neurology* (2nd ed., pp. 332–372). New York, NY: Oxford University Press.

De Renzi, E. (2000). Disorders of visual recognition. *Seminars in Neurology, 20*, 479–485.

Doricchi, F., Thiebaut de Schotten, M., Tomaiuolo, F., & Bartolomeo, P. (2008). White matter disconnections and gray matter dysfunctions in visual neglect: Gaining insights into the brain networks of spatial awareness. *Cortex, 44*, 983–995.

Farah, M. (1994). Perception and awareness after brain damage. *Current Opinion in Neurobiology, 4*, 252–255.

Fink, G., Marshall, J., Halligan, P., & Dolan, R. (1999). Hemispheric asymmetries in global/local processing are modulated by perceptual salience. *Neuropsychologia, 37*, 31–40.

Fox, C., Iaria, G., & Barton, J. (2008). Disconnection in prosopagnosia and face processing. *Cortex, 44*, 996–1009.

Freud, S. (1891). *Zur auffasung der aphasien*. Vienna, Austria: Franz Deuticke.

Haxby, J., Gobbini, M., Furey, M., Ishai, A., Schouten, J., & Pietrini, P. (2001). Distributed and overlapping representations of faces and objects in ventral temporal cortex. *Science, 293*(5539), 2425–2430.

Heilman, K., Watson, R. & Valenstein, E. (1979). Neglect and related disorders. In K. Heilman & E. Valenstein (Eds.), *Clinical neuropsychology* (pp. 268–307). New York, NY: Oxford University Press.

Jackson, G., Shepherd, T., Mueller, S., Husain, M., & Jackson, S. (2006). Dorsal simultanagnosia: An impairment of visual processing or visual awareness? *Cortex, 42*(5), 740–749.

James, T., Culham, J., Humphrey, G., Milner, A., & Goodale, M. (2003). Ventral occipital lesions impair object recognition but not object-directed grasping: An fMRI study. *Brain, 126*, 2463–2475.

Kase, C., Troncoso, J., Tapia, F., et al. (1977). Global spatial disorientation. *Journal of the Neurological Sciences, 34*, 267–278.

Kinsbourne, M., & Warrington, E. (1963). A study of visual perseveration. *Journal of Neurology, Neurosurgery, and Psychiatry, 26*, 468–475.

Leek, E., d'Avossa, G., Tainturier, M., Roberts, D., Yuen, S., Hu, M., et al. (2012). Impaired integration of object knowledge and visual input in a case of ventral simultanagnosia with bilateral damage to area V4. *Cognitive Neuropsychology, 29*(7/8), 569–583.

Lissauer, H. (1890). Ein fall von seelenblindheit nebst einem beitrage zur theorie derselben. *Archive fur Psychiatrie und Nervenkrankheiten, 21*, 222–270.

Marr, D. (1980). Visual information processing: The structure and creation of visual representations. *Philosophical Transactions of the Royal Society of London Series B, 290*(1038), 199–218.

McCarthy, R., & Warrington, E. (1986). Visual associative agnosia: A clinico-anatomical study of a single case. *Journal of Neurology, Neurosurgery, and Psychiatry, 49*, 1233–1240.

Meadows, J. (1974). Disturbed perceptron of colors associated with localized cerebral lesions. *Brain, 97*, 615–632.

Milner, A., Perrett, D., Johnston, R., Benson, P., Jordan, T., Heeley, D., et al. (1991). Perception and action in "visual form agnosia." *Brain, 114*, 405–428.

Mishkin, M., Ungerleider, L., & Macko, K. (1983). Object vision and spatial vision: Two cortical pathways. *Trends in Neuroscience, 6*, 414–417.

Nachson, I. (1995). On the modularity of face recognition: The riddle of domain specificity. *Journal of Clinical and Experimental Neuropsychology, 17*(2), 256–275.

Pavese, A., Coslett, H. B., Saffran, E. M., & Buxbaum, L. (2002). Limitations of attentional orienting: Effects of abrupt visual onsets and offsets on naming two objects in a patient with simultanagnosia. *Neuropsychologia, 40*(7), 1097–1103.

Ramon, M., & Rossion, B. (2010). Impaired processing of relative distances between features and of the eye region in acquired prosopagnosia—Two sides of the same holistic coin? *Cortex, 46*, 374–389.

Rapcsak, S. (2003). Face memory and its disorders. *Current Neurology and Neuroscience Reports, 3*(6), 494–501.

Riddoch, M., Chechlacz, M., Mevorach, C., et al. (2010). The neural mechanisms of visual selection: The view from neuropsychology. *Annals of the New York Academy of Sciences, 1191*, 156–181.

Riddoch, M., & Humphreys, G. (1987). A case of integrative agnosia. *Brain, 110*, 1431–1462.

Riddoch, M., & Humphreys, G. (2003). Visual agnosia. *Neurologic Clinics, 21*, 501–520.

Riddoch, M., Humphreys, G., Akhtar, N., Allen, H., Bracewell, R., & Schofield, A. (2008). A tale of two agnosias: Distinctions between form and integrative agnosia. *Cognitive Neuropsychology, 25*(1), 56–92.

Rizzo, M., & Hurtig, R. (1987). Looking but not seeing: Attention, perception, and eye movements in simultanagnosia. *Neurology, 37*, 1642–1648.

Rizzo, M., Smith, V., Pokorny, J., & Damasio, A. (1993). Color perception profiles in central achromatopsia. *Neurology, 43*(5), 995–1001.

Rossion, B., Schiltz, C., & Crommelinck, M. (2003). The functionally defined right occipital and fusiform "face areas" discriminate novel from visually familiar faces. *Neuroimage, 19*(3), 877–883.

Spiridon, M., & Kanwisher, N. (2002). How distributed is visual category information in human occipito-temporal cortex? An fMRI study. *Neuron, 35*(6), 1157–1165.

Ungerleider, L., & Mishkin, M. (1982). Two cortical visual systems. In D. J. Ingle, M. A. Goodale, & R. J. Mansfeld (Eds.), *Analysis of visual behavior* (pp. 549–586). Cambridge, MA: MIT Press.

Vallar, G. (2001). Extrapersonal visual unilateral spatial neglect and its neuroanatomy. *Neuroimage, 14*, S52–S58.

Vallar, G., & Perani, D. (1986). The anatomy of unilateral neglect after right hemisphere stroke lesions: A clinical CT scan correlation study in man. *Neuropsychologia, 24*, 609–622.

Vallar, G., & Perani, D. (1987). The anatomy of spatial neglect in humans. In M. Jeannerod (Ed.), *Neurophysiological and neuropsychological aspects of spatial neglect* (pp. 235–258). Amsterdam: North-Holland.

Vecera, S., & Behrmann, M. (1997). Spatial attention does not require preattentive grouping. *Neuropsychology, 11*, 30–43.

Verdon, V., Schwartz, S., Lovblad, K., Hauert, C., & Vuilleumier, P. (2010). Neuroanatomy of hemispatial neglect and its functional components: A study using voxel-based lesion–symptom mapping. *Brain, 133*, 880–894.

Verrey, L. (1888). Hémiachromatopsie droite absolue. Conservation partielle de la perception lumineuse et des formes. Ancien kyste hémorrhagique de la partie inférieure du lobe occipital gauche. *Archives d'Ophtalmologie, 8*, 289–300.

8

Higher-Order Sensory Processing

Higher-order sensory processing may be considered as much cognitive in nature as it may be considered in the perceptual domains. In fact, some consider that there is only an artificial or no separation between the perceptual and cognitive domains. Some investigators have suggested that the same neural regions function in both perception and cognition, suggesting that these may not represent clearly separable entities.

Conceptualization of cognitive operations that probe higher-order sensory processing such that both activation and lesion studies demonstrate a consistent anatomical correlate to a cognitive unit would allow for establishing cognitive–anatomic units (CAUs) that are definable and reproducible. Recognition of a familiar entity within a single cognitive domain has been investigated for similar units in multiple sensory domains to determine if common recognition units exist across domains. This delineation of cognitive recognition units can best be accomplished in conjunction with the investigation of recognition deficits, such as the sensory agnosias.

Sensory agnosias are disorders in which individuals are unable to recognize items presented to them in a specific modality (e.g., auditory, visual, and tactile) but are able to recognize them if presented in the other unaffected modalities. To diagnose an agnosia requires that the peripheral sensory system of the modality being studied be intact. Previously, lesions in the primary sensory cortices could not be involved for a diagnosis of agnosia to be made. However, recent functional neuroimaging studies have shown that perceptual cortices are engaged in higher-order processing other than imagery and are integral to information processing outside of simple perceptual encoding (Kamitani & Tong, 2005).

The most extensive studies of agnosias are the visual agnosias and their subtypes that were discussed in Chapter 7. This could be secondary to the occurrence of lesions that result in agnosias being more common in visual agnosia. This notion is supported by the fact that typically bilateral lesions are necessary to cause an agnosia, and the visual "what" system is located in areas where watershed infarctions, typically from cardiac events, occur. Nevertheless, the presence and localizations to the sensory agnosias are of importance to theories of brain organization. It appears that the initial processing for a sensory modality, after the cortex first receives input from the periphery (primary sensory cortex), includes more complex interpretation of the sensory perceptual signal. This occurs regularly across all modalities. Primary sensory cortices are typically organized functionally along the lines of the peripheral nervous system input. For example, the acoustic nerve delivers input in terms of frequencies, not the integrated sound we hear as presented in the environment. The primary auditory cortex also has what is referred to as a tonotopic organization structured anatomically along the lines of the frequency input it receives from the periphery. Following this initial perceptual input at the primary perceptual cortices, the secondary association cortices, for the most part, process the raw signal from primary cortices into more complex representations, which more closely resemble what was first experienced in the periphery. In general, likely secondary to the speed required to process information about the environment as expeditiously as possible for survival purposes, the cortices that perform this higher-order sensory processing—that is, converting peripheral sensory signals into meaningful internal brain representations—are typically located next to or within close proximity of the primary sensory cortex. With this general framework of perceptual–cognitive processing in mind, we next explore recognition of entities within the auditory domain.

AUDITORY AGNOSIAS AND COGNITIVE PROCESSING

There are four major different types of auditory agnosias: general auditory agnosia, pure word deafness, environmental sound agnosia, and amusia. The latter three are described in more detail in this chapter. In addition, the reader is referred to an excellent review of central auditory disorders, including agnosias, by Goll et al. (2010).

In the auditory domain, there are clear examples of lesions in the peri-primary auditory cortex region associated with auditory perceptual deficits. Twenty-one patients who had lesions in auditory cortical and subcortical structures (the auditory cortex, the auditory thalamus, or the acoustic radiation) were studied for central auditory processing deficits. Lesions of the auditory cortex led to a contralateral impairment in discrimination thresholds in the acoustic parameters of frequency, intensity, and tone duration. This represents a more perceptual deficit in sound (Biedermann et al., 2008). The following discussion details a higher-order auditory agnosia—pure word deafness.

Word Deafness (Auditory Word Agnosia)

Spoken words can be thought of as a highly characteristic and meaningful category of auditory objects. The selective auditory agnosia associated with the inability to recognize this specific subset of auditory stimuli—words—is called pure word deafness (PWD). This phenomenon is best explained as a deficit of auditory temporal resolution in the speech spectral range that underlies the impaired discrimination of speech sounds. Speech perception is thought to be processed in its early stages bilaterally in the brain. The left and right hemispheres can both perform speech perceptual processing, even in left hemisphere speech- and language-dominant individuals (Hickok & Poeppel, 2007).

PWD is characterized by an inability to comprehend individual spoken words. These individuals typically try to understand spoken language with the use of lip reading and contextual cues, but these are only compensatory aids. Repetition of words is markedly impaired. Discrimination of pairs of phonemes or syllables as to whether they are the same or different is impaired. Word pair discrimination and word comprehension are also notably impaired. In contrast, speech production and comprehension of written language are normal. In the purest form of the deficit, environmental sound and music perception, two other auditory subtypes of stimuli, are relatively intact.

Several plausible accounts have been posited for PWD. The lesions that typically have led to PWD have included those in the bilateral superior temporal lobes (Figure 8.1) (Turkeltaub & Coslett, 2010), left temporal lobe (Lichtheim, 1885; Saffran et al., 1976; Wang et al., 2000), and, rarely, right temporal lobe (Roberts et al., 1987). The proposal put forth to account for how these lesions affect cognition is that bilateral superior temporal lesions are required to impede auditory perceptual data from reaching regions where auditory word forms and meaning are processed.

Initial accounts of PWD from a disconnection approach emerged based on a proposed disconnection between auditory input and auditory "word forms" stored in Wernicke's area (Geschwind, 1965). Wernicke's area was assumed to not be involved in these lesions to allow for the storage of the auditory word forms themselves to be intact and for the preserved speech production noted in these patients.

Most of the cases of PWD in the literature that supported the disconnection model reported bilateral superior temporal gyrus lesions. A lesion in the left superior temporal region can be positioned to include cortical areas and underlying white matter such that the white matter disruption prevents transmission of auditory information from the right hemisphere to reach Wernicke's area. A lesion can be placed in other regions of the brain as long as it prevents auditory perceptual information from reaching Wernicke's area, which would result in the disconnection needed by that model. This is demonstrated by the case of a 55-year-old right-handed man who presented with a persistent PWD following a left thalamic hemorrhage. The lesion affected predominantly white matter of the temporal and parietal lobes, with Wernicke's area largely preserved. It was proposed that PWD exhibited by the patient was secondary to isolation of Wernicke's area from incoming auditory information, with the lesion affecting the association fibers from the right auditory area traveling across the corpus callosum and of the left auditory radiations (Takahashi et al., 1992). Slevc et al. (2011) reported on patient NL, who had PWD with a left-sided lesion involving the superior temporal gyrus, supramarginal gyrus, and angular gyrus (Figure 8.2). Diffusion tensor imaging suggested that NL's cross-callosal projections were relatively intact, implying that PWD can arise from a unilateral lesion even in the presence of intact cross-hemispheric connectivity.

An extension of the cognitive neuroscience approach to this syndrome is to further delineate cognitive units beyond "word recognition." There

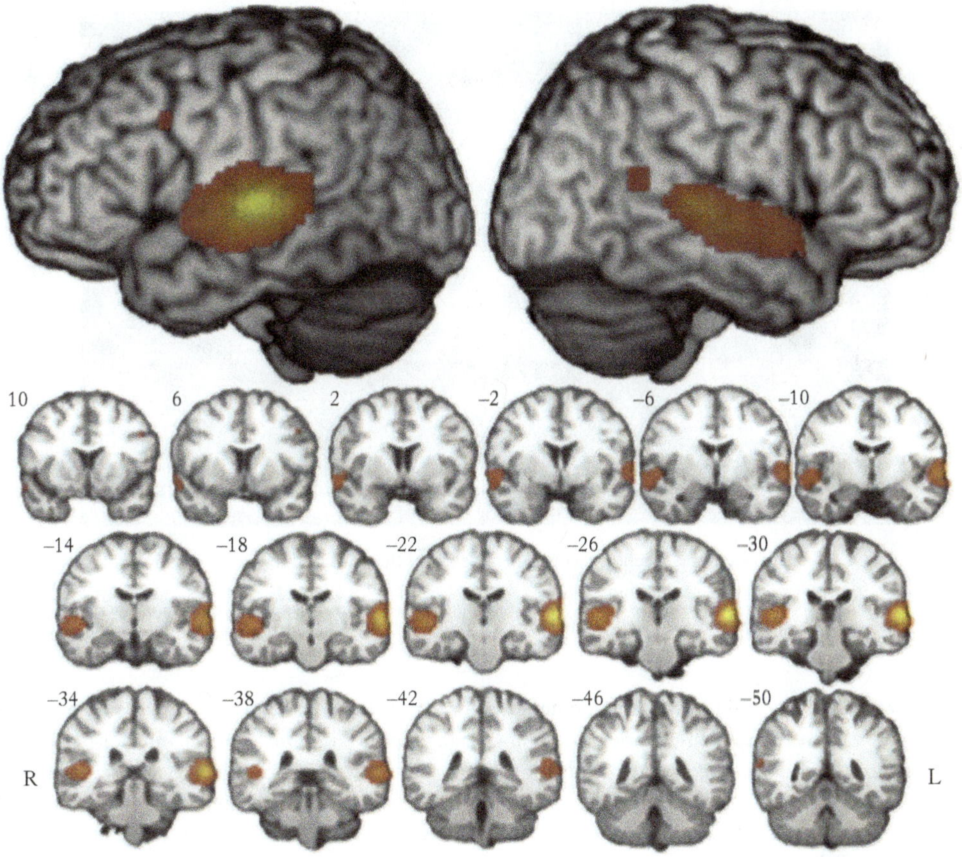

FIGURE 8.1: Bilateral regions where lesions are detected (yellow-orange color) in patients with pure word deafness. The lesions are centered on the superior temporal gyri in both hemispheres.

Source: Adapted from Turkeltaub and Coslett (2010).

are processes engaged in speech perception for lexical stimuli that are shorter than a complete word. A meta-analysis of 23 functional magnetic resonance imaging (MRI) experiments identified brain areas engaged in auditory speech perception of speech sounds that are smaller than whole, complete words (referred to as sublexical speech sounds). The speech sounds consist of vowels, consonants, or nonword syllables. Using a technique for evaluating whether there are common regions of activation across functional imaging studies (activation likelihood estimation), a speech processing network was identified. Bilateral superior temporal cortices perform acoustic analysis of speech and nonspeech auditory stimuli, the middle aspects of the left posterior superior temporal sulcus are engaged in phonetic and phonological analysis, and the left inferior parietal lobule is involved in detection of differences between different groups of phonemes (Turkeltaub & Coslett, 2010). (To clarify, phonetics is the study of the physical properties of speech sounds (acoustic properties and physiology of how to make the sounds with the oropharynx), whereas phonology is the abstract representation of sounds stored in the brain.) Re-evaluation of the early studies of PWD along with additional lesion studies will aid in establishing these regions as CAUs with this more fine-grained description of cognitive units and anatomic specificity provided. Given that PWD studies are rare and the findings from the studies reported thus far have been couched in terms of the disconnection model, the consistent finding at this point is that bilateral superior temporal gyrus lesions disrupt performance of the acoustic analysis of auditory speech stimuli resulting in the clinical syndrome of PWD.

Environmental Sound Agnosia

Nonverbal sound agnosia, also referred to as environmental sound agnosia, is a rare neuropsychological

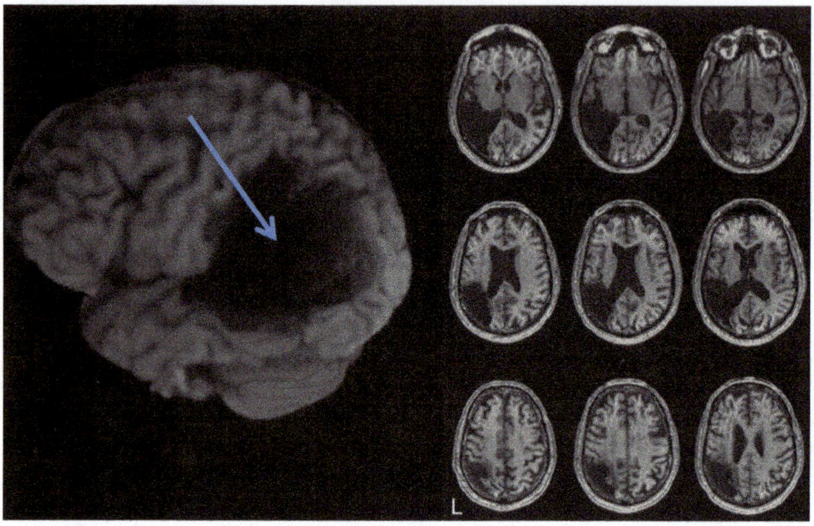

FIGURE 8.2: Left-sided lesion in a patient with pure word deafness that included the superior temporal, supramarginal, and angular gyri (blue arrow points to the lesion).
Source: Slevc et al. (2011).

disorder that is characterized by an isolated deficit in being unable to recognize environmental (nonspeech) sounds despite normal hearing. In addition, these patients have normal speech/word recognition and auditory comprehension.

It is unclear what the underlying physiological characteristics (sound perceptual characteristics) are that define this group of nonspeech sounds that can account for the agnosia. Environmental sounds can collectively span a broad range of spectrotemporal characteristics, and thus specific dysfunction in a region encoding for specific sound frequencies appears unlikely to account for the agnosia. Subsequent discovery of more specific nonverbal sound agnosias related to sounds of similar spectrotemporal features might occur and give rise to more selective deficits, but these have not yet been identified.

Although selective deficits of environmental sound perception (without involvement of other sound categories) are rare, they have been described in association with, in general, bilateral temporal or subcortical lesions; less frequently, unilateral lesions have also been reported. For example, environmental sound agnosia has been linked to a left hemisphere infarct to posterior middle and superior temporal gyri and inferior parietal lobe cortical regions (Saygin et al., 2003, 2010), bilateral putaminal hemorrhage involving the fibers from the medial geniculate body to the temporal lobes (Taniwaki et al., 2000), and right hemisphere damage (superior temporal gyrus, inferior parietal lobe, and the parietal operculum) (Schnider et al., 1994). These lesions have spanned the perisylvian regions bilaterally, particularly the superior temporal gyrus and inferior parietal lobule regions, without specific localization. This is noted in contrast to the PWD accounts that are typically localized to the superior temporal gyri. Thus, the number of cases is too scant and there is a lack of specificity to make a firm localization.

Amusia

Impaired discrimination of musical instrument sounds has been documented in patients with what is termed music agnosia or amusia. Music as a category of stimuli contains distinct aspects, including instrumental sounds, melodies, and written music. In terms of the sound aspects of music, there are characteristic spectrotemporal properties, and most amusias are perceptually based, arising from specific deficits in processing components of music (e.g., melody vs. rhythm; Omar et al., 2010; Vignolo, 2003).

Amusia had been associated in general with auditory cortex and/or frontal lobe damage; however, there is no clear evidence of hemispheric lateralization (Sarkamo et al., 2009). Apperceptive agnosia for music has been described following resection of a right temporoparietal tumor with the

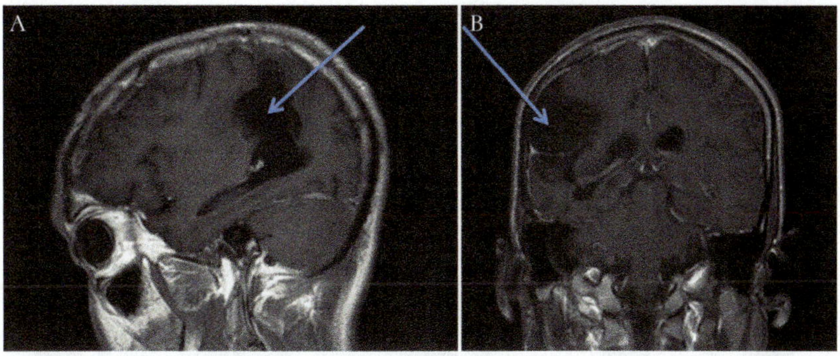

FIGURE 8.3: Post-resection T1 MRI brain image in the sagittal (A) and coronal (B) plane showing focal damage to the posterior third of the superior temporal gyrus. The inferior parietal lobule (supramarginal and angular gyri) was also involved (blue arrows point to lesions).

Source: Baird et al. (2014).

patient subsequently demonstrating an inability to discriminate musical scales and musical rhythm. The patient was intact for recognizing his favorite songs, famous titles of songs, the emotional connotations of songs, and temporal metric organization (Figure 8.3) (Baird et al., 2014). In one study, 20 patients with middle cerebral artery (MCA) aneurysms (right, left, and bilateral) and 20 controls were tested on music recognition measures. In the left MCA lesioned group, there were 2 patients with apperceptive musical agnosia with impairment on musical discrimination and perception tasks, with impaired long-term memory for music associated with lesions in the right superior temporal lobe and insula (Ayotte et al., 2000). A case report of another patient demonstrated intact performance on recognition of environmental sounds, pitch discrimination, rhythm discrimination, and meter discrimination. The patient was impaired on the discrimination and recognition of familiar songs. This pattern of performance was associated with bilateral infarction of the temporal poles (Figure 8.4) (Satoh et al., 2005).

Currently, there are no clear localizations for music knowledge or operations performed on musical knowledge. There is considerable variability not only in the anatomic correlates of amusias but also in the variability of the types of musical stimulus characteristics that contribute to this lack of localizations.

TACTILE OBJECT PROCESSING AND AGNOSIA

An item recognition disorder in the somatosensory system is termed tactile agnosia. The disorder is marked by an inability of an individual to identify objects when manipulated with his or her hands, while there are no defects in the perceptual sensory touch system (including light touch, pressure, temperature, and kinesthetic sensory detection). In addition, these patients can recognize the same objects when presented to them through other, unaffected modalities.

As in the case of visual agnosia, two subdivisions have been proposed for tactile agnosia: apperceptive and associative tactile agnosias. Apperceptive tactile agnosia is defined by the inability to discriminate the tactile features of objects (weight, roughness, etc.). Associative tactile agnosia represents an impairment in tactile object recognition with spared elementary tactile perceptual sensory and discrimination abilities.

The initial localizations were based on case studies such as a patient reported by Endo et al. (1992) who had tactile agnosia in only his right hand, secondary to a subcortical lesion in the left angular gyrus region. The contention was that the lesion resulted in a disconnection of somatosensory association parietal lobe cortices from semantic memory regions in the temporal lobe. This finding was extended by the case of a patient with bilateral tactile recognition deficits diagnosed as bilateral tactile agnosia with bilateral lesions in the subcortical regions of the angular gyrus (Figure 8.5) (Nakamura et al., 1998). Tomberg and Desmedt (1999) reported a case of tactile agnosia resulting from a lesion in the contralateral parietal cortex (left postcentral gyrus), a region that has been proposed to be where sensory input from the finger joints is represented. Reed and Caselli (1994) described a unilateral tactile agnosia patient with an associated

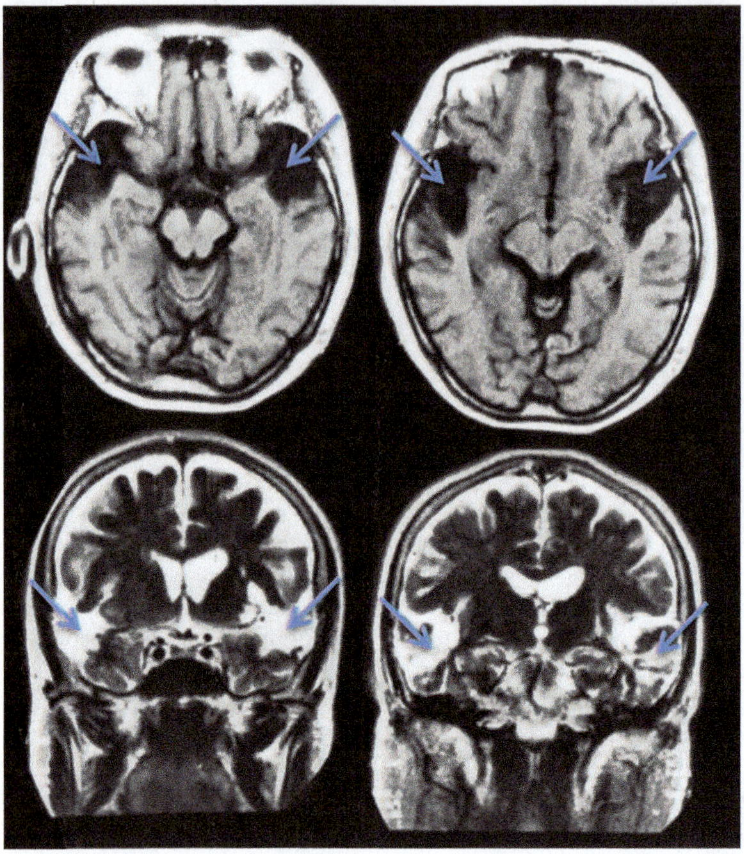

FIGURE 8.4: MRI of a patient acquired 17 years after the onset of amusia (blue arrows point to lesions). The top two images show T1 axial images, and the lower two are coronal T2 images (radiological convention). Lesions are located in the temporal poles bilaterally and include the bilateral superior and middle temporal gyri, with some minor involvement of the left insula.

Source: Satoh et al. (2005).

lesion in the left inferior parietal lobule, including Brodmann areas 39 and 40. A more in-depth assessment of this patient with unilateral tactile agnosia revealed that this deficit can occur with intact tactile spatial ability and manual shape exploration. That these domains are spared but the subject still cannot perform tactile object recognition suggests that this deficit could be the result of a specific loss of tactile representations of shape or tactile features of objects. This argues for the existence of a system specialized for tactile shape representations for tactile recognition (Reed et al., 1996).

Bohlhalter et al. (2002) studied two cases of unilateral apperceptive tactile agnosia. Both patients were impaired in detecting tactile characteristics (e.g., roughness) of objects, with one patient also impaired at perceiving gross tactile characteristics (e.g., length) of objects. These perceptual deficits were associated with lesions in the postcentral gyrus in both patients and in the secondary somatosensory area (SII) and the posterior parietal cortex in the more severely affected patient. These results demonstrated that the underlying failure in apperceptive tactile agnosia is mainly impaired perception of detailed tactile properties of objects due to a lesion of primary sensory cortex (Figures 8.6 and 8.7) and, in the patient with extension of the lesion into the posterior parietal cortex, there is also disruption in the cognitive process of encoding of gross tactile characteristics. These findings further refined the cognitive roles of the tactile/somatosensory recognition system into at least two cognitive units of tactile information processing.

Further analysis of these two subjects and one additional patient with apperceptive tactile agnosia of the right hand from a left parietal lesion was

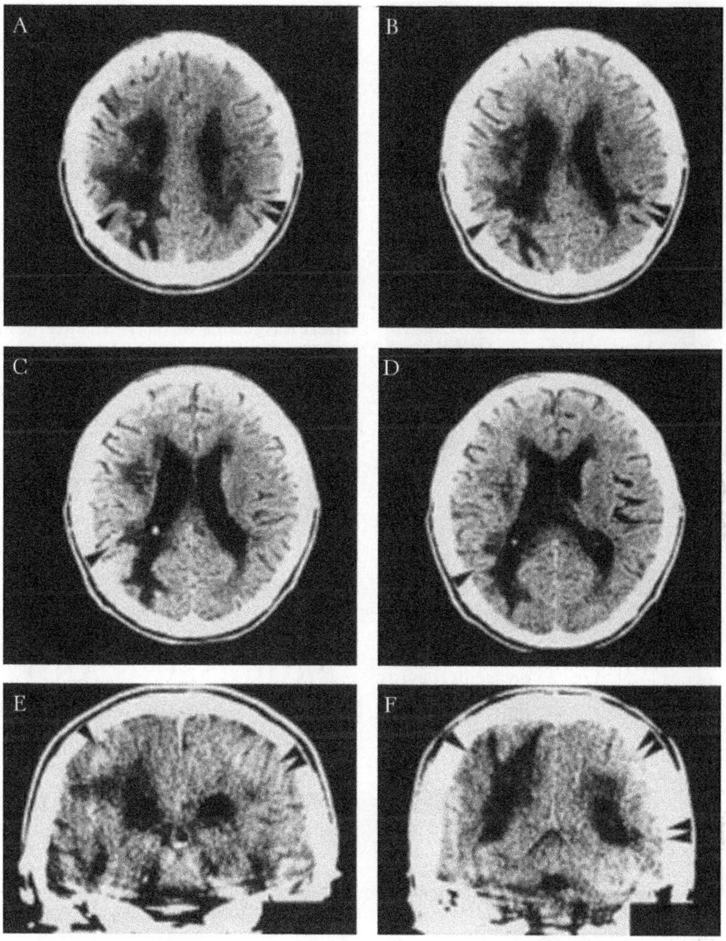

FIGURE 8.5: CT scan images of a patient with bilateral tactile agnosia demonstrating bilateral lesions in the subcortical regions of the angular gyri (black arrowheads point in direction of regions of involvement).

Source: Nakamura et al. (1998).

performed using probabilistic cytoarchitectonic mapping of three-dimensional MR images of the whole brain (Homke et al., 2009). The analysis suggested that (1) the postcentral gyrus performs elementary sensory information processing for texture recognition and (2) the posterior parietal regions process kinesthetic information for shape recognition. Thus, the involvement of Brodmann areas 4a, 4p, 3a, 3b, 1, 2 (postcentral gyrus regions) and areas IP1 and IP2 (posterior parietal regions) of the intraparietal sulcus can be delineated into the subfunctions of texture and shape recognition of the tactile system (Figure 8.8) (Homke et al., 2009).

Another account for the cognitive units underlying tactile recognition is also consistent with the clinical findings of apperceptive and associative tactile agnosia. Tactile object recognition consists of interpreting tactile information and associating that information with previously acquired tactile semantic knowledge to determine if the tactile information is consistent with that of an object representation (Endo et al., 1992; Platz, 1996). Platz suggested that semantic meaning representations needed for tactile object identification are present for each modality (Hart & Gordon, 1992). In this framework, apperceptive tactile agnosia would be the result of a selective disruption of interpreting tactile sensory information, and associative tactile agnosia occurs because of a disconnection between cortical regions processing tactile sensory information and a semantic memory store (Endo et al., 1992; Nakamura et al., 1998).

Anatomically, the lesions detected suggest that somatosensory association cortices of both parietal

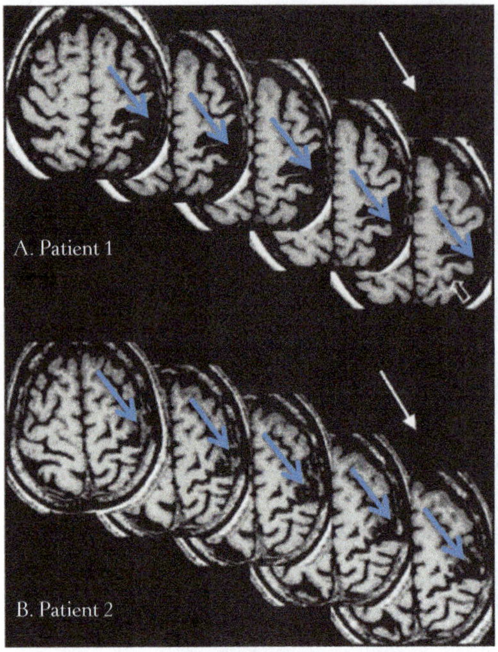

FIGURE 8.6: Lesions located in the postcentral gyrus (blue arrows) in two patients with tactile agnosia.

Source: Bohlhalter et al. (2002).

lobes is where tactile information is processed and that these need to be bilaterally disconnected from the inferior temporal areas of both hemispheres, where semantic memory stores have been proposed to be stored, to develop tactile agnosia (Ross, 2008). This would purportedly lead to an associative tactile agnosia. A left parietal lesion that disrupted the regions engaged in higher-order processing of tactile information would result in apperceptive tactile agnosia (Crutch et al., 2005). Furthermore, because there are cases of both unilateral and bilateral tactile agnosia, it was proposed that most subjects have bilateral representations of tactile information processing so that a lesion results in contralateral tactile agnosia. In the few cases in which it appears that the left hemisphere is specialized as the single store of tactile semantic knowledge for object recognition, lesions in the left parietal area can result in bilateral tactile agnosia.

TASTE/OLFACTORY PROCESSING AND AGNOSIA

Taste, olfaction, and trigeminal nerve stimulation determine flavor. Agnosia for the senses of taste and smell has been difficult to identify clearly with regard to whether deficits are the result of dysfunction of higher-order cognitive dysfunction as

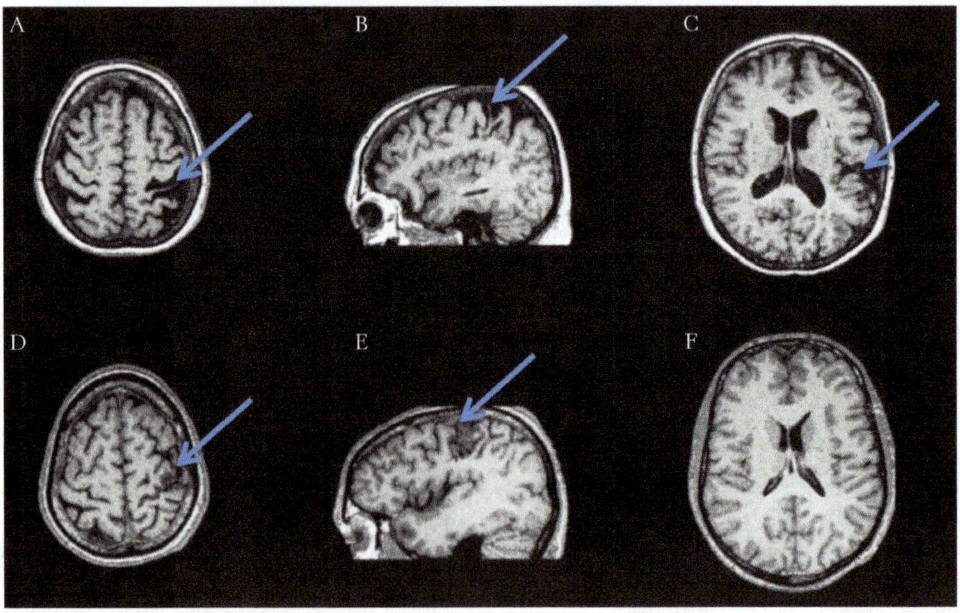

FIGURE 8.7: MRIs of the postcentral gyrus lesions in two individuals with tactile agnosia (one patient on each row, with the first column in axial view, the second column in sagittal view, and the third column in axial view at another plane) (blue arrows designate lesion).

Source: Bohlhalter et al. (2002).

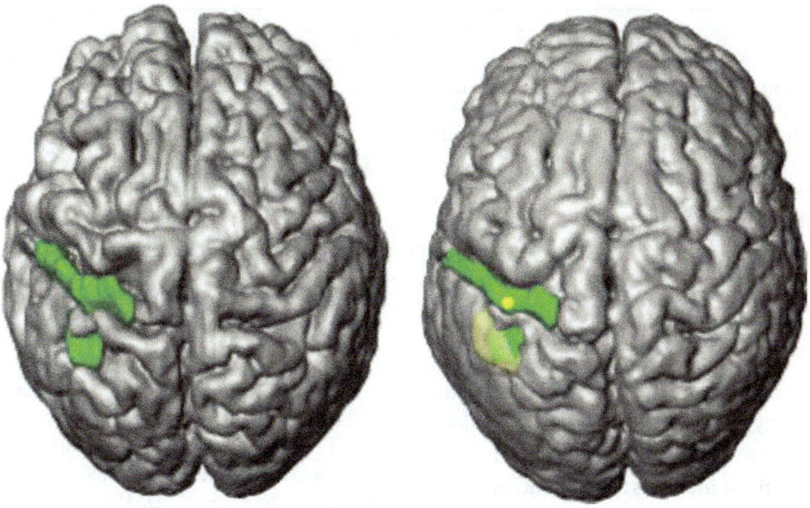

FIGURE 8.8: Two patients who have tactile agnosia with surface rendering of their lesions in the postcentral gyri on 3-D brain reconstructions. The more anterior green region is the postcentral gyrus, and the more posterior green and yellow region is the posterior parietal cortex, which is engaged in shape recognition.

Source: Homke et al. (2009).

opposed to a perceptual impairment. Taste receptors on the taste buds of the tongue consist of five major sense detections: sweet, sour, salty, bitter, and umami (detected through receptors for glutamate and commonly found in monosodium glutamate and in foods high in glutamate—seafood, cured meats, and aged cheeses). Where these five taste qualities are encoded in the neocortex as flavors and how they are organized are not well understood. Brain regions that have been implicated in organizing flavor knowledge include the anterior insula and pyriform cortex, the anterior temporal lobe, and the orbitofrontal cortex (Piwnica-Worms et al., 2010; Rolls, 2005; Savic, 2002; Small et al., 2001, 2004). The specific roles that these regions play in the representation and/or processing of taste and olfaction have not been clearly identified. Further investigations using functional imaging studies are indicated to delineate better representational and processing correlates for taste and smell and how these systems are segregated in the brain. Lesions in the areas that are proposed to be engaged in these senses are not commonly occurring, and thus functional studies will likely provide a much clearer map as to how functions in taste and smell are organized cortically.

CONCLUSIONS

Although cases of sensory agnosias are uncommon, the localizations associated with agnosias have important neurobiological significance. Previously described localizations have been centered on functions related to the lateralization and localization of speech mechanisms and memory functions whose localization is linked to an anatomically anchored, primitive brain structure—the Papez circuit. The sensory agnosias exhibit a unique pattern of localization in that (1) higher-order perceptual processing exists with CAUs in multiple domains; (2) anatomically they are located adjacent to or neighboring the primary sensory cortices; and (3) typically, disruption of the processing requires bilateral lesions due to the sensory cortices having bilateral primary sensory cortical representations. This unique set of conditions that is present across sensory modalities represents a set of neurobiological principles that underlie the CAUs (see Table 8.1 for CAUs) that are present across these modalities, typically for object recognition, following initial perceptual processing.

The configuration of the anatomic regions in the CAUs is related to the shape or conformation of the primary perceptual cortical region, the nature of the perceptual domain and its processing, and the other regions to which the perceptual domain preferentially connects. The visual system, for example, utilizes for higher processing relatively large, bilateral regions because there is extensive processing of all of the visual information that is required for processing a scene. These regions can be relatively far away

TABLE 8.1: SENSORY AGNOSIAS SUMMARY

Brain Region	Function
Bilateral superior temporal gyrus	Performance of the acoustic analysis of auditory speech stimuli → pure word deafness
Somatosensory association cortices in the parietal lobes (postcentral gyrus)	Elementary processing for texture recognition → apperceptive tactile agnosia
Posterior parietal regions	Processing kinesthetic information for shape recognition → apperceptive tactile agnosia

from the primary sensory cortices because visual the stimulus is typically not transient thus allowing time for analyses and it extends to the language system where it most interacts. On the other hand, the auditory higher-order processing system utilizes smaller regions directly surrounding the primary auditory cortices; the regions are neighboring both primary auditory cortices and the language system, which is its main system of interaction; and the regions are circumscribed and close to its targets because sound stimuli are transient. Because these form key neurobiological principles of brain localization, they are discussed further in Chapter 14.

REFERENCES

Ayotte, J., Peretz, I., Rousseau, I., Bard, C., & Bojanowski, M. (2000). Patterns of music agnosia associated with middle cerebral artery infarcts. *Brain, 123,* 1926–1938.

Baird, A., Walker, D., Biggs, V., & Robinson, G. (2014). Selective preservation of the beat in apperceptive music agnosia: A case study. *Cortex, 53,* 27–33.

Biedermann, F., Bungert, P., Doerrscheidt, G., von Cramon, Y., & Ruebsamen, R. (2008). Central auditory impairment in unilateral diencephalic and telencephalic lesions. *Audiology and Neurotology, 13,* 123–144.

Bohlhalter, S., Fretz, C., & Weder, B. (2002). Hierarchical versus parallel processing in tactile object recognition: A behavioural–neuroanatomical study of aperceptive tactile agnosia. *Brain, 125,* 2537–2548.

Crutch, S., Warren, D., Harding, L., & Warrington, E. (2005). Computation of tactile object properties requires the integrity of praxic skills. *Neuropsychologia, 43,* 1792–1800.

Endo, K., Miyasaka, M., Makishita, M., Yanagisawa, N., & Sugishita, M. (1992). Tactile agnosia and tactile aphasia: Symptomatological and anatomical differences. *Cortex, 28,* 445–469.

Geschwind, N. (1965). Disconnection syndromes in animals and man. *Brain, 88,* 237–294, 585–644.

Goll, J. C., Crutch, S. J., & Warren, J. D. (2010). Central auditory disorders: toward a neuropsychology of auditory objects. *Current opinion in neurology, 23*(6), 617.

Hart, J., & Gordon, B. (1992). Neural subsystems for object knowledge. *Nature, 359,* 60–64.

Hickok, G., & Poeppel, D. (2007). The cortical organization of speech processing. *Nature Reviews Neuroscience, 8*(5), 393–402.

Homke, L., Amunts, K., Bonig, L., Fretz, C., Binkofski, F., Zilles, K., et al. (2009). Analysis of lesions in patients with unilateral tactile agnosia using cytoarchitectonic probabilistic maps. *Human Brain Mapping, 30,* 1444–1456.

Kamitani, Y., & Tong, F. (2005). Decoding the visual and subjective contents of the human brain. *Nature Neuroscience, 8,* 679–685.

Lichtheim, L. (1885). On aphasia. *Brain, 7,* 433–484.

Nakamura, J., Endo, K., Sumida, T., & Hasegawa, T. (1998). Bilateral tactile agnosia: A case report. *Cortex, 34,* 375–388.

Omar, R., Hailstone, J., Warren, J., et al. (2010). The cognitive organization of music knowledge: A clinical analysis. *Brain, 133,* 1200–1213.

Piwnica-Worms, K., Omar, R., Hailstone, J., & Warren, J. (2010). Flavour processing in semantic dementia. *Cortex, 46*(6), 761–768.

Platz, T. (1996). Tactile agnosia: Casuistic evidence and theoretical remarks on modality-specific meaning representations and sensorimotor integration. *Brain, 119,* 1565–1574.

Reed, C., & Caselli, R. (1994). The nature of tactile agnosia: A case study. *Neuropsychologia, 32,* 527–539.

Reed, C., Caselli, R., & Farah, M. (1996). Tactile agnosia: Underlying impairment and implications for normal tactile object recognition. *Brain, 119,* 875–888.

Roberts, M., Sandercock, P., & Ghadiali, E. (1987). Pure word deafness and unilateral right temporo-parietal lesions: A case report. *Journal of Neurology, Neurosurgery, and Psychiatry, 50*(12), 1708–1709.

Rolls, E. (2005). Taste, olfactory and food texture processing in the brain, and the control of food intake. *Physiology and Behaviour, 85,* 45–56.

Ross, E. (2008). Sensory-specific amnesia and hypoemotionality in humans and monkeys: Gateway for developing a hodology of memory. *Cortex, 44,* 1010–1022.

Saffran, E., Marin, O., & Yeni-Komshian, G. (1976). An analysis of speech perception in word deafness. *Brain and Language, 3*(2), 209–228.

Sarkamo, T., Tervaniemi, M., Soinila, S., et al. (2009). Cognitive deficits associated with acquired amusia after stroke: A neuropsychological follow-up study. *Neuropsychologia, 47*, 2642–2651.

Satoh, M., Takeda, K., Murakami, Y., Onouchi, K., Inoue, K., & Kuzuhara, S. (2005). A case of amusia caused by the infarction of anterior portion of bilateral temporal lobes. *Cortex, 41*, 77–83.

Savic, I. (2002). Brain imaging studies of the functional organization of human olfaction. *Neuroscientist, 8*, 204–211.

Saygin, A., Dick, F., Wilson, S., et al. (2003). Neural resources for processing language and environmental sounds: Evidence from aphasia. *Brain, 126*, 928–945.

Saygin, A., Leech, R., & Dick, F. (2010). Nonverbal auditory agnosia with lesion to Wernicke's area. *Neuropsychologia, 48*, 107–113.

Schnider, A., Benson, D., Alexander, D., & Schnider-Klaus, A. (1994). Nonverbal environmental sound recognition after unilateral hemispheric stroke. *Brain, 117*, 281–287.

Slevc, L., Martin, R., Hamilton, A., & Joanisse, M. (2011). Speech perception, rapid temporal processing, and the left hemisphere: A case study of unilateral pure word deafness. *Neuropsychologia, 49*(2), 216–230.

Small, D., Voss, J., Mak, E., Simmons, K., Parrish, T., & Gitelman, D. (2004). Experience-dependent neural integration of taste and smell in the human brain. *Journal of Neurophysiology, 92*, 1892–1903.

Small, D., Zatorre, R., Dagher, A., Evans, A., & Jones-Gotman, M. (2001). Changes in brain activity related to eating chocolate: From pleasure to aversion. *Brain, 124*, 1720–1733.

Takahashi, N., Kawamura, M., Shinotou, H., Hirayama, K., Kaga, K., & Shindo, M. (1992). Pure word deafness due to left hemisphere damage. *Cortex, 28*(2), 295–303.

Taniwaki, T., Tagawa, K., Sato, F., & Iino, K. (2000). Auditory agnosia restricted to environmental sounds following cortical deafness and generalized auditory agnosia. *Clinical Neurology and Neurosurgery, 102*, 156–162.

Tomberg, C., & Desmedt, J. (1999). Failure to recognize objects by active touch (astereognosia) results from lesion of parietal-cortex representation of finger kinaesthesis. *Lancet, 354*, 393–394.

Turkeltaub, P., & Coslett, H. (2010). Localization of sublexical speech perception components. *Brain and Language, 114*, 1–15.

Vignolo, L. (2003). Music agnosia and auditory agnosia: Dissociations in stroke patients. *Annals of the New York Academy of Sciences, 999*, 50–57.

Wang, E., Peach, R., Xu, Y., Schneck, M., & Manry, C. (2000). Perception of dynamic acoustic patterns by an individual with unilateral verbal auditory agnosia. *Brain and Language, 73*(3), 442–455.

9

Executive Functions/Cognitive Control Functions

The topic of this chapter is the cognitive domain with the most elusive name. Originally, the functions were referred to as frontal lobe functions, which evolved into executive functions and are now referred to as cognitive control functions. In parallel to the evolving label of these functions, the definition of the cognitive units that comprise these functions has been evolving, as well as their corresponding anatomic locations. In addition, these anatomic locations have expanded to extend beyond the frontal lobe. As a result, the cognitive control domain represents the most evolving area in cognitive neuroscience.

One approach to investigating executive/cognitive control functions throughout the years has been to link deficits in neuropsychological test performance with anatomic localizations, without much success. In a meta-analytic review, Alvarez and Emory (2006) could not find consistent correlations between the neuropsychological tests of the Wisconsin Card Sort, phonemic verbal fluency (e.g., "Say as many words as you can that begin with the letter 'F'; you have one minute"), and the Stroop Color–Word Interference tests with isolated focal lesions. Part of the lack of anatomic correlation with test performance stems from the "frontal lobe" neuropsychological tasks consisting of multiple cognitive units.

Consequently, we proceed with describing functional–anatomic correlates of what are referred to as "cognitive control functions" because these are based on more clearly delineated cognitive operations. *Cognitive control functions* refer to a group of processes that direct, configure, or modulate processing in different cognitive domains in accordance with what the task in each domain demands. These functions appear to be particularly necessary when the cognitive processing stream of a task that leads to a specific targeted action is in conflict with a more habitual processing stream (Hommel et al., 2002; Miller & Cohen, 2001). As noted in the definition, cognitive control functions operate as ancillary functions to other cognitive tasks that are to be performed. Thus, isolating cognitive control operations has been and can be difficult secondary to having to isolate them within another task.

Serving an ancillary role aiding in performance of other tasks leads to the need to define whether cognitive control operations are effective in only one cognitive domain ("domain-specific") or can be effective as control functions across multiple cognitive domains ("domain-general"). These terms are defined as follows: (1) A domain-specific cognitive operation designates a function (selection, shifting, etc.) that is engaged in only one cognitive domain (e.g., language, episodic memory, and working memory); (2) a domain-general cognitive operation refers to an operation that can perform that same function in multiple domains. Localization of cognitive control functions is thus delineated as to whether these cognitive–anatomic units (CAUs) function in one or multiple cognitive domains.

Cognitive control operations can often be engaged as part of a network of regions performing a complex task involving multiple cognitive units, which may require control circuits to monitor or regulate the network to produce a resultant output. Another facet to consider is that it has been proposed that rather than localized to circumscribed regions, cognitive control units may be associated anatomically with global, nondifferentiated regions located primarily in the frontal lobes, as opposed to well-differentiated, selective circumscribed anatomic regions (Stuss, 2006). The amount and location of regions that a global adaptive system is engaged by a cognitive unit are proposed to depend on the complexity and demands of the unit: Increased complexity of the cognitive unit leads to an increased involvement of a region and/or more extensive regions being engaged.

Thus, the two proposed models of the anatomic correlates of cognitive control processes are: (1) organized similarly to most of the other CAUs described as circumscribed anatomic units with regional specialization or as (2) a general undifferentiated cognitive domain that can recruit brain regions depending on the complexity of the cognitive unit. What has been derived experimentally does support the proposal in that cognitive control units appear to be supported by circumscribed, specialized regions and others are best characterized as recruiting regions to perform the operation from a more nondifferentiated area, typically located in the frontal lobes.

With these factors in mind, we delineate the defined cognitive control functions and their anatomic correlates when lesions overlapping in specific regions show that an area is essential to implementing a specific type of control unit.

ENERGIZATION, MONITORING, AND TASK SETTING

Stuss (2011) and colleagues have worked extensively on delineating those discrete frontal lobe regions that control specific cognitive control operations through multiple studies. The conclusion of those evaluations was that there is no specific central executive cognitive unit that was isolatable, but that there were three cognitive control units associated with specific frontal lobe anatomic regions: dorsomedial frontal for energization, left dorsolateral frontal for task setting, and right dorsolateral frontal for monitoring. The energization unit is defined as the process of initiation and sustaining of any response. Impairment of energization results in performing slower on tasks requiring a speeded response, decreased ability to sustain responses, and an overall inability to initiate and sustain responses. This is reflected in poor performance on vigilance tasks, continual attention tasks, choice reaction time tasks, and tasks required to continually generate a targeted response (letter fluency and category fluency). This domain-general function (see Chapter 4 for semantic retrieval, which possibly engages this function in lexical semantics) is associated with lesions to superior medial frontal lobes, including Brodmann areas (BAs) 24, 9, and 6. Task setting is an attentional process that refers to the ability to set criteria to make successful task decisions. The cognitive unit of task setting or criterion setting can also be characterized as performing an "if–then" function. Task performance that could be most affected if this unit were impaired included the Wisconsin Card Sorting Test, response inhibition, and list learning (errors of false positives). The anatomical correlate includes the left lateral frontal lobe region including BAs 9 and 46. The monitoring cognitive unit is defined as the process of checking the task one is performing over time as a quality control function and then adjusting behavior if needed. If monitoring is impaired, it can lead to variable task performance, an increase in all error types (false positive and false negative), difficulty keeping track of the count of stimuli in a task (e.g., the *n*-back task), and overall poor on-line monitoring of performance across multiple tasks. Patients who have disruption with this cognitive unit have lesions in the right lateral frontal lobe region, including involvement of BAs 44–46, 9, and 47/12.

For approximately the past two decades, Stuss, Alexander, and colleagues have investigated fractionation of cognitive control functions into CAUs using a variety of statistical techniques. The three surviving CAUs from the investigations of this group are the result of comprehensive analyses of multiple cognitive control units, adding strength to the consistency of the CAUs reported. The following sections discuss cognitive control circuits that are typically identified by targeted investigations of the one unit to be identified.

INHIBITION

Several regions in the frontal lobe, including the left superior medial prefrontal cortex and right inferior frontal cortices, have been implicated in studies as having major roles in the function of inhibition. Response inhibition is required in a multitude of tasks, best exemplified in the Go/NoGo task. In this task, the subject must respond quickly (e.g., typically with a button push) to Go stimuli trials and then not respond to the NoGo stimuli trials. The ratio of Go versus NoGo trials can be manipulated to vary the difficulty of inhibition required. A higher number of Go versus NoGo trials biases the subject to more likely make a Go response on each trial. Thus, inhibiting a Go response for the rare NoGo trial becomes much more difficult as the ratio of the number of Go trials increases and the number of NoGo trials decreases. By using a neuropsychological test composed of one task with 25% NoGo trials (improbable NoGo) and the other with 25% Go trials (improbable Go), Picton et al. (2007) found that lesions in the superior medial frontal regions, compared to controls and lesions in other frontal areas, were associated with more false alarms during improbable NoGo trials (referred to as commission errors of pushing the button when the trial is NoGo—do not push). Molenberghs et al. (2009) used a task consisting of presenting one digit at a time (1–9) up to 25 times with the subject to respond by pushing a button for all digits except "3." This task was administered to 44 stroke patients, and task performance was compared to lesion location using voxel-based lesion symptom mapping (VBLSM). Those with lesions of the right inferior frontal gyrus had a significantly increased commission error rate.

A variation of the response inhibition task is called the stop-signal task. In the stop-signal task, a motor response (the default response) should be made immediately upon the moment when a cue (Go signal; e.g., a square on the screen) is presented. However, a different cue (Stop signal; e.g., a beeping sound) is randomly introduced at various time intervals after the onset of the Go cue. The longer the interval (stop-signal delay), the harder it is to inhibit the response. The ability of inhibitory control is thus indexed by how much delay can be tolerated to maintain a certain level of successful inhibition, measured for each individual as the stop signal reaction time (SSRT) (shorter SSRT indicates more effective inhibitory control). Aron et al. (2003) showed that increasing damage to the right inferior frontal cortex resulted in increasingly impaired performance (slower SSRT) on a stop-signal task. The dysfunctional right inferior frontal cortex was proposed to lead to commission errors because of the loss of impaired inhibitory control, with the damaged right inferior frontal cortex not able to respond in the time needed to identify the stop signal stimulus and stop the "Go" response (Aron et al., 2004b).

Therefore, there is evidence that both the superior medial frontal gryus (including supplementary motor and pre-supplementary motor areas) and the right inferior frontal cortex are central to inhibitory functions, as implemented within an associative frontal–striatal network that includes a subcortical structure, the subthalamus nucleus (Aron et al., 2004b, 2014). Lesion studies confirm that inhibition and the right inferior frontal cortex represent a CAU that is domain-general in that this same region and the inhibition function are also engaged in other cognitive domains; for example, neuropsychological tests of task switching engage this inhibitory operation.

It is important to note that other investigators who have assessed performance in a Go/NoGo task have suggested that response inhibition is also impaired with lesions to the left inferior frontal gyrus (Swick et al., 2008). Given that these patients can also be aphasic, this localization has been difficult to establish, and further studies are needed before it is clearly a consistent localization.

SUSTAINED ATTENTION

The Go/NoGo task(s) in which a response is made to one stimulus but not another and that is conducted over an extensive period of time requires sustained attention to perform a persistent response. This type of task is used in clinical settings to detect continued attentional deficits, also known as deficits of vigilance (continuous performance task and sustained attention to response task; Molenberghs et al., 2009).

The behavioral performance marker of sustaining attention across time when using a Go/NoGo task is indexed differently from inhibitory control. The performance marker is omission errors (failing to make a motor response when required) and reaction time variability, particularly as the task becomes longer. In the same study mentioned in the previous section, Molenberghs et al. (2009) assessed whether sustained attention was associated with a particular brain region. They found that those with lesions of the middle third of the right inferior frontal sulcus (IFS) were unable to utilize errors to adjust for future responses. This finding suggested that the middle third of the right IFS is involved in online readjustment of attentional resources for vigilance performance (Figure 9.1). However, this was found only in six patients, and at the individual level, the finding did not reach significance in any of the six patients compared to controls. Thus, as additional data become available, this finding may be considered more consistent. In a similar vein, Picton et al. (2007), using a Go/NoGo task (as mentioned in the previous section) requiring sustained attention, found that patients with lesions to the right anterior cingulate and the right ventrolateral prefrontal cortex demonstrated reaction time variability during Go trials—a marker of an impairment in sustained attention that warrants further investigation.

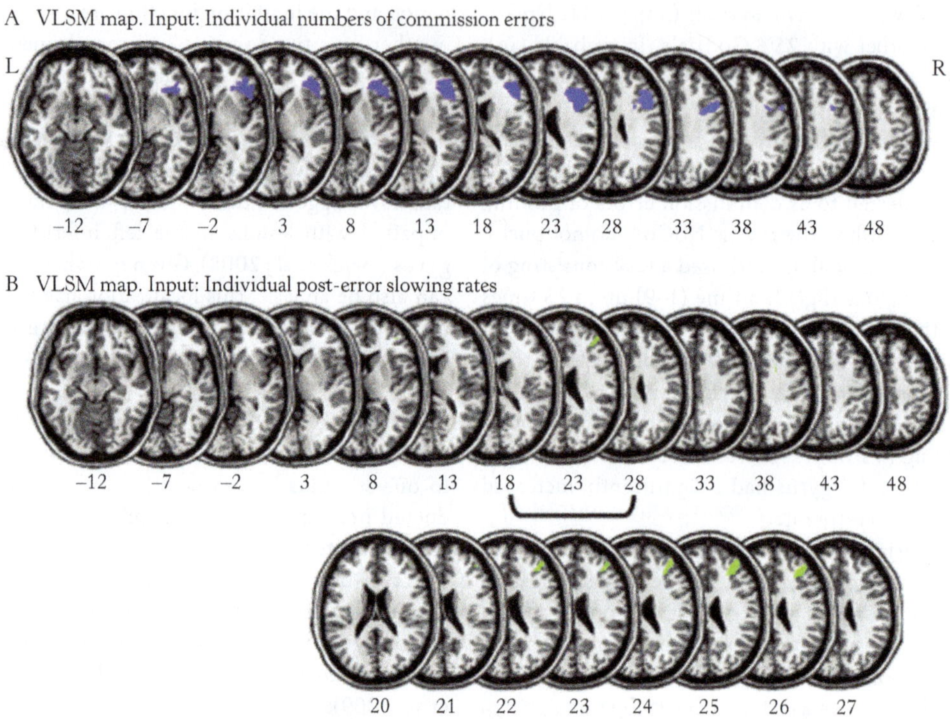

FIGURE 9.1: Lesion–symptom map using VLSM with (A) commission error rate with lesion location as input ($p < .05$, Bonferroni corrected) and (B) post-error slowing as the input with lesion location.

Source: Molenberghs et al. (2009).

TASK SWITCHING AND INTERFERENCE

Tsuchida and Fellows (2013) studied 45 patients with focal prefrontal lobe damage and 50 normal, matched controls who had all performed an attention-shifting task, the Stroop Interference Test, and a spatial search task. In the attention-shifting task, for each trial they presented a series of number–letter pairs. In each trial, there was a cue on whether the subjects should read the number or the letter out loud as fast as they can. The trial types were interwoven between number cue and letter cue, in a sequence such as letter–letter–number–number–letter–letter and so on. The measure used to assess performance in the task is based on the cost of reaction time between task-switching and task-nonswitching trials. The Stroop Interference Test emphasizes the ability to overcome inherent interference in stimuli. The task requires subjects to say aloud the ink color in which words are printed. The words are color names (e.g., green, red, and blue). The difficulty arises in that the color word name does not match the ink color in which the word is printed (e.g., the word "green" is written in red ink). VBLSM was performed on the lesion group and showed that damage to the left ventrolateral prefrontal cortex, centered in the inferior frontal gyrus, is associated with impaired performance on both the attention shifting and the interference tasks (Figure 9.2). The spatial search task did not associate with any specific brain regions but was weakly correlated with most regions of the frontal lobe, except the left ventrolateral prefrontal cortex.

This well-performed study demonstrated that two cognitive operations were both supported by the same anatomic region. As mentioned in the introductory chapters, one region can encode for the two functions by the neurons in the region firing in different frequencies (e.g., gamma rhythm for one function and theta rhythm for another function) and/or if some of the neurons in this region are engaged in one function and other neurons are engaged in the other function. This latter account in essence signifies that the present tools for anatomic localization are inadequate to distinguish between these two groups of neurons in this one region. It is hoped that future investigative techniques will

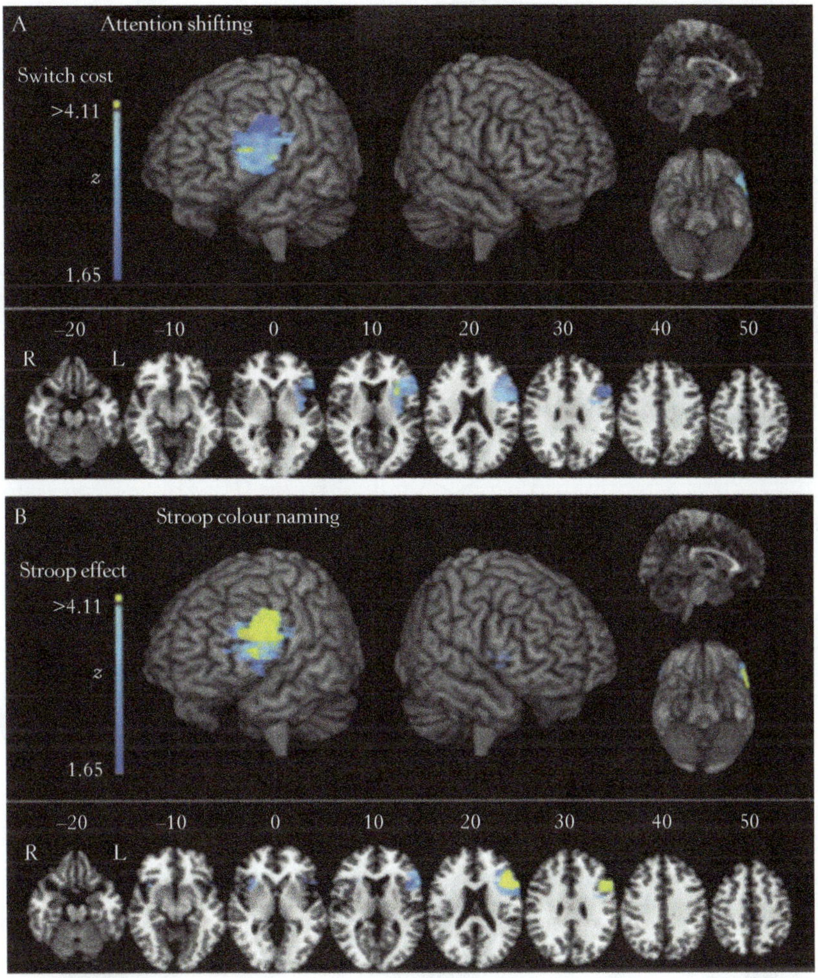

FIGURE 9.2: VBLSM lesion map for (A) the attention shifting task and (B) the Stroop interference task. The blue region designates a *t*-test thresholded at $p < .05$, uncorrected with yellow from regions with Bonferonni correction.

Source: Tsuchida and Fellows (2013).

allow for a distinction between the anatomic units. The findings may also reflect the fact that the definition of the cognitive units proffered is incorrect and that there is one underlying cognitive unit that is engaged in both of these neuropsychological tasks (e.g., possibly a general switching operation), which is not evident at this point. Further investigations into delineating finer-grained cognitive operations may prove fruitful in isolating a common cognitive unit to both tasks.

These types of findings highlight the challenges of defining the component processes of cognitive control functions and their anatomic correlates. Although absence of evidence is not evidence of absence, the diffuse anatomic correlation with the spatial search task may also support the notion that some cognitive control functions may best be encoded anatomically as part of a general undifferentiated system located predominantly in the frontal lobes.

Another version of the task-switching test used by Aron et al. (2004b) showed that lesions of the right inferior frontal cortex disrupted patients' ability to inhibit irrelevant information when having to switch set, consistent with the right inferior frontal lesions' inducement of errors in the Go/NoGo and stop-signal tasks (Figure 9.3). Furthermore, lesions to the left middle frontal gyrus were also associated with impaired set switching ability, which may well be a different cognitive unit located in a different region that is needed to perform this particular version of the task. Compared

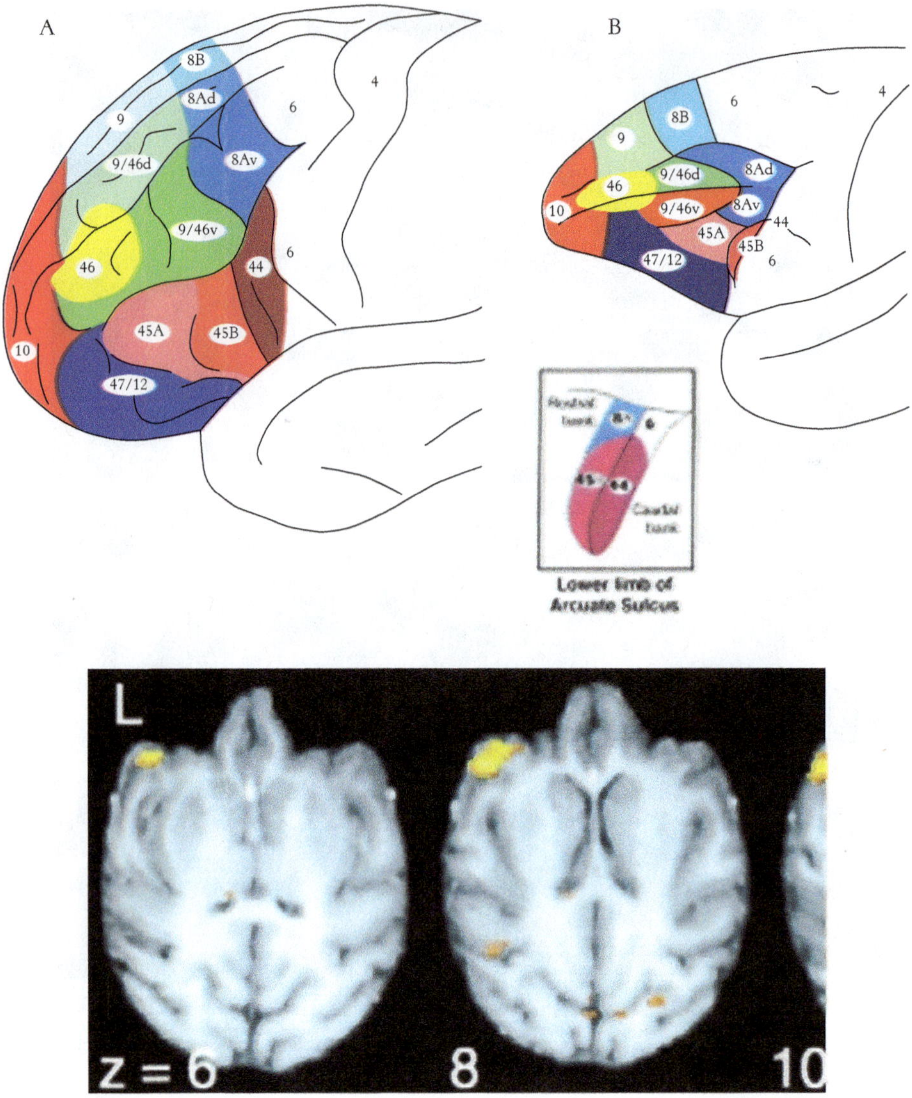

FIGURE 9.3 (Top) Cytoarchitectonic map of lateral surface of prefrontal lobe. Brodmann areas are designated by the colored, numbered (BA numbers) regions. (Bottom) Activation from fMRI studies identifying regions associated with set shifting on the Wisconsin Card Sorting Test.

Source: Aron et al. (2004).

to the findings in Tsuchida and Fellows (2013), it is important to note that there exists subcomponents in task-switching/interference performance that may vary dependent on experimental design and demands. A consistent localization is currently not possible. Studies defining the cognitive units and anatomic correlates must consider the demands of the task, and its complexity may influence the involvement of the cognitive unit and the extent of the anatomic region that may be recruited to support that unit.

DECISION-MAKING

Impaired decision-making and its associated medial orbitofrontal pathology have long been linked with the clinical symptoms of risky behavior and lack of regard for long-term consequences (Shallice & Burgess, 1991). Bechara et al. (1994) developed the Iowa Gambling Task to assess this function and associated brain regions, which has now been used extensively in both normal and impaired populations. The task consists of a subject making a series of card selections that lead to winning and/or losing money. There are multiple card decks, with different combinations of cards: Some decks have higher possible gains but also a corresponding higher number of losses, whereas other decks have lower gain/lower loss cards. Patients with medial orbitofrontal lesions (for orbitofrontal anatomy, see Figure 9.4) preferred the riskier decks and made riskier decisions, without evidence of an effective anticipation of losses (Bechara et al., 1994, 1996, 1998).

These findings showed that lesions involving the medial orbitofrontal cortex (OFC) are correlated with impaired decision-making. However, others have questioned the role that the extent and laterality of the OFC lesion play in decision-making. For example, Manes et al. (2002) conducted a study using three decision-making tests and concluded that lesions restricted to just the OFC did not result in decision-making impairments (see also Bechara, 2004). There are few isolated lesions of the medial OFC, so large lesion studies have not been forthcoming. However, it appears that the preponderance of evidence supports the claim that OFC damage leads to impairment in integrating information to assess potential reward outcomes in decision-making (Figure 9.4) (Wallis, 2007).

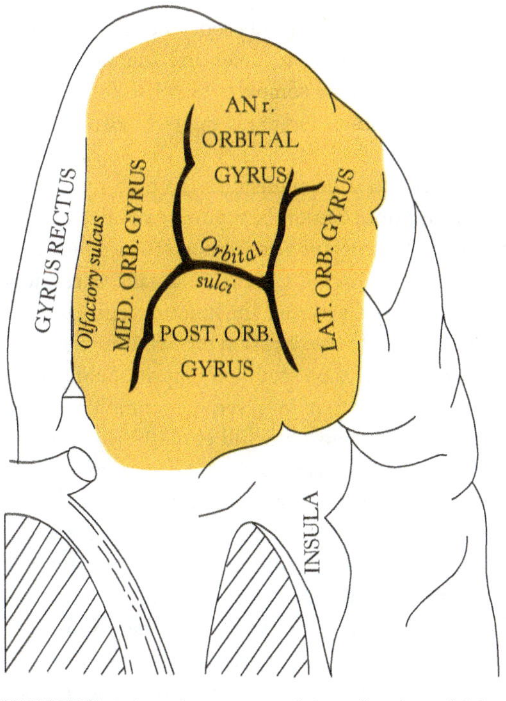

FIGURE 9.4: Inferior view of the orbitofrontal lobe. The figure shows the main sulci of the orbitofrontal region.
Source: http://www.wikipedia.org.

To further clarify if this localization was specific to the function of decision-making as opposed to a cognitive control function in general, the CAU of orbitofrontal cortex with decision-making was assessed in a large study of lesion patients who had received a variety of tests engaging cognitive control functions. One of these was the Wisconsin Card Sorting Test (Heaton, 1981), which is a popular neuropsychological assessment of cognitive control functions that requires task (set) switching and inhibition, along with the other cognitive operations. The task uses cards with multiple types of cues on them (shape, color, number, etc.), and the subject must determine by what cue the examiner wants him or her to sort the cards. After the subject decides how each card is to be sorted, the examiner tells the subject if it was sorted correctly or not. Once the subject determines how to successfully sort the cards and is told "correct," he or she can continue to sort 10 successive cards in a row by that same criteria with the examiner saying "yes" each time. On the 11th straight successful trial, the examiner says "incorrect." At this point, the subject is supposed to inhibit continuing to sort by that criteria, and the subject must then be mentally flexible enough to shift set to try a new sort criteria. This set shifting occurs several times throughout the task after 10 correct successive sorts in a row occur. Another task requiring cognitive control functions is Trailmaking Test (TMT) Part B, which consists of a subject connecting circles on a page by drawing a continuous line between the circles as fast as he or she can. Inside the circles are letters and numbers. In TMT B, the subject connects the circles while alternating between letters and numbers sequentially (e.g., 1-A-2-B-3-C. . . .). In contrast, TMT A is normally used as a visual motor speed task, with its implementation quite similar to that of TMT B but requiring only numbers in sequence. Performance on both tasks of the TMT is measured by the amount of time it takes to finish drawing the line. TMT B strongly engages the function of flexibility of shifting. If TMT B is impaired and TMT A is intact, then the deficit is in flexibility of shifting. If both TMT A and B are impaired, then the deficit could be in shift flexibility or could be slow reaction times in both tasks due to reduced processing speed.

Glascher et al. (2012) assessed several of the previously discussed functions and localizations with a VBLSM study of 165 individuals with lesions of the prefrontal cortex (out of 344 people with lesions included in the study) who had performed

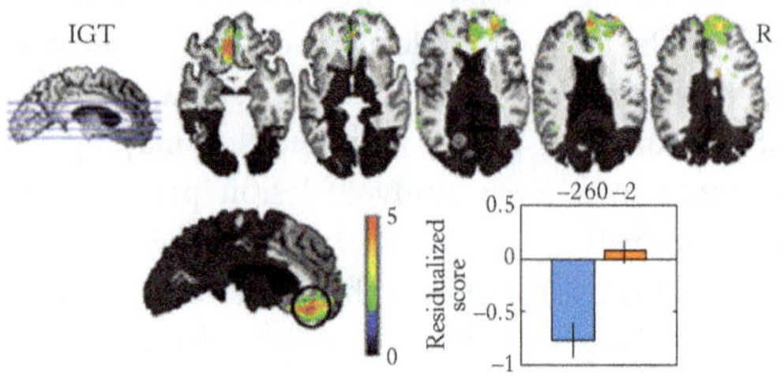

FIGURE 9.5: Results from lesion overlap analysis of a test of value-based decision-making. These VBLSM results are at $p < .05$, FDR corrected with color representing increased significance. These findings show the orbitofrontal lobe to be highly associated with decision-making in the Iowa Gambling Test.

Source: Glascher et al. (2012).

neuropsychological tests emphasizing cognitive control mechanisms—the Wisconsin Card Sorting Test (set switching/inhibition), TMT (attention/flexibility of switching cost: time used in TMT B minus TMT A), Stroop Test (response inhibition/interference), and the Iowa Gambling Test (decision-making). Lower performance on the TMT was associated with damage to a focal region of left rostral anterior cingulate cortex (ACC), whereas lower performance on the Wisconsin Card Sorting Test was associated with damage to a slightly more anterior region of the ACC and left medial superior frontal gyrus, along with other brain regions. Lower Stroop Test performance was associated with left dorsal lateral prefrontal cortex (DLPFC) damage (overlapping with the middle frontal gryus). More important, value-based decision-making engaged in the Iowa Gambling Test was associated with lesions involving the orbitofrontal, ventromedial, and frontopolar cortices (Figure 9.5). These studies as a group suggest that the DLPFC and ACC appear to be engaged in cognitive control functions, with the ACC appearing to play a key role in flexibly shifting between cognitive tasks and response sets (TMT and Wisconsin Card Sorting Test). This ACC localization may emerge as a CAU if more consistent lesion findings support its association with the function of shifting between cognitive sets. This lesion study further confirms that disrupting the OFC can play an integral role in impairing decision-making.

MEMORY CONTROL

Another role for cognitive control mechanisms is to mediate a variety of functions in different memory systems to store, retrieve, or access memories. One region that has been implicated in semantic memory functions is the left inferior frontal gyrus (IFG). The left IFG was shown in functional neuroimaging studies to be engaged in controlled access to retrieving/selecting semantic knowledge in a variety of tasks, including making simple semantic decisions and performing semantic classifications compared to other types of classifications (Devlin et al., 2003; Gabrieli et al., 1998; Otten & Rugg, 2001; Poldrack et al., 1999; Thompson-Schill et al., 1997). For example, in one of these studies, subjects performed three semantic tasks during functional magnetic resonance imaging (fMRI): (1) a semantic-generation task that required subjects to read a word naming an object and generate a related verb to that object, with high selection (e.g., many possible options of associated actions) and low selection (e.g., few possible choices of associated actions) stimuli included as objects; (2) a semantic classification task requiring subjects to classify pictures of objects (one type of high selection classification is to classify 10 pictures by a given feature (big, light, expensive, etc.) and another easier low selection classification in which 10 pictures were to be classified only by their name (bird, ball, etc.)); and (3) a semantic comparison task in which subjects make semantic comparisons between a target word and probes along a particular feature dimension (e.g., color and function) (high selection condition compares target to four probes and low selection compares target to two probes) (Thompson-Schill et al., 1997). The activation in the left IFG was dependent on the high versus low selection demands, not the type of semantic decision being made. This was also interpreted to reflect that the selection process, not the retrieval process, was supported by this region. The functional importance of the left IFG in the selection process is further corroborated by a lesion study (Thompson-Schill et al., 1998) showing that in a verb-generation task (as in task 1 in Thompson-Schill et al., 1997), left IFG lesions were associated with increased impairment, compared to controls and other frontal lesions, in the high selection condition but not the low selection condition. In addition, lesions to the left IFG disrupt semantic selection processes, suggesting that this region is essential to these functions (Martin & Cheng, 2006; Metzler, 2001). However, evidence is emerging that this region may not be related only to selection processes in semantic memory but also to selection in episodic memory and other cognitive domains. It appears that selection

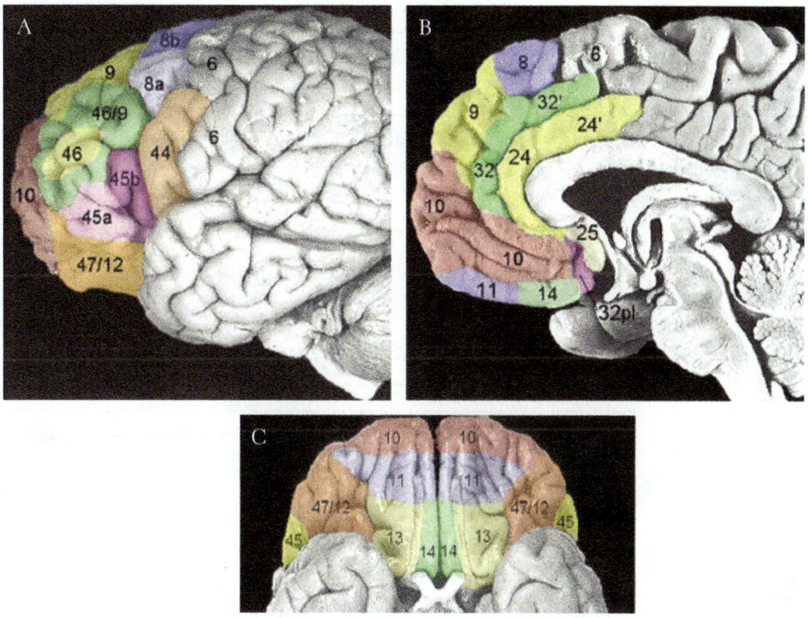

FIGURE 9.6: Brodmann areas of the prefrontal cortex. BA 45 is the region associated with retrieval selection processes. *Source:* Ridderinkhof et al. (2004).

processes are mediated by middle aspects of the left IFG (BA 45) and that this selection function is a domain-general process to select between multiple competing options in multiple tasks and domains (for anatomic location, see Figure 9.6) (Badre & Wagner, 2007; Robinson et al., 2010).

THEORY OF MIND

Theory of mind, a key concept in social cognition, refers to an individual's ability to understand the mental state of others and relate how it differs from their own mental state. The mental state characteristics that are typically included in the theory of mind concept are intentions, beliefs, emotional states, wants, and desires (Siegal & Varley, 2002). For this complex cognitive activity, there are obviously multiple brain regions engaged in theory of mind processing (Stuss et al., 2001; Weed, 2008), including, but not limited to, the anterior corpus callosum (Baird et al., 2006), right prefrontal cortex (Brunet et al., 2000), medial prefrontal, language regions (Rizzolatti et al., 2001), superior temporal gyrus, right inferior parietal lobe, right temporo-parietal junction (Ruby & Decety, 2001), precuneus, and amygdala (Adolphs, 1999; Shaw et al., 2004).

One particular region that has been implicated in a specific theory of mind deficit is the ventromedial frontal lobe. Shamay-Tsoory et al. (2007) administered affective theory of mind and cognitive theory of mind questions to 49 lesioned patients and 44 healthy controls. In the theory of mind task, the subjects are shown a cartoon outline of a face and four colored pictures of objects. In the affective theory of mind questions, the subject must infer what the individual in the picture is feeling; in the cognitive theory of mind questions, the inference to be determined is what the individual is thinking. The subject's task is to point to the correct object answer based on a sentence that appears at the top of the screen and available cues from the face, such as eye gaze and facial expression (e.g., the image to which the face is referring; "Yoni [name of the character] loves the orange") (Figure 9.7). There are two main conditions—"cognitive" and "affective"—based on the type of mental inferences that the subject has to make from the stimuli. In the cognitive condition, both facial expression and the verbal cue are emotionally neutral, whereas in the affective conditions, both cues provide affective information. Both positive and negative affective statements are used (e.g., statements such as "Yoni loves the orange" and "Yoni does not love the orange") (see Figure 9.7).

Shamay-Tsoory et al. (2007) found that whereas the cognitive theory of mind task did not have a clear single anatomic correlate in the lesioned patients, the affective theory of mind task had a significant

First Order	Second Order–directed toward picture	Figure 2 Second Order–directed straight ahead
Cognitive ToM (24 trials)		
Cog1 12 trials	Cog2 6 trials	Cog2 6 trials
Yeni is thinking of ______ 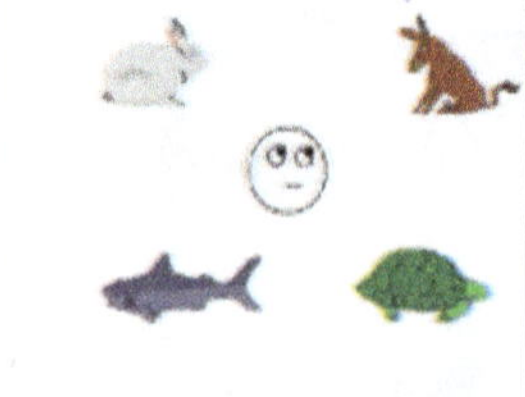	Yeni is thinking of the fruit that ______ wants 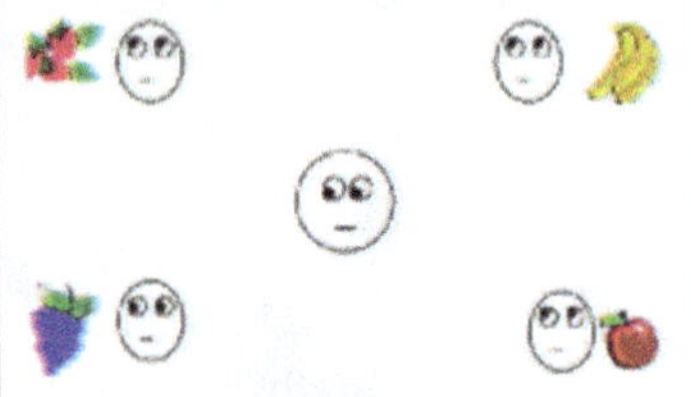	Yeni is thinking about the toy that ______ wants 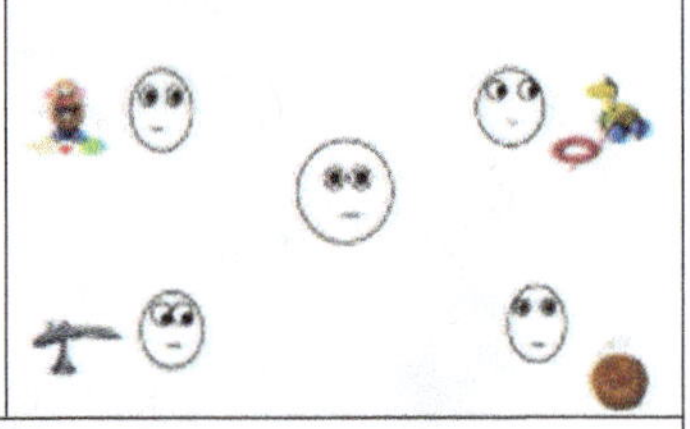
Affective ToM (24 trials)		
Aff1 12 trials	Aff2 6 trials	Aff2 6 trials
Yeni loves ______ 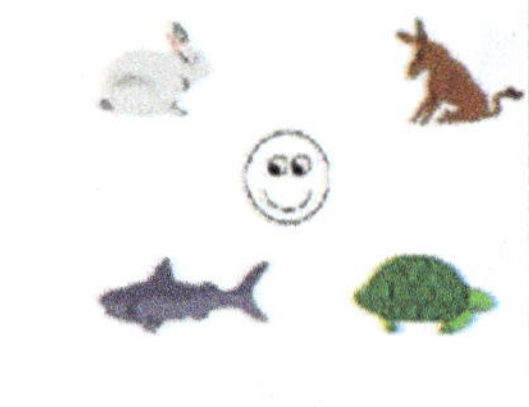	Yeni loves the toy that ______ loves 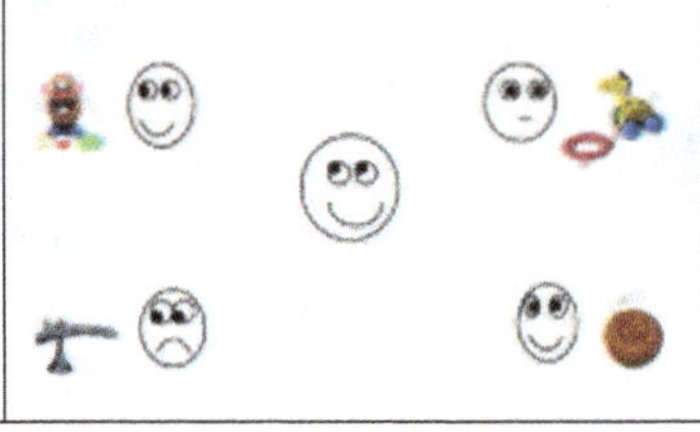	Yeni loves the toy that ______ does not love 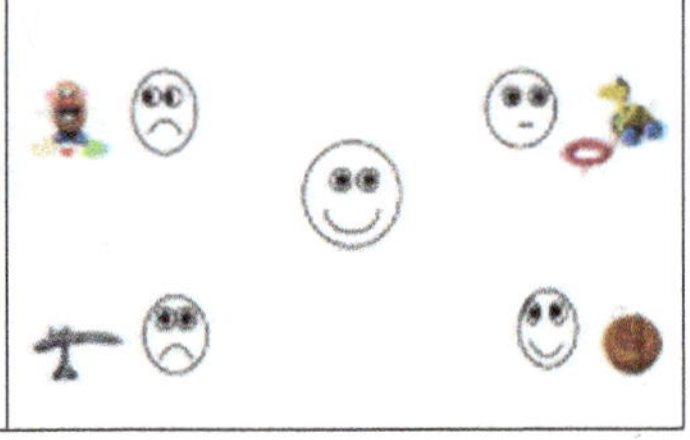

FIGURE 9.7: Examples of theory of mind stimuli.
Source: Shamay-Tsoory et al. (2007).

correlation with ventromedial frontal lobe damage (BA mesial 8, 9, 10, 24, and 32) (Figure 9.8) (see also Shamay-Tsoory et al., 2003, 2006; Stone et al., 1998).

There remain several cognitive control functions that have been delineated from a cognitive unit perspective but have not been associated with a specific anatomic localization. Some of these cognitive operations have not been localized because there is not a clear anatomic correlate; however, as mentioned previously, other operations are associated with a generalized global adaptive anatomic system that can contribute to multiple cognitive control functions. Resources that are recruited from this global system of anatomic regions are dependent on the complexity and demands of the cognitive control operations. Another plausible reason for a lack of localization of cognitive control operations is the small number of cases of lesioned patients reported for each function.

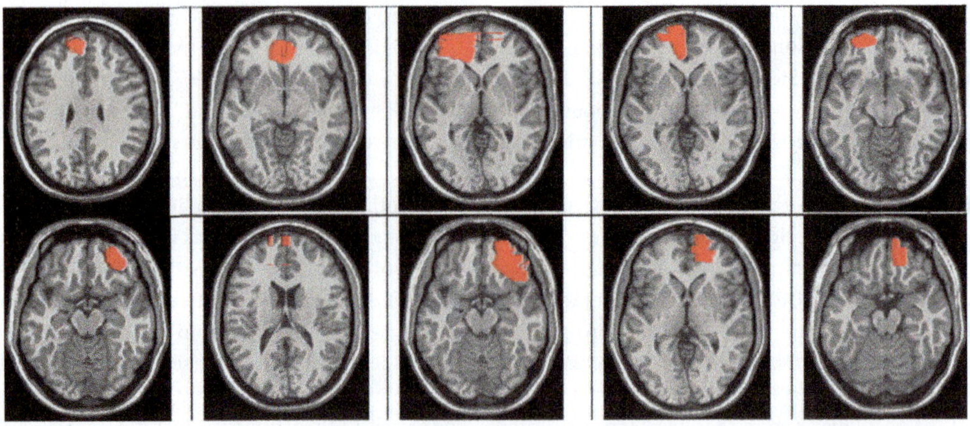

FIGURE 9.8: Map of lesions of patients with impaired affective theory of mind and ventromedial frontal lobe lesions.
Source: Adapted from Shamay-Tsoory et al. (2007).

TABLE 9.1: COGNITIVE CONTROL SUMMARY

Brain Region	Function
Superior medial frontal lobe (BA 24, 9, 6)	"Energization" (domain—general)
Right lateral frontal lobe (BA 44–46, 9, 47/12)	Monitoring (domain—general)
Left lateral frontal lobe (BA 9, 46)	Task setting (domain—general)
Right inferior frontal cortex	Response inhibition (domain—general)
Orbitofrontal cortex	Integrating information to assess potential reward outcomes in decision-making
Left inferior frontal gyrus (middle)	Selecting between multiple competing options (domain—general)
Ventromedial frontal lobe	Affective theory of mind

For some other cognitive control functions for which a larger number of cases were reported, there is a somewhat inconsistent pattern of localization. Two examples with inconsistent localizations are multitasking, which has been associated with BA 10 (Roca et al., 2011), and the right frontal pole being associated with prospective (time-based) memory in multiple domains (words and pictures) (Volle et al., 2011). Future studies of these functional–anatomic correlates may lead to convincing associations.

Overall, it appears that cognitive control functions likely are encoded in two different anatomic systems: (1) circumscribed anatomic regions forming CAUs as noted when detectable (see Table 9.1 for CAUs) and (2) an undifferentiated, generalized global adaptive anatomic system that can recruit resources (regions) from this global system depending on the complexity and demands of the cognitive control operation. This appears to be a unique combination of anatomic alternatives for a set of cognitive operations. In addition, cognitive control functions are unique in that their roles in tasks are typically ancillary to the main outcome of the tasks and are engaged to provide oversight of the tasks or maximize performance. Given that this role in oversight and enhancement of overall task performance can range dramatically based on the complexity of the task, a system that allows for recruitment of brain regions based on a factor such as complexity is optimal for a system tasked with optimizing complex task outcomes, with no upper limits on task complexity.

REFERENCES

Adolphs, R. (1999). Social cognition and the human brain. *Trends in Cognitive Sciences, 3*, 469–479.

Alvarez, J., & Emory, E. (2006). Executive function and the frontal lobes: A meta-analytic review. *Neuropsychology Review, 16*(1), 17–42.

Aron, A., Fletcher, P., Bullmore, E., Sahakian, B., & Robbins, T. (2003). Stop-signal inhibition disrupted by damage to right inferior frontal gyrus in humans. *Nature Neuroscience, 6*, 115–116.

Aron, A., Monsell, S., Sahakian, B., & Robbins, T. (2004a). A componential analysis of task-switching deficits associated with lesions of left and right frontal cortex. *Brain, 127*(Pt. 7), 1561–1573.

Aron, A., Robbins, T., & Poldrack, R. (2004b). Inhibition and the right inferior frontal cortex. *Trends in Cognitive Sciences, 8*(4), 170–177.

Badre, D., & Wagner, A. (2007). Left ventrolateral prefrontal cortex and the cognitive control of memory. *Neuropsychologia, 45*, 2883–2901.

Baird, A., Dewar, B., Critchley, H., Dolan, R., Shallice, T., & Cipolotti, L. (2006). Social and emotional functions in three patients with medial frontal lobe damage including the anterior cingulate cortex. *Cognitive Neuropsychiatry, 11*(4), 369–388.

Bechara, A. (2004). The role of emotion in decision-making: Evidence from neurological patients with orbitofrontal damage. *Brain and Cognition, 55*, 30–40.

Bechara, A., Damasio, A., Damasio, H., & Anderson, S. (1994). Insensitivity to future consequences following damage to human prefrontal cortex. *Cognition, 50*, 7–15.

Bechara, A., Damasio, H., Tranel, D., & Anderson, S. (1998). Dissociation of working memory from decision making within the human prefrontal cortex. *Journal of Neuroscience, 18*, 428–437.

Bechara, A., Tranel, D., Damasio, H., & Damasio, A. (1996). Failure to respond autonomically to anticipated future outcomes following damage to prefrontal cortex. *Cerebral Cortex, 6*, 215–225.

Brunet, E., Sarfati, Y., Hardy-Bayle, M., & Decety, J. (2000). A PET investigation of the attribution of intentions with a nonverbal task. *Neuroimage, 11*, 157–166.

Devlin, J., Matthews, P., & Rushworth, M. (2003). Semantic processing in the left inferior prefrontal cortex: A combined functional magnetic resonance imaging and transcranial magnetic stimulation study. *Journal of Cognitive Neuroscience, 15*(1), 71–84.

Gabrieli, J., Poldrack, R., & Desmond, J. (1998). The role of left prefrontal cortex in language and memory. *Proceedings of the National Academy of Sciences of the USA, 95*(3), 906–913.

Glascher, J., Adolphs, R., Damasio, H., Bechara, A., Rudrauf, A., Calamia, M., et al. (2012). Lesion mapping of cognitive control and value-based decision making in the prefrontal cortex. *Proceedings of the National Academy of Sciences of the USA, 109*(36), 14681–14686.

Heaton, R. (1981). *A manual for the Wisconsin Card Sorting Test.* Odessa, FL: Psychological Assessment Resources.

Hommel, B., Ridderinkhof, K., & Theeuwes, J. (2002). Cognitive control of attention and action: Issues and trends. *Psychological Research, 66,* 215–219.

Manes, F., Sahakian, B., Clark, L., Rogers, R., Antoun, N., Aitken, M., et al. (2002). Decision-making processes following damage to the prefrontal cortex. *Brain, 125,* 624–639.

Martin, R., & Cheng, Y. (2006). Selection demands versus association strength in the verb generation task. *Psychonomic Bulletin & Review, 13*(3), 396–401.

Metzler, C. (2001). Effects of left frontal lesions on the selection of context-appropriate meanings. *Neuropsychology, 15*(3), 315–328.

Miller, E., & Cohen, J. (2001). An integrative theory of prefrontal cortex function. *Annual Review of Neuroscience, 24,* 167–202.

Molenberghs, P., Gillebert, C., Schoofs, H., Dupont, P., Peeters, R., & Vandenberghe, R. (2009). Lesion neuroanatomy of the sustained attention to response task. *Neuropsychologia, 47,* 2866–2875.

Otten, L., & Rugg, M. (2001). Task-dependency of the neural correlates of episodic encoding as measured by fMRI. *Cerebral Cortex, 11*(12), 1150–1160.

Picton, T., Stuss, D., Alexander, M., Shallice, T., Binns, M., & Gillingham, S. (2007). Effects of focal frontal lesions on response inhibition. *Cereb Cortex, 17*(4), 826–838.

Poldrack, R., Wagner, A., Prull, M., Desmond, J., Glover, G., & Gabrieli, J. (1999). Functional specialization for semantic and phonological processing in the left inferior prefrontal cortex. *Neuroimage, 10*(1), 15–35.

Ridderinkhof, K., van den Wildenberg, W., Segalowitz, S., & Carter, C. (2004). Neurocognitive mechanisms of cognitive control: The role of prefrontal cortex in action selection, response inhibition, performance monitoring, and reward-based learning. *Brain and Cognition, 56,* 129–140.

Rizzolatti, G., Fogassi, L., & Gallese, V. (2001). Neurophysiological mechanisms underlying the understanding and imitation of action. *Nature Reviews Neuroscience, 2,* 661–670.

Robinson, G., Shallice, T., Bozzali, M., & Cipolotti, L. (2010). Conceptual proposition selection and the LIFG: Neuropsychological evidence from a focal frontal group. *Neuropsychologia, 48,* 1652–1663.

Roca, M., Torralva, T., Gleichgerrcht, E., Woolgar, A., Thompson, R., Duncan, J., et al. (2011). The role of area 10 (BA 10) in human multitasking and in social cognition: A lesion study. *Neuropsychologia, 49,* 3525–3531.

Ruby, P., & Decety, J. (2001). Effect of subjective perspective taking during simulation of action: A PET investigation of agency. *Nature Neuroscience, 4,* 546–550.

Shallice, T., & Burgess, P. (1991). Deficits in strategy application following frontal lobe damage in man. *Brain, 114,* 727–741.

Shamay-Tsoory, S., & Aharon-Peretz, J. (2007). Dissociable prefrontal networks for cognitive and affective theory of mind: A lesion study. *Neuropsychologia, 45,* 3054–3067.

Shamay-Tsoory, S., Tibi-Elhanany, Y., & Aharon-Peretz, J. (2006). The ventromedial prefrontal cortex is involved in understanding affective but not cognitive theory of mind stories. *Social Neuroscience, 1*(3/4), 149–166.

Shamay-Tsoory, S., Tomer, R., Berger, B., & Aharon-Peretz, J. (2003). Characterization of empathy deficits following prefrontal brain damage: The role of the right ventromedial cortex. *Journal of Cognitive Neuroscience, 15,* 324–337.

Shaw, P., Lawrence, E., Radbourne, C, Bramham, J., Polkey, C., & David, A. (2004). The impact of early and late damage to the human amygdala on "theory of mind" reasoning. *Brain, 127,* 1535–1548.

Siegal, M., & Varley, R. (2002). Neural systems involved in "theory of mind." *Nature Reviews Neuroscience, 3,* 463–471.

Stone, V., Baron-Cohen, S., & Knight, R. (1998). Frontal lobe contributions to theory of mind. *Journal of Cognitive Neuroscience, 10,* 640–656.

Stuss, D. (2006). Frontal lobes and attention: Processes and networks, fractionation and integration. *Journal of the International Neuropsychological Society, 12,* 261–271.

Stuss, D. (2011). Functions of the frontal lobes: Relation to executive functions. *Journal of the International Neuropsychological Society, 17,* 769–765.

Stuss, D., Gallup, G., & Alexander, M. (2001). The frontal lobes are necessary for "theory of mind." *Brain, 124,* 279–286.

Swick, D., Ashley, V., & Turken, A. (2008). Left inferior frontal gyrus is critical for response inhibition. *BMC Neuroscience, 9,* 102.

Thompson-Schill, S., D'Esposito, M., Aguirre, G. K., & Farah, M. J. (1997). Role of left prefrontal cortex in retrieval of semantic knowledge: A re-evaluation. *Proceedings of the National Academy of Sciences of the USA, 94,* 14792–14797.

Thompson-Schill, S., Swick, D., Farah, M., D'Esposito, M., Kan, I., & Knight, R. (1998). Verb generation in patients with focal frontal lesions: A neuropsychological test of neuroimaging findings. *Proceedings of the National Academy of Sciences of the USA, 95*(26), 15855–15860.

Tsuchida, A., & Fellows, L. (2013). Are core component processes of executive function dissociable within the frontal lobes? Evidence from humans with focal prefrontal damage. *Cortex, 49,* 1790–1800.

Volle, E., Gonen-Yaacovi, G., Costello, A., Gilbert, S., & Burgess, P. (2011). The role of rostral prefrontal cortex in prospective memory: A voxel based lesion study. *Neuropsychologia, 49,* 2185–2198.

Wallis, J. (2007). Orbitofrontal cortex and its contribution to decision-making. *Annual Review of Neuroscience, 30,* 31–56.

Weed, E. (2008). Theory of mind impairment in right hemisphere damage: A review of the evidence. *International Journal of Speech-Language Pathology, 10*(6), 414–424.

10

Working Memory

Working memory has long been considered a part of the group of functions that were discussed in Chapter 9—executive/frontal lobe/cognitive control functions. The working memory system has been extensively studied in humans as well as animals (Procyk & Goldman-Rakic, 2006) using functional neuroimaging and lesion studies (Courtney, 2004; Lee & D'Esposito, 2012). In addition, the neural circuitry has been further elaborated by delineating that the major neurotransmitter system underlying this system is dopamine (Gao & Goldman-Rakic, 2003). As such, it is discussed separately from other cognitive control functions.

The term *working memory* is typically misunderstood and confused with other terms. Working memory refers to a brain system that provides *temporary* storage and processing of information for a brief period of time. A clear example is when one is given a phone number to remember from an information operator and then must dial the number quickly immediately after hanging up with the operator before forgetting it. Working memory also functions as an ancillary operation to other cognitive domains. At times, the information held in temporary storage in working memory is necessary for other cognitive domains and tasks, such as language comprehension, episodic memory, and reasoning.

The working memory system allows an individual to temporarily store and manipulate information over a brief period of time. The most commonly used cognitive framework to account for how a working memory system operates is through three cognitive units: the central executive, which is assumed to be an attention-controlling system, and two "slave" systems termed the visuospatial sketch pad, which manipulates visual images, and the phonological loop, which stores and rehearses speech-based information (Figure 10.1) (Baddeley, 1992). This general framework of three major cognitive units has not changed considerably since first proposed by Baddeley. There has been further elaboration of cognitive subunits within each unit, which is described next.

The three key cognitive subunits that have been explored extensively for functional–anatomic correlates are storage, rehearsal/maintenance, and control processes. These cognitive subunits have been delineated as follows. The internal representations of information in working memory can be held by *rehearsal* of the information to prevent the contents of storage from being lost and have it remain accessible. *Storage* refers to the "holding" of information in a store for use. *Control processes* allow for manipulation of the information in the store. The rehearsal and store subunits are described for both the visuospatial sketchpad and phonological loop units, and control processes theoretically can be specific for each of these two units or shared across components and have been attributed to the central executive.

Clinical assessments of working memory have focused on the auditory storage and manipulation of information capacity of an individual. This is typically measured for an individual by how many units of information he or she can receive aurally and immediately repeat back. The most commonly used test to assess this is the Digit Span test from the WAIS-IV (Wechsler Adult Intelligence Scale IV; Wechsler, 2008). In the first part of the task, subjects are told numbers at a rate of one per second and asked to repeat them back to the examiner when the number string is completed. The longest string of numbers that a subject can repeat forward is called his or her forward span and is a marker of the individual's ability to register information. In the second part of the task, subjects are given a string similarly, but they must repeat the numbers backwards. The longest string of numbers repeated backwards in the correct order is referred to as an individual's backward span. This is viewed more as a measure of the working memory storage capacity of an individual because this includes the subject's ability to manipulate the information. There was also a visual version of the Digit Span task; however,

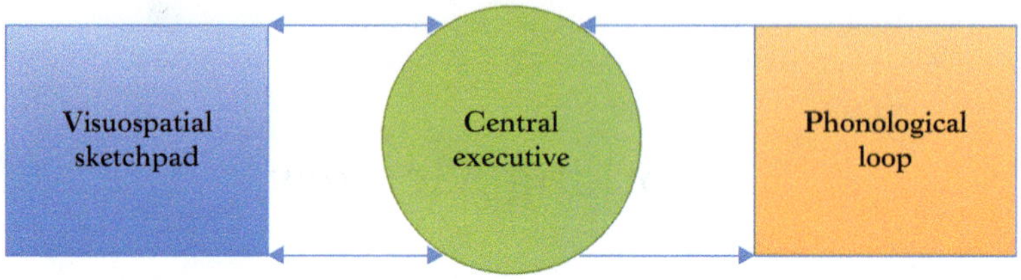

FIGURE 10.1: The three key components of Baddeley's model of working memory include the phonological loop for rehearsing an auditory input, visuospatial sketchpad for rehearsing a visual stimulus, and the central executive that can interact with either system to manipulate the stimulus.

Source: Baddeley (1992).

this was difficult to administer and has not been used extensively. Although this typically administered neuropsychological test measures working memory capacity as a whole, it does not address the cognitive units (phonological loop, visuospatial sketchpad, and central executive) or subunits (storage, rehearsal, and control processes) individually. It is assumed, but not validated except when done concurrently with functional magnetic resonance imaging (fMRI), that in performing a task such as the auditory Digit Span, the phonological loop is used as an auditory rehearsal process to maintain information. The visual Digit Span purported rehearses information to be maintained by visualizing the information using the visuospatial sketchpad. These assignations can only be inferred from Digit Span task performance because they are not assessed directly by the task.

Another neuropsychological type of assessment test that is being used more extensively in functional neuroimaging studies, but still assesses several aspects of the working memory system, is the *n*-back test (Kane et al., 2007). In this test, a subject is presented with a series of letters visually, one at a time, and then must indicate when a letter appears if it matches the letter that appeared *n* trials previously (with *n* being one, two, or three letters back in the series). The *n*-back task provides a continuous measure of a subject's ability to (1) process and monitor a series of stimuli; (2) maintain activation of relevant items; (3) discard recent, irrelevant information; and (4) make comparisons between various items in the series to identify a correct match. Thus, this task examines maintenance, manipulation, and monitoring of stimuli in working memory (Kane et al., 2007). Unfortunately, this test has not yet been normed for use as a clinical test.

TABLE 10.1: WORKING MEMORY SUMMARY

Brain Region	Function
Left DLPFC and underlying white matter	Manipulation of both verbal and spatial representations in working memory
Superior parietal lobule and its underlying white matter (left or right)	Manipulation and rearrangement of both verbal and spatial information in working memory

Another set of assessment tools are delay tasks, which consist of giving a subject information to hold/remember and varying the time delay between when the information was presented and when they must retrieve it and give the information back to the examiner. The amount of delay time that a person can hold the information is the best metric of rehearsal or maintenance abilities in assessing these cognitive subunits of working memory.

The third cognitive subunit, control processes of working memory, varies widely depending on the variety of tasks being asked of a subject and thus is not typically assessed as an independent clinical measure. For the control processes that have been evaluated within a clinical or research setting, functional–anatomic correlates are described later. Some of the control processes within working memory may be selective to a specific modality (e.g., auditory and visual) or general control processes that operate in multiple modalities.

The cognitive–anatomic units (CAUs; see Table 10.1) delineated for working memory are outlined here.

WORKING MEMORY NEURAL SYSTEMS

Extending from functional neuroimaging studies, the dorsolateral prefrontal cortex (DLPFC) plays a key role in working memory and was thus the logical place to assess for functional–anatomic correlates. Although it would have been proposed from fMRI studies that the DLPFC would support a CAU, initial studies of unilateral PFC lesions did not consistently disrupt storage or rehearsal processes in working memory (D'Esposito & Postle, 1999; D'Esposito et al., 2006). One of the reasons proposed for the lack of a unilateral lesion resulting in a deficit was that storage of information could be occurring in other brain regions and that rehearsal performance may rely on both hemispheres (D'Esposito et al., 2006; Muller & Knight, 2006).

Using a large sample of patients from the Vietnam Head Injury Study (VHIS; Barbey et al., 2013), investigators found that unilateral left DLPFC was not necessary for working memory maintenance, monitoring, or tasks that measure working memory performance. The study did find that the left DLPFC was essential for manipulating representations in working memory, as evidenced by patients' impairments on verbal manipulation. This was seen in relation to performance on the letter–number sequencing task and for spatial manipulation on the spatial span backwards task (Figure 10.2) (Barbey et al., 2013). The findings are most consistent with the DLPFC being multimodal (verbal and visual) for monitoring and manipulating information (Petrides, 2005). The authors noted that the lesions in these patients were not limited to the DLPFC but also included involvement of the superior longitudinal fasciculus, frontal aslant tract, and frontostriatal white matter tracts. It was proposed that for left DLPFC lesions to induce a deficit, these underlying white matter tracts need be included in the lesion. These tracts, if disrupted, can disconnect the DLPFC from key regions engaged in working memory and other functions such as the superior parietal cortex (superior longitudinal fasciculus), ventrolateral PFC from the bilateral medial premotor (frontal aslant tract), and DLPFC from the basal ganglia (frontostriatal tracts).

The importance of white matter involvement in lesions providing a "disconnection" between cortical regions in networks needs be considered in assessing for consistent lesion-deficit correlations, and this does appear to play a key factor in working memory (Barbey et al., 2013; Sepulcre et al., 2009). The lack of assessment for white matter involvement in other studies may lead to the inconsistency between findings across studies when white matter was involved in some studies and not in others.

Thus, the left DLPFC and underlying white matter were found to be associated with manipulation of both verbal and spatial representations to form a CAU, once an adequate sample from the VHIS study could be analyzed. In assessing for other regions engaged in working memory, patients from the VHIS registry were further explored. Individuals with significant damage to the superior parietal lobule (SPL) in either hemisphere ($n = 19$), a neurologically healthy group ($n = 55$), and patients with lesions that did not include the SPL in either hemisphere ($n = 146$) were administered a battery of

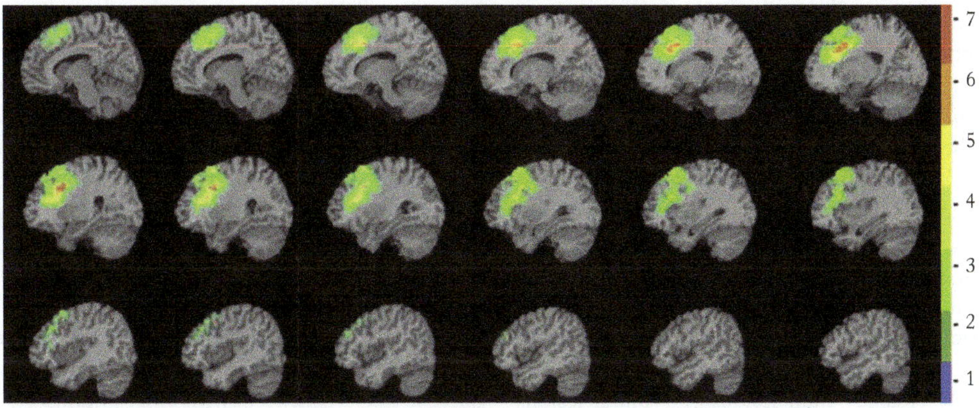

FIGURE 10.2: Lesion overlap map for DLPFC patients ($n = 7$) associated with disruption of spatial manipulation in working memory. The color indicates the number of patients with lesion extent to that region: Red designates greatest overlap and is in DLPFC in BA 9. The sagittal slices progress from the midline (top left) to the lateral left hemisphere (bottom right).

Source: Barbey et al. (2013).

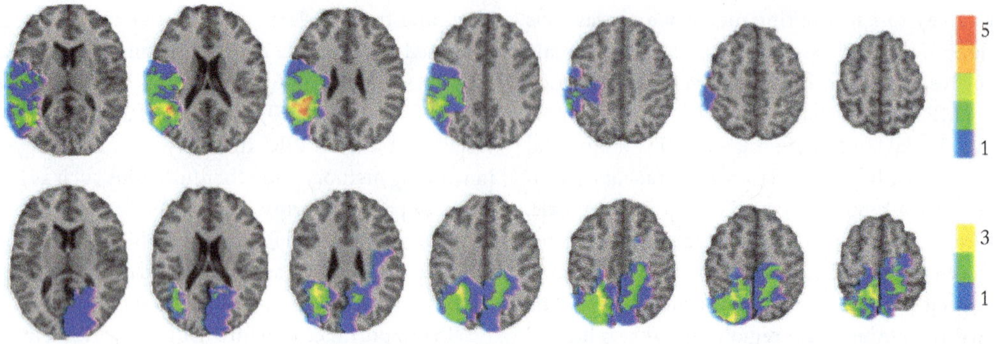

FIGURE 10.3: Lesion overlaps of right parietal lobe patients (n = 6) associated with disruption to manipulation and rearrangement of verbal and visual information in working memory. Color represents the number of overlapping lesions in a region. Lesion overlap on the right is shown in the top row; lesions are in the right IPL lateral and inferior to the intraparietal sulcus. The bottom row shows overlap for focal superior parietal lobe lesion patients, with overlap largely superior and medial to the intraparietal sulcus.

Source: Koenigs et al. (2009).

working memory tasks. This study found that those individuals with either right or left SPL damage displayed deficits in the manipulation and rearrangement of information within working memory but not the simple retention and retrieval of information in working memory (Figure 10.3). This localization was present for this cognitive unit for manipulation of multiple stimulus modalities, including auditory–verbal and visual–spatial stimuli, rendering it a multimodality CAU processing unit. As in the previous instance, it was noteworthy that the SPL lesions included both the gray matter and the underlying white matter of that region, which connects the SPL to the frontal lobes. Taken together, the overall finding is that a CAU consisting of the SPL and its underlying white matter connections is essential for the manipulation and rearrangement of information (both auditory and visual) in working memory (Koenigs et al., 2009).

The superior frontal gyrus (SFG) region had also been thought to be essential for working memory, although the nature of its involvement remained unclear. A key lesion study investigating the role of the SFG in working memory compared the performance of 8 patients with left prefrontal lesions restricted to the SFG with that of a group of 11 healthy control subjects and two groups of patients with other focal brain lesions (prefrontal lesions sparing the SFG (n = 5) and right parietal lesions (n = 4)) on a group of working memory n-back tasks using stimuli from different modalities and complexity. Patients with a left SFG lesion had selective working memory impairments for monitoring and manipulation functions across all modalities compared to the other groups, with the lateral and posterior portion of the SFG (mostly Brodmann area 8) appearing to be the key region within the SFG (Figure 10.4) (Boisgueheneuc et al., 2006). This was not a universal finding, however, because another group study of frontal lobe lesion patients found spatial and object 2-back impairments in 4 patients with damage affecting broad regions of (primarily left) lateral PFC but not SFG (n = 5) (Muller et al., 2002).

To aid in clarifying this issue, Tsuchida and Fellows (2009) studied 27 patients with focal prefrontal damage and 29 controls on n-back test performance. Analytic methods included qualitative lesion analyses, voxel-based lesion–symptom mapping (VBLSM) methods, and "lesion-defined" groupwise comparisons with the consensus from this study being that lesions involving the dorsal anterior cingulate cortex (ACC) and adjacent dorsal frontomedial cortex led to impairment on n-back tasks (Tsuchida & Fellows, 2009). The consistent error on these tasks was increased false positives, suggesting that this region may be involved in adjusting response bias (in this case, a bias toward not making any errors so that even if subjects were not sure if the item was n-back, they would say yes). Because this is consistent with other findings associated with dorsal ACC damage and the ability to stop a potential response, it appears likely that these adjacent regions—left superior frontal gyrus, dorsal ACC, and dorsal frontomedial cortices adjacent to ACC—may be involved in controlling response bias

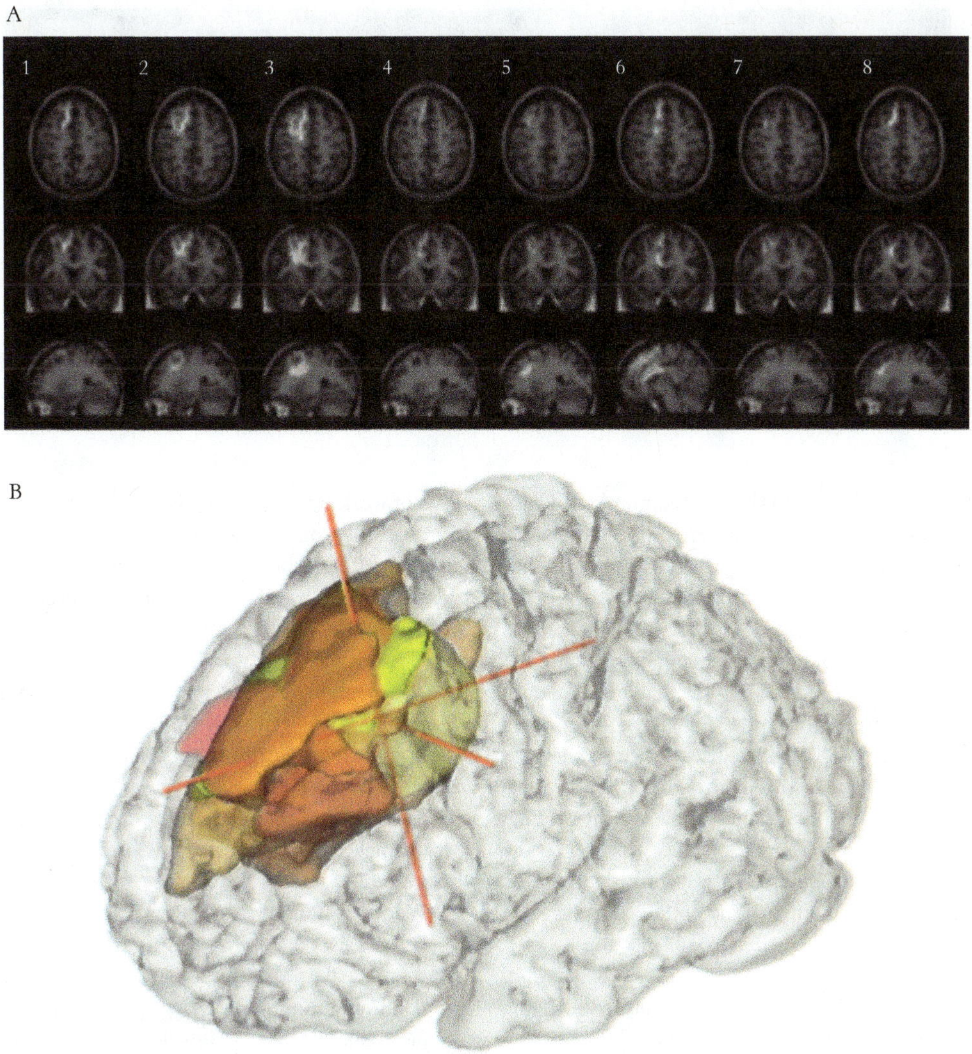

FIGURE 10.4: Lesion diagram and overlay of eight patients with SFG lesions. Panel A shows the extent of the lesions on (from top to bottom) axial, coronal, and sagittal MRI. Panel B shows three-dimensional overlap mapping of the eight lesions. The left SFG was found to be involved in all of the patients who had an associated general disruption in monitoring and manipulating working memory functions.

Source: Boisgueheneuc et al. (2006).

in working memory decisions. Overall, the data are not clear with regard to what role these dorsal midline structures play in working memory.

Regions related to other control operations, such as inhibiting irrelevant information from working memory, have also been investigated. Using the VBLSM approach, 61 stroke patients (31 right-sided and 30 left-sided) were investigated with a task in which "to-be-remembered" targets were presented together with task-irrelevant items. There was lesion overlap in the left putamen for patients with an impairment in hindering irrelevant information from entering working memory (Figure 10.5). These findings support models of working memory incorporating frontal lobe and basal ganglia structures whereby the basal ganglia structures, like the putamen, play a gatekeeping role by allowing only relevant information to enter prefrontal cortex circuits, where this information is then actively maintained in working memory (Baier et al., 2010). This is quite likely because the basal ganglia performs similar functions in other cognitive and motor

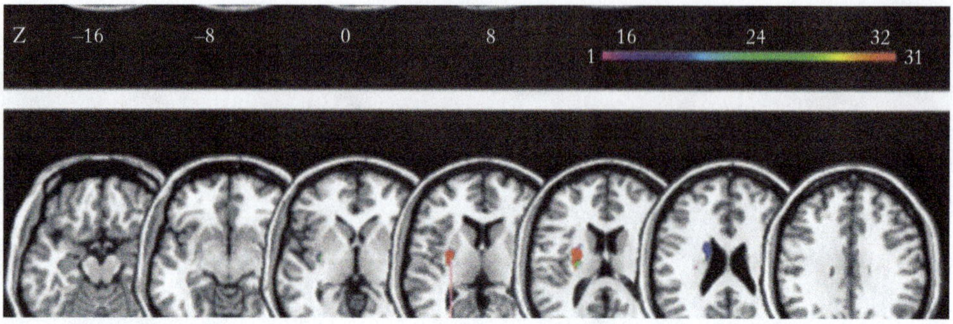

FIGURE 10.5: Patients with left-sided brain lesions were analyzed using VBLSM to assess performance on a modified delayed match-to-sample working memory task. Lesions of the putamen were associated with deficits in filtering ability.
Source: Baier et al. (2010).

tasks. However, due to the limited number of cases cited thus far and the number of individuals who have basal ganglia lesions but have not been shown to have this deficit, this will have to be further studied to determine if and where this specific basal ganglia localization of function should be attributed.

Control operations of working memory have also been associated with frontal cortical regions. Again, patients from the VHIS registry were studied and included veterans with a history of penetrating head injuries (n = 199), a neurologically healthy group of Vietnam veterans (n = 54), and a comparison group of brain-injured veterans with prefrontal cortex damage but without orbitofrontal cortex involvement (n = 40). When this group was administered a number of working memory tasks, Barbey et al. (2011) found that patients with lesions in the medial orbitofrontal cortex (Figure 10.6) were impaired on working memory tests that require the coordination of maintenance, manipulation, and monitoring processes (as assessed by total errors for 1-back, 2-back, and 3-back). This was interpreted as showing that the medial orbitofrontal cortex is essential for control functions underlying the coordination of working memory maintenance, manipulation, and monitoring processes (n-back task). However, this region was not found to be essential on pure tests of working memory maintenance (span tasks) or manipulation (span tasks and letter–number sequencing). Although these findings appear to be wide ranging and nonspecific, the authors proposed that the medial orbitofrontal region appears to be coordinating and integrating two or more of the component processes of the working memory system (Barbey et al., 2011). This is an important operation theoretically within a network system and needs to be explored further in relation to working memory and other cognitive domains to better ascertain how complex systems are controlled in cognition.

Working memory can be utilized on its own as a task or as a set of cognitive units as part of a larger task (e.g., "Call information to get the pizza parlor's phone number and order a large pepperoni pizza"). As such, one must also consider how the working memory cognitive units function within their own network to complete a dedicated working memory task and if those functions and their interrelationships differ if working memory is part of a larger network(s) to perform a more complex task(s). This must be considered in determining the consistent cognitive anatomic associations and may contribute to the lack of some inconsistent associations up to this point.

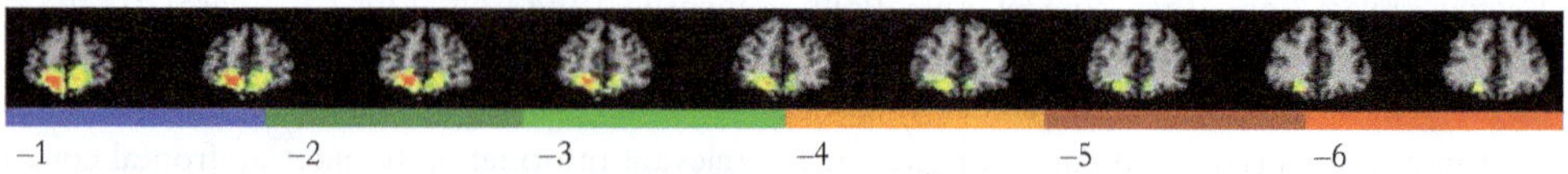

FIGURE 10.6: Lesion overlap of patients with medial orbitofrontal involvement. Color indicates the number of subjects with damage to a given voxel, showing maximal overlap occurring in the medial orbitofrontal cortex. (The right hemisphere is on the left side of the figure.)
Source: Barbey et al. (2011).

For example, it has been proposed that when part of another task involving other domains, working memory may be recruiting modality-specific working memory units (Martin & Chao, 2001). Working memory has been considered to be a part of the group of frontal lobe/cognitive control functions as noted previously. As such, one can postulate that working memory functions or aspects of certain functions may well be encoded as part of the an undifferentiated, generalized global adaptive anatomic system that can recruit resources (regions) from this global system depending the complexity and demands of the cognitive control operation (see Chapter 9). This has not been conclusively established for working memory; however, it is worth consideration as to why a set of functions that have been so deeply studied in both animals and humans, including delineation of dopamine as the major neurotransmitter engaged in the system's functioning, has not been consistently localized as to this point. Because general localizations to regions of the frontal and parietal lobes have been established for aspects of working memory units, assessing localizations as a function of how they change with changing complexity of a task. Further studies along these lines may lead to a clearer understanding of the type of anatomic localization these cognitive units have. It is important to consider that this is just one hypothesis; others are being considered to better understand the cognitive anatomic associations underlying working memory.

REFERENCES

Baddeley, A. (1992). Working memory. *Science, 255,* 556–559.

Baier, B., Karnath, H.-O., Dieterich, M., Birklein, F., Heinze, C., & Muller, N. (2010). Keeping memory clear and stable—The contribution of human basal ganglia and prefrontal cortex to working memory. *Journal of Neuroscience, 30*(29), 9788–9792.

Barbey, A., Koenigs, M., & Grafman, J. (2011). Orbitofrontal contributions to human working memory. *Cerebral Cortex, 21*(4), 789–795.

Barbey, A., Koenigs, M., & Grafman, J. (2013). Dorsolateral prefrontal contributions to human working memory. *Cortex, 49,* 1195–1205.

Boisgueheneuc, F., Levy, R., Volle, E., Seassau, M., Duffau, H., Kinkingnehun, S., et al. (2006). Functions of the left superior frontal gyrus in humans: A lesion study. *Brain, 129,* 3315–3328.

Courtney, S. (2004). Attention and cognitive control as emergent properties of information representation in working memory. *Cognitive, Affective, & Behavioral Neuroscience, 4*(4), 501–516.

D'Esposito, M., Cooney, J., Gazzaley, A., Gibbs, S., & Postle, B. (2006). Is the prefrontal cortex necessary for delay task performance? Evidence from lesion and FMRI data. *Journal of the International Neuropsychological Society, 12*(2), 248–260.

D'Esposito, M., & Postle, B. R. (1999). The dependence of span and delayed-response performance on prefrontal cortex. *Neuropsychologia, 37*(11), 1303–1315.

Gao, W., & Goldman-Rakic, P. (2003). Selective modulation of excitatory and inhibitory microcircuits by dopamine. *Proceedings of the National Academy of Sciences of the USA, 100*(5), 2836–2841.

Kane, M., Conway, A., Miura, T., & Colflesh, G. (2007). Working memory, attention control, and the *n*-back task: A question of construct validity. *Journal of Experimental Psychology: Learning, Memory, and Cognition, 33,* 615–622.

Koenigs, M., Barbey, A., Postle, B., & Grafman, J. (2009). Superior parietal cortex is critical for the manipulation of information in working memory. *Journal of Neuroscience, 29*(47), 14980–14986.

Lee, T., & D'Esposito, M. (2012). The dynamic nature of top-down signals originating from prefrontal cortex: A combined fMRI–TMS study. *Journal of Neuroscience, 32*(44), 15458–15466.

Martin, A., & Chao, L. (2001). Semantic memory and the brain: Structure and processes. *Current Opinion in Neurobiology, 11*(2), 194–201.

Muller, N., & Knight, R. (2006). The functional neuroanatomy of working memory: Contributions of human brain lesions studies. *Neuroscience, 139,* 51–58.

Muller, N., Machado, L., & Knight, R. (2002). Contributions of subregions of the prefrontal cortex to working memory: Evidence from brain lesions in humans. *Journal of Cognitive Neuroscience, 14*(5), 673–686.

Petrides, M. (2005). Lateral prefrontal cortex: Architectonic and functional organization. *Philosophical Transactions of the Royal Society of London B: Biological Sciences, 360*(1456), 781–795.

Procyk, E., & Goldman-Rakic, P. (2006). Modulation of dorsolateral prefrontal delay activity during self-organized behavior. *Journal of Neuroscience, 26*(44), 11313–11323.

Sepulcre, J., Masdeu, J., Pastor, M., Goni, J., Barbosa, C., Bejarano, B., et al. (209). Brain pathways of verbal working memory: A lesion–function correlation study. *Neuroimage, 47,* 773–778.

Tsuchida, A., & Fellows, L. (2009). Lesion evidence that two distinct regions within prefrontal cortex are critical for *n*-back performance in humans. *Journal of Cognitive Neuroscience, 21*(12), 2263–2275.

Wechsler, D. (2008). *Wechsler Adult Intelligence Scale—Fourth edition: Technical and interpretive manual.* San Antonio, TX: Pearson.

11

Emotional Organization

The previous chapters focused on specific units within a cognitive domain that were typically delineated experimentally and then associated with anatomic regions via activation and lesion studies to determine if a consistent dysfunction of that cognitive unit is associated with that lesion. This chapter on emotional states extends from initial observations of disrupted behaviors detected in patients with psychiatric disorders more so than experimental investigations of deconstructed subunits of an emotion in a reductionist manner. As a result, this chapter on emotion is more symptom- or syndrome-driven in terms of the behavioral phenomena associated with anatomic correlates. The reasons for this approach are addressed throughout the chapter, but in general, it is due to behavioral/emotional states being supported more by a balance between interconnected neurotransmitter systems than are cognitive systems. Also, the field is still evolving as emotional processing is delineated into more finer-grained units that can be isolated and associated with anatomic regions, networks, or transmitter systems.

In addition, compared to the other localizations in this book, those reported in this chapter for psychiatric disorders and emotional dysfunction do not consistently lead to the psychiatric disorder associated with it unless otherwise noted in Table 11.1. There is not as clear of a cognitive–anatomic unit (CAU)-type relationship of circumscribed lesion localization and behavioral dysfunction for emotional states as there is for cognitive states. In general, the localizations described here for emotional states apply if the dysfunction occurs acutely (or subacutely) after a brain lesion. In many instances, a lesion in the areas described does not lead to disruption of the emotional state.

There have been numerous reports of psychiatric disorders developing after focal brain lesions, which initially were not routinely localized to a specific region. In the 1980s, the work of Robinson and colleagues on affective disorders associated with strokes provided one of the first proposed laterality-based accounts of mood dysfunction. They proposed that left hemisphere strokes were associated with depression and that right-sided lesions were associated with manic disorders (Robinson et al., 1983, 1984). Further studies of affective and other psychiatric disorders with brain lesions have led to several proposed anatomic correlates and are described in the following sections.

DEPRESSION

As noted previously, the initial localization of mood dysfunction with focal lesions was a broad generalization that, if developing a mood disorder after a stroke, left hemisphere strokes result in a depressive disorder and right hemisphere strokes result in manic symptoms (Robinson et al., 1983, 1984). It is important to emphasize the factor of "if a mood disorder develops."

Again, several reasons have been offered as to why mood dysfunction does not correlate as consistently as those of cognition, including but not limited to the following: (1) The symptom complexes that group to define psychiatric disorders are best described by (and treated using) dysfunctional neurotransmitter systems; (2) these neurotransmitter systems, except regions that are major nuclei of transmitter production/transmission, do not organize anatomically by focal regions; (3) pre-existing status of neurotransmitter levels/systems plays a significant role in the development of emotional dysfunction when an acute insult occurs; and/or (4) the interaction between the multiple different neurotransmitter systems and the equilibrium developed to maintain an emotional state can lead to variable results after a lesion. Neurotransmitter levels and the equilibrium with other transmitter systems play a major role in the outcome of lesions that affect the emotional systems, particularly mood.

TABLE 11.1: EMOTION SUMMARY

Brain Region	Function
Subgenual prefrontal cortex/ventral anterior cingulate cortex	Depression
Pallidum (globus pallidus and the ventral pallidum)	Depression
Right caudate or thalamus	Mania
Caudate; orbitofrontal cortex	OCD
Basal ganglia	Apathy
Medial orbitofrontal region and connections	Apathy
Ventromedial frontal lobe	Disinhibition*
Bilateral temporal lobes	Kluver–Bucy syndrome*

*Similar to other chapters in that lesion reliably results in dysfunction noted.

Considering that a left hemisphere stroke did not routinely lead to depression, this laterality-based approach led to a lack of enthusiasm in applying these findings clinically. In addition, there was a lack of clarity at the time as to whether the mood dysfunction was secondary to an emotional response of the patient to the "deficit" that he or she had experienced—a loss of neurological function, occupation, and social function. Robinson and colleagues went on to demonstrate that post-stroke depression was associated with left hemisphere anterior lesions, and the more severe the depression, the more involvement of the frontal pole (Robinson et al., 1983, 1984). This last point that frontal lobe volume correlates with the degree of depression argues against the notion of a response to a deficit being the etiology of the depression in these individuals, even if a larger frontal lobe lesion may have resulted in more functional neurological deficit. For example, a possible worsening of a neurological condition (a more severe aphasia) was taken into account in these later studies.

These initial gross localizations were followed by more extensive investigations. For example, a population-based study of 142 patients with strokes were assessed in the hospital in the relatively acute state after the incident and then were followed longitudinally 1 or 2 years later for the presence of depressive symptoms and lesion location. The findings immediately after the strokes validated the previous claims of Robinson et al. (1983, 1984) that as a group initially following a stroke, depressive symptoms were more likely to be associated with having a left hemisphere stroke, being near the left frontal pole, and depression severity associated with lesion volume in the immediate setting. However, 1 or 2 years post-stroke, depression was associated with right hemisphere lesion volume and proximity of the lesion to the occipital pole (Shimoda & Robinson, 1999; see also Narushima et al., 2003). These types of studies that showed shifting anatomical correlates of mood disruption over time cast further skepticism over a localizationist approach to mood disorders, particularly if striving for a standard of consistent localizations of focal brain regions with specific mood dysfunction. Subsequent studies uncovered different regions associated with depression (Singh et al., 2000) or found no correlations of lesion and depression (Carson et al., 2000). An extensive meta-analysis of the literature up to that time found no strong evidence even of left hemispheric lesion laterality being associated with depression (Bhogal et al., 2004).

An alternative account has been proposed that white matter hyperintensities (WMH) and lacunar infarcts are associated with the development of depression in older subjects and that these lesions must first be present for the development of depression after a cortical/subcortical lesion occurs in older individuals. In a study of 626 older subjects, depressive symptoms were correlated with WMH in the frontal and temporal lobes but not WMH in the occipital or parietal lobes, basal ganglia lacunar strokes, or lacunar strokes in other regions (O'Brien et al., 2006). These widespread white matter correlates with depression need to be further investigated and better specified if they are going to be considered as a more consistent correlate.

Overall, these initial gross localizations by hemisphere or lobe for depression appeared inconclusive. Further investigations have shown more specific and consistent localizations of mood dysfunction with focal lesions. This newer evidence for the association of specific brain regions with mood dysfunction extends from a variety of studies. One specific focal region, the ventral anterior cingulate

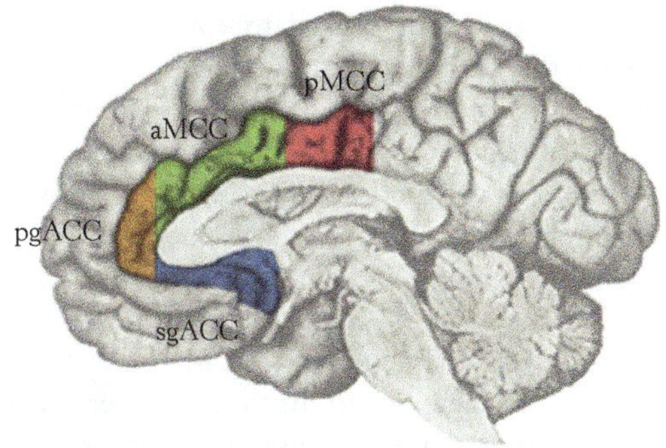

FIGURE 11.1: The area in blue designates the subgenual anterior corpus callosum.

Source: http://www.nature.com.

cortical region (also referred to as the prefrontal cortex ventral to the genu of the corpus callosum) (Figure 11.1), has been investigated with a variety of neuroinvestigative techniques, each consistently demonstrating abnormalities in this region being associated with clinical symptoms of depression. Postmortem histopathology evaluations of patients with depressive disorders in the prefrontal region ventral to the corpus callosum have shown decreased gray matter volume, which consisted of glia cell loss without neuronal cell loss (Drevets et al., 1998). This region's association with depression has been confirmed in neuroimaging studies of patients with mood disorders who had abnormal blood flow to this ventral anterior cingulate region (Drevets et al., 1997). Magnetic resonance imaging (MRI) morphometric measures also supported this localization when reduced gray matter volume was reported in the ventral anterior cingulate of bipolar patients compared to controls (Figure 11.2). The clearest morphometric evidence that neuronal loss in this region is associated with depressive symptoms is from a postmortem analysis of 60 subjects with major depressive disorder, bipolar disorder, or schizophrenia. The findings in these postmortem brains were reduced neuronal size in cortical layer 1 in the caudal orbitofrontal cortex in bipolar disease and in layer 3 in major depression with no cellular loss noted in those with schizophrenia, suggesting this region's involvement in only affective disorders and not psychiatric disorders in general (Cotter et al., 2005). An account for why damage to this subgenual anterior cingulate cortex (ACC) region could result in depressive symptoms has been put forth suggesting that dysfunction in this region can lead to abnormal autonomic responses to emotional

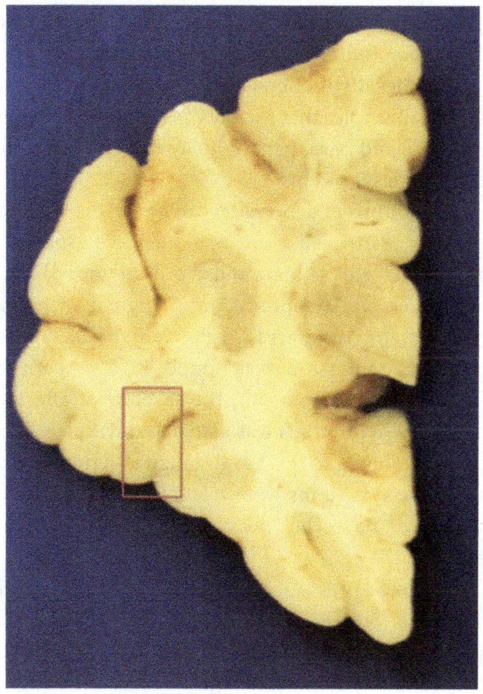

FIGURE 11.2: Coronal section through the right hemisphere of a formalin-fixed brain showing the level at which the caudal orbitofrontal cortex was sampled. The square box encloses the lateral wall of the orbitofrontal sulcus.

Source: Cotter et al. (2005).

experiences, an inability to experience emotion related to issues that are ordinarily emotional, and/or an inability to use information regarding punishment or reward in social situations (Bechara et al., 1994).

Even with the morphometric studies noted that demonstrate an association between mood and the subgenual ACC region, there are few studies showing that a lesion in that region consistently results in depression compared to CAUs of cognitive function. Thus, although there is an association between depressive symptoms and subgenual ACC, it is not listed in Table 11.1 as a CAU, which signifies that when a lesion does occur in the subgenual ACC, no consistent cognitive/behavioral deficit is being detected.

Other regions with a similar pattern of localization that are implicated in depression have emerged from frontal–subcortical circuits, particularly basal ganglia structures. In a study of 70 patients with strokes, a logistic regression analysis showed that those with lesions in the pallidum of the basal ganglia had a markedly increased risk of post-stroke depression (odds ratio = 7.2) (Vataja et al., 2004).

Further distinctions have been made regarding the possible roles that each of these regions (pregenual ACC and basal ganglia) play in depression and depressive symptoms.

Symptoms of depression can be viewed in terms of those associated more with affective aspects of depression (e.g., sadness and depressed mood) compared to those symptoms more aligned with apathy (e.g., loss of interest). In a study of 243 stroke patients, depression was found in 126 patients (51.9%). More important, the severity of affective depressive symptoms was associated with left frontal lobe (but not the basal ganglia) damage, and apathetic symptoms were related to bilateral basal ganglia damage (but not the frontal lobe) (Hama et al., 2007).

As noted previously with regard to hemispheric lateralization for mood dysfunction, it has been suggested that lesions in the previously described cortical and subcortical regions (e.g., the subgenual prefrontal cortex/ventral anterior cingulate cortex and pallidum) may be inadequate to result in post-stroke depression but that depression can develop after an acute stroke in those regions only if there had been significant accumulation of white matter microvascular lesions prior to the acute stroke (Santos et al., 2009). In addition, many of the symptoms associated with depression (e.g., fatigue, sleep disturbances, memory and attention deficits, and reduced thinking) after stroke are also present in post-stroke patients who do not have depression. Thus, in assessing for functional–anatomic localizations of mood, it is essential to assess for the entire pattern of symptoms to confirm the presence of a significant, clinical depressive disorder (Gainotti et al., 1999) and to assess the pattern of lesions to networks associated with emotional state.

Limbic–Cortical– Striatal–Pallidal–Thalamic Circuit

Studies have investigated depression after lesions involving a circuit of regions engaged in mood regulation referred to as the limbic–cortical–striatal–pallidal–thalamic (LCSPT) circuit, which is formed by connections between the orbital and medial prefrontal cortex, amygdala, hippocampus, ventromedial striatum of the basal ganglia (nucleus accumbens and olfactory tubercle), mediodorsal and midline thalamic nuclei, and ventral pallidum (Ongur et al., 2003). The LCSPT circuit initially was related to emotional behavior on the basis of the anatomical connectivity between the regions in the circuit and connections to structures that control emotional responses. Dysfunction within the circuit alters transmission in various ways and can produce the pathological emotional symptoms (Drevets et al., 2004; Nauta & Domesick, 1984). The orbital and medial prefrontal cortices involved in the LCSPT circuit have extensive connections to limbic and visceral control structures (hypothalamus and periaqueductal gray) (Ongur & Price, 2000; Saleem et al., 2008). This is referred to as the visceromotor system, and it is particularly involved in mood and emotion, as well as the visceral reactions to emotional stimuli. Pharmacological, neurosurgical, and deep brain stimulation treatments for mood disorders appear to suppress pathological activity within visceromotor network structures such as the subgenual anterior cingulate cortex, amygdala, and ventral striatum (Drevets & Price, 2005; Drevets et al., 2002). Permanent lesions that affect this circuit can be associated with depression. In a study of 68 stroke patients, 21 patients (31%) were found to have major depressions with larger lesions (~3000 mm^3) in the LCSPT circuit, with the ventral (BA24) and dorsal anterior cingulate cortex (BA32) and subgenual cortex (BA25) being the regions of the circuit most associated with depression (Terroni et al., 2011), consistent with the findings discussed previously.

Overall, the optimal localizations that appear to be associated with depression if it occurs after an acute event are the ventral anterior cingulate (subgenual) cortical region and the pallidum of the basal ganglia (globus pallidus and the ventral pallidum). An individual with a lesion in these regions may have a higher probability of developing depression if he or she has a previous history of white matter hyperintensities consistent with microvascular disease.

ANXIETY

Focal lesions that result in the production of an anxiety state have only recently been investigated. One study evaluated 73 patients 3 months post-stroke to assess for the prevalence of anxiety and found that 21% of these patients met criteria for clinically significant disorders. Further analysis revealed that the presence of a left hemisphere lesion was a significant predictor of who would develop an anxiety disorder (Barker-Collo, 2007); however, more specific localization beyond hemispheric was not performed.

The hippocampus has been implicated in studies of emotional states. Previous studies have suggested that the hippocampus is functionally subdivided into dorsal and ventral regions, each associated with a distinct set of behaviors. Dorsal hippocampus has been proposed to be engaged in learning and memory, with the ventral hippocampus appearing to have a preferential role in anxiety-related behaviors. The latter's role in emotional processing is also distinct from that of the amygdala, which is associated specifically with fear (Bannerman et al., 2004). In a study of 182 Vietnam War veterans with penetrating brain injuries, a voxel-based lesion–symptom mapping analysis showed a significant association between anxiety and lesions in cortical and limbic areas of the left hemisphere, including the mesial temporal lobe structures of the hippocampus, parahippocampal gyrus, amygdala, and insula, along with the fusiform gyrus and the inferior occipital lobe. These localizations were verified with further comparison to a control group of combat veterans without brain injury (Figure 11.3) (Knutson et al., 2013).

Other candidate regions associated with the development of anxiety are other temporal lobe structures and the thalamus. A study that assessed 26 patients with acute middle cerebral artery infarction at 1 week and 1 month post-stroke found that the right superior and middle temporal gyri were associated with anxiety at 1 month after stroke (Ku et al., 2013). Sixty-eight patients with previous ischemic thalamic strokes were examined along with 34 age-matched controls who only had a history of previous transient ischemic attacks. Those with posterior thalamic lesions were noted to have elevated anxiety levels. The anxiety was postulated to extend from damage to the connections between the medial pulvinar and extrathalamic regions involved in affective processing (Lindermann et al., 2013).

For the localizations associated with anxiety, further studies are necessary for any of these findings related to anxiety to be considered consistent correlations because, again, a lesion in the candidate regions does not always result in increased anxiety. In addition, anxiety is not always assessed after brain lesions, and including assessment may also increase the ability to further localize lesions to this mood disorder.

MANIA

The incidence of mania following acute stroke is very low, approximately 1% (Starkstein et al., 1991). Although rare in occurrence, there has been relative consistency regarding the location of the lesion associated with these manic conditions. Thus, it is the same situation as for depression: When post-lesion

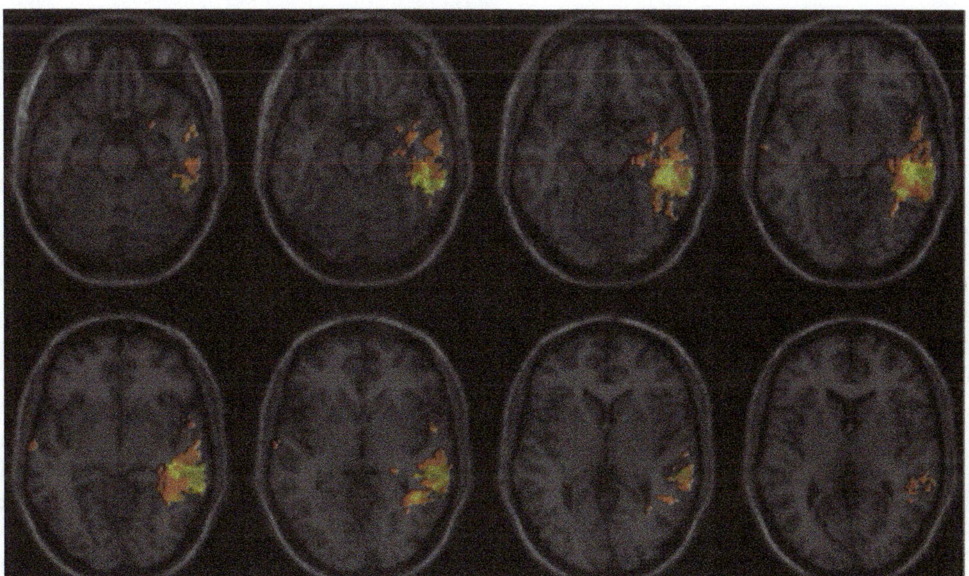

FIGURE 11.3: Color indicates brain regions where the association between lesion location and NRS anxiety score is statistically significant.

Source: Knutson et al. (2013).

mania occurs, the lesion is in a relatively consistent location. Conversely, a lesion in these locations does not consistently result in mania.

The regions that have been most consistently associated with mania are subcortical structures. Specifically, in a study of 19 patients with post-stroke mania, Starkstein et al. (1991) found that those who experienced both mania and depression had lesions involving the right caudate or right thalamus (see also Vuilleumier et al., 1998). The thalamic localization has been further confirmed in individual studies. A young man with bilateral dorsomedial nuclei infarcts (Figure 11.4) presented after the lesions occurred with temporary manic symptoms consisting of restlessness, mood elevation, a tendency for pleasurable activities, inflated self-esteem, sexual disinhibition, and a reduced need for food and sleep. As in previous cases with thalamic lesions and mania, these patients also demonstrate a significant episodic memory impairment from the thalamic lesion due to the extent of the lesion involving regions of the Papez circuit. It has been proposed that this lesion results in manic behavior by disrupting frontosubcortical connections—specifically the right orbitofrontal–thalamic loop, which is involved in mood regulation, and the dorsolateral prefrontal–thalamic loop, which mediates cognitive control functions (Benke et al., 2002).

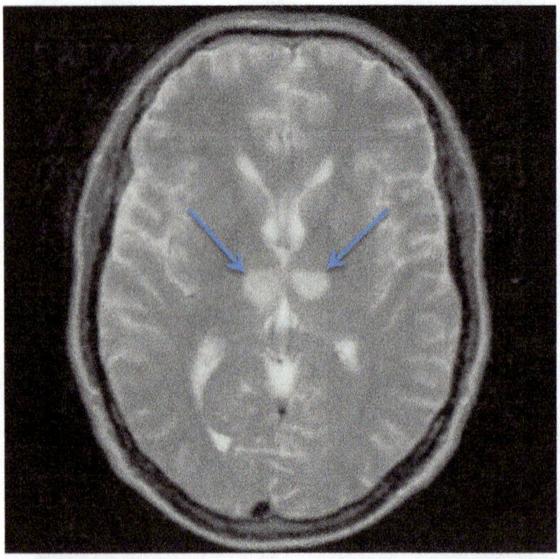

FIGURE 11.4: MRI showing bilateral ischemic lesion, including both dorsomedial thalami; the lesion also includes parts of the intralaminar and anterior nuclei.

Source: Benke et al. (2002).

OBSESSIVE–COMPULSIVE DISORDER

Obsessive–compulsive disorder (OCD), characterized by intrusive thoughts that lead to ritualized or stereotypical motor behavior, has been associated with dysfunction of frontal and/or basal ganglia regions. Patients with frontal lobe lesions in general have been reported to have increased compulsive behaviors but not necessarily significant in occurrence to qualify as a clinical disorder; However, for present purposes, the focus here is on lesions resulting in the full psychiatric disorder of OCD.

One early indication of localization of OCD symptoms came from neuroimaging of the response to treatment. Successful treatment with selective serotonin reuptake inhibitors has been shown to reduce markers of neural activity in the caudate and orbitofrontal cortices as OCD symptoms are diminished (Baxter et al., 1992). These findings led to multiple investigations to delineate the group of brain regions involved in OCD (Figure 11.5), and lesion studies have suggested some specific functions that these regions support and how they may be implicated in OCD. The two key regions that continued to be implicated with further studies were the caudate or the orbitofrontal cortices (for review, see Huey et al., 2008).

Basal ganglia lesions, typically caudate, have resulted in OCD-like syndromes in multiple reported cases (Berthier et al., 1996; Chacko et al., 2000; Laplane et al., 1989). This is true whether the patients' etiology was stroke, degenerative disease (Huntington's disease), or post-infectious (Cummings & Cunningham, 1992; Swedo et al., 1998). It was postulated from these studies that caudate disruption leads to dysregulation of the orbitofrontal cortex in which obsessive thoughts have been proposed to be generated, leading to overproduction of these intrusive thoughts.

The involvement of the orbitofrontal region and its possible role in OCD also extend from data collected on leukotomies performed in this region as a treatment for patients with OCD. A leukotomy is a neurosurgical procedure that consists of disrupting the connections between the anterior parts of the frontal lobes of the brain to treat psychiatric disorders that were refractive to medication management (Freeman & Watts, 1939). Irle et al. (1998) reported that in the 16 OCD patients who had been treated with ventromedial frontal leukotomy (Figure 11.6), the subsequent disruption of the white matter

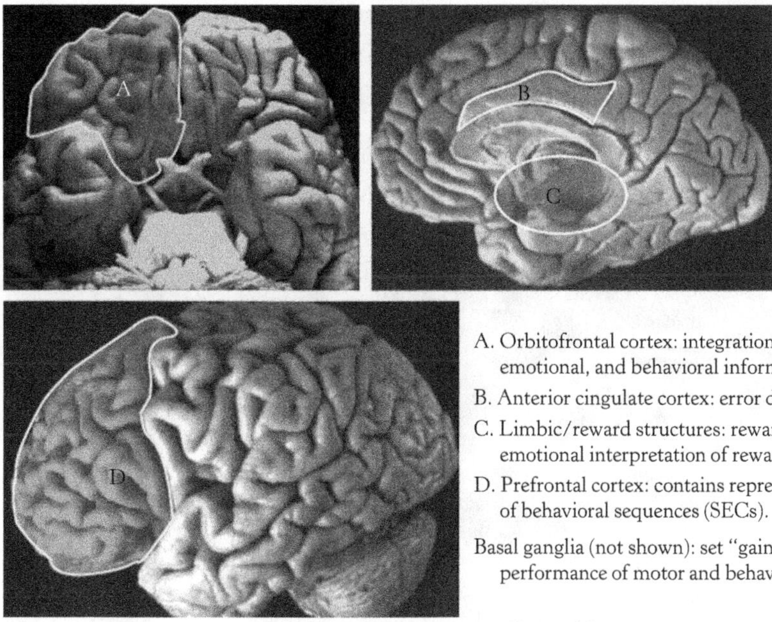

A. Orbitofrontal cortex: integration of reward, emotional, and behavioral information
B. Anterior cingulate cortex: error detection
C. Limbic/reward structures: reward signal and emotional interpretation of reward signal
D. Prefrontal cortex: contains representations of behavioral sequences (SECs).
Basal ganglia (not shown): set "gain" for performance of motor and behavioral sequences

FIGURE 11.5: Regions associated with obsessive–compulsive disorder.
Source: Huey et al. (2008).

pathways from the orbitofrontal lobe to the basal ganglia reduced OCD symptoms.

A proposed mechanism for compulsive behaviors extends from animal studies, which have shown that disruption of the orbitofrontal cortex in animals results in their continual performance of repetitive behaviors. These repetitive behaviors would continue to occur even without reward given for the behavior. It was thus hypothesized that a normally functioning orbitofrontal region allows for disengagement from repetitive behaviors. The role of the basal ganglia in this circuit was proposed to perform gating operations to stop unproductive behaviors (O'Reilly & Frank, 2006; for review, see Ramsey et al., 2011), and that if lesions to this gating were to occur, there would develop repetitive behaviors that would continue unchecked. Gating in this behavioral and neural sense is when a neural circuit allows in or redirects/inhibits a signal from passing from one region to another for processing. In the case of compulsive, repetitive behaviors, dysfunctional gating most likely leads to not allowing a specific behavior to be resolved and move to other behaviors, but the impaired gating keeps the behavior in a repetitive cycle. Impaired gating could also refer to allowing a behavior into a repetitive neural loop as opposed to normally blocking it from entering that type of circuit. Further mapping of these circuits will allow for better specification of whether this is an impaired gating mechanism and the aspects of gating that are disrupted to lead to circuitous, repetitive behaviors. This level of specifying an emotional dysfunction in terms of a neural mechanism should be considered a prototype to strive for because this account of a dysfunctional behavior as a recurring electrical loop located in specific regions lends itself to a therapeutic intervention with electrical stimulation disrupting the repetitive loop. It is important to note that lesions in the caudate and/or orbitofrontal cortex do not routinely result in OCD.

KLUVER–BUCY SYNDROME

Kluver–Bucy syndrome, a disorder consisting of hypersexuality, hyperorality, and hyperaggressiveness, was originally described secondary to bilateral anterior temporal lobe lesions in monkeys (Kluver & Bucy, 1939). It has also been described in humans in association with bilateral lesions to the medial temporal lobes (Marlowe et al., 1975; Terzian & Ore, 1955) with the assertion that one of the key structures disrupted that leads to these behaviors is the amygdalae in the medial temporal lobes.

Kluver–Bucy syndrome has been reported in a variety of clinical conditions, including bilateral temporal lobectomy (Terzian & Ore, 1955), Pick's disease (Cummings & Duchen, 1981),

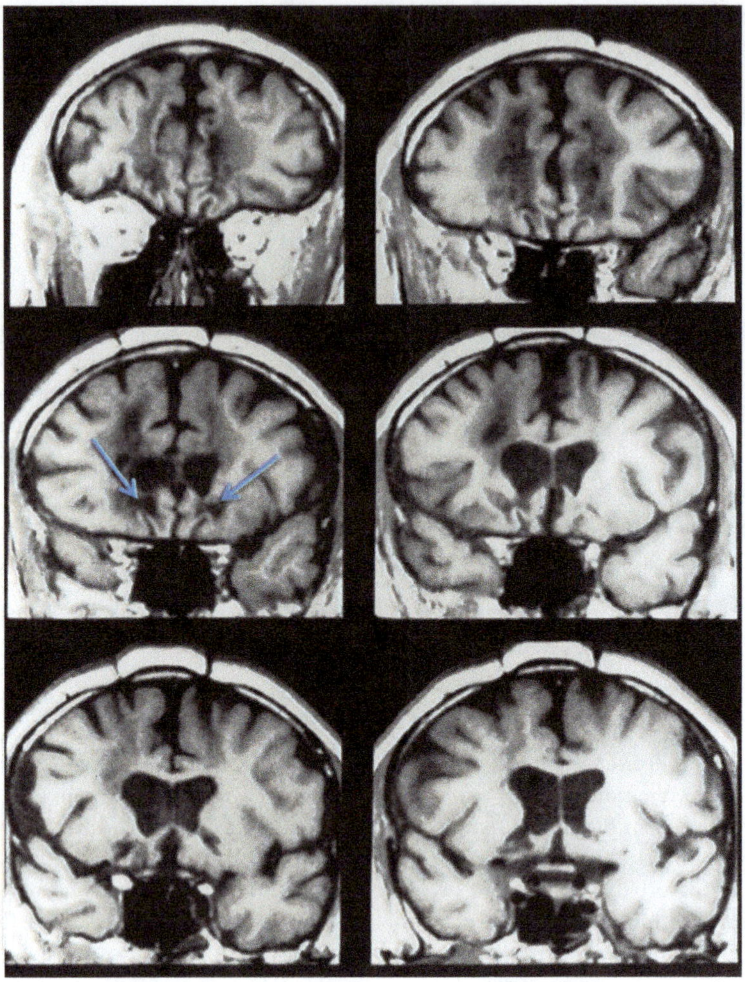

FIGURE 11.6: MRI scans of a subject show a lesion in the ventromedial frontal region associated with OCD.

Source: Irle et al. (1998).

traumatic brain injury (Gerstenbrand et al., 1983; Hardy & Aldridge, 1981), herpes simplex encephalitis (Chutorian & Antunes, 1981), epilepsy (Nakada et al., 1984), systemic lupus erythematosus (Oliveira et al., 1989), anoxic encephalopathy (Sandson et al., 1988), frontotemporal degeneration (Filley & Cullum, 1993), mycoplasma pneumonia (Daxboeck, 2006), and Alzheimer's disease with amygdala involvement (Kile et al., 2009).

In the majority of the previously mentioned cases, the patients had bilateral temporal lobe damage, typically medial temporal involvement. As opposed to the other emotion state–anatomic lesion correlations discussed in this chapter in which the lesion does not consistently produce the emotional state disruption, in the case of Kluver–Bucy syndrome, bilateral medial temporal lesions including the amygdala do lead in a relatively consistent manner to the behavioral disruptions described.

The only other region suggested to be associated with Kluver–Bucy syndrome is the thalamus. A patient developed Kluver–Bucy syndrome after small bilateral ischemic lesions in the thalami. It was proposed that this resulted from disruption of the pathways connecting the dorsomedial thalami with the prefrontal cortices and with other limbic regions (Müller et al., 1999). Further disconnection cases will need to be reported for this to be considered a consistent localization.

FRONTAL APATHY

Marin (1991) described apathy as a psychiatric disorder characterized by reduced goal-directed behavior (lack of effort and initiative), reduced goal-directed cognition (decreased interests, lack of plans and goals, and lack of concern), and flat affect/ emotional indifference.

One set of reports identified apathy as a disorder based on its emergence as a relatively isolated cognitive dysfunction after patients underwent prefrontal lobotomy for treatment of aggressive and/or disinhibited behavior. In a classic article by Walter Freeman and James Watts (1936) that reviewed 48 cases of prefrontal lobectomy, the authors came to the following conclusion about the frontal lobes:

> They assemble the available data, synthesize them, plan a course of action with the ideal in mind, and, equipped with energy of response and with appropriate affective tone, project the individual into the future, direct him toward his goal—and criticize his shortcomings.

The underlying mechanisms responsible for apathy have been divided into disruption of one or both of two processing circuits: "emotional" and "auto-activation" (Levy & Dubois, 2006). Apathy due to disturbances of "emotional" processing refers to disruptions in the circuitry between the orbitomedial prefrontal cortex and basal ganglia (e.g., ventral striatum, ventral pallidum, and caudate). Disruption of "auto-activation" processing refers to the inability to self-initiate actions contrasting with a relatively spared ability to generate externally driven behavior. It is responsible for the most severe form of apathy, and in most cases the lesions affect bilaterally the associative and limbic territories of the internal portion of the globus pallidus. In both situations, the capacity of the frontal cortex to select, initiate, maintain, and shift programs of actions is impaired.

One key clinical condition that can result in damage to these circuits is rupture of an anterior communicating artery aneurysm, which can result in damage to the orbitomedial prefrontal cortices and present with amnesia and a personality change described as flattening of affect (Greene et al., 1995). The other conditions that can present with apathy are dementing illnesses. Patients with frontotemporal dementia (FTD), particularly those with behavioral variant social and executive deficits (bvFTD), are associated with a significant breakdown in goal-directed motivated behavior secondary to disruption of cortical–basal ganglia circuits, which also results in social and executive function deficits (Eslinger et al., 2012). In another study of 62 patients with FTD, severity of apathy was found to be correlated with atrophy in the right dorsolateral prefrontal cortex (Zamboni et al., 2008). Individuals with the previously noted lesions and/ or conditions do not reliably develop apathy; rather, if apathy is detected relatively acutely in an individual or occurs progressively with a degenerative condition, the conditions noted are likely etiologies.

FRONTAL DISINHIBITION

In 1848, a tamping iron penetrated 25-year-old Phineas Gage's face and skull, which led to a marked change in his personality. This previously affable, hard-working man became socially inappropriate and remarkably irresponsible (Damasio et al., 1994). The penetrating lesion associated with his lack of inhibition damaged the left orbitofrontal cortex, mesial frontal cortices, and anterior cingulate gyrus and also the right mesial orbital region, polar frontal cortices, and anterior cingulate gyrus. The white matter core of the frontal lobes was more extensively damaged in the left hemisphere than in the right hemisphere. This finding led to the proposal that decision-making within the social domain—leading to disinhibited behavior when dysfunctional—is dependent on the ventromedial frontal region, with the finding of disinhibition occurring relatively consistently after a lesion to the region.

Frontal lobe dysfunction may underlie the excessively impulsive and risky behavior observed in a range of neurological disorders. Gambling tasks were used as a probe to examine these behavioral tendencies in a sample of patients who had sustained focal damage and demonstrated elements of disinhibition. In an extensive study of patients with frontal lobe lesions, those with non-frontal lobe lesions, and control subjects, risk-taking performance strategies were found to be associated with left ventrofrontal lobe lesions. It was proposed that left ventromedial frontal lobe lesions resulted in disruption of the reward-based aspects of decision-making that lead to increased risk-taking (Floden et al., 2008). There is also confirmation of this localization and an increased incidence of occurrence of disinhibition in dementing illnesses. In a study of 157 patients with neurodegenerative disease, social disinhibition was associated with orbitofrontal atrophy (Krueger et al., 2011).

Another set of regions have been implicated in a lack of inhibition from a study of 62 patients with FTD. In that patient group, the severity of disinhibition correlated with atrophy in the right nucleus accumbens, right superior temporal sulcus, and right mediotemporal limbic structures (Zamboni et al., 2008). Further studies supporting this localization are needed to confirm that it is a consistent finding.

It is of note that the regions referred to as the medial aspects of the ventral frontal lobes and their connections are associated with two distinctly different disorders: apathy and disinhibition. The localization of the regions associated with these two conditions has not been exact enough to be able to clearly tease apart differing frontal lobe regions that may be distinctly associated with each condition, or there may be regions of neurons and/or firing patterns in these regions to account for both types of behavioral symptoms. In addition, there is a great deal of variability in the anatomic organization of this region in normal individuals. However, the most likely reason why lesions in close proximity in the ventral frontal lobe can lead to such differing conditions is that it is not just the frontal lesions themselves but also the connections to other, likely different, brain regions that are disrupted with each of these two types of frontal lesions, leading to different disconnections resulting in different behavioral outcomes.

As noted at the beginning of the chapter, most of the behavior/emotional state associations with anatomic correlates do not have the same type of relationships as do the CAUs described in other chapters. Also, when lesions resulting in emotional state changes do occur, the resultant behavioral changes are typically not of a single behavioral unit but, rather, collections of co-occurring behavioral symptoms. This is secondary to the behavioral/emotional state systems being defined more so by networks of regions related to the regions sharing the same neurotransmitter. This has led to terrific gains in treatment from medications that modulate an entire neurotransmitter system. Greater delineations of these emotional states into dissociable behavioral units (e.g., OCD symptoms) will noticeably advance our understanding of behavior and possibly lead to further advancements in developing options to modulate dysfunctional behavior.

REFERENCES

Bannerman, D., Rawlins, J., McHugh, S., et al. (2004). Regional dissociations with the hippocampus—Memory and anxiety. *Neuroscience and Biobehavioral Reviews, 28*, 273–283.

Barker-Collo, S. (2007). Depression and anxiety 3 months post-stroke prevalence and correlates. *Archives of Clinical Neuropsychology, 22*(4), 519–531.

Baxter, L., Schwartz, J., Bergman, K., et al. (1992). Caudate glucose metabolic rate changes with both drug and behavior therapy for obsessive–compulsive disorder. *Archives of General Psychiatry, 49*, 681–689.

Bechara, A., Damasio, A., Damasio, H., & Anderson, S. (1994). Insensitivity to future consequences following damage to human prefrontal cortex. *Cognition, 50*, 507–515.

Benke, T., Kurzthaler, I., Schmidauer, C., Moncayo, R., & Donnemiller, E. (2002). Mania caused by a diencephalic lesion. *Neuropsychologia, 40*, 245–252.

Berthier, M., Kulisevsky, J., Gironell, A., et al. (1996). Obsessive–compulsive disorder associated with brain lesions: Clinical phenomenology, cognitive function, and anatomic correlates. *Neurology, 47*, 353–361.

Bhogal, S., Teasell, R., Foley, N., & Speechley, M. (2004). Lesion location and poststroke depression: Systematic review of the methodological limitations in the literature. *Stroke, 35*, 794–802.

Carson, A., MacHale, S., Allen, K., Lawrie, S., Dennis, M., House, A., et al. (2000). Depression after stroke and lesion location: A systematic review. *Lancet, 356*, 122–126.

Chacko, R., Corbin, M., & Harper, R. (2000). Acquired obsessive–compulsive disorder associated with basal ganglia lesions. *Journal of Neuropsychiatry and Clinical Neurosciences, 12*, 269–272.

Chutorian, A., & Antunes, J. (1981). Klüver–Bucy syndrome and herpes encephalitis: Case report. *Neurosurgery, 8*(3), 388–390.

Cotter, D., Hudson, L., & Landau, S. (2005). Evidence for orbitofrontal pathology in bipolar disorder and major depression, but not in schizophrenia. *Bipolar Disorder, 7*, 358–369.

Cummings, J., & Cunningham, K. (1992). Obsessive–compulsive disorder in Huntington's disease. *Biological Psychiatry, 31*, 263–270.

Cummings, J., & Duchen, L. (1981). Kluver–Bucy syndrome in Pick disease: Clinical and pathologic correlations. *Neurology, 31*(11), 1415–1422.

Damasio, H., Grabowski, T., Feank, R., et al. (1994). The return of Phineas Gage: Clues about the brain from the skull of a famous patient. *Science, 264*(5162), 1102–1105.

Daxboeck, F. (2006). Mycoplasma pneumoniae central nervous system infections. *Current Opinion in Neurology, 19*(4), 374–378.

Drevets, W. C., & Price, J. L. (2005). Neuroimaging and neuropathological studies of mood disorders. *Biology of depression: From novel insights to therapeutic strategies*, 427–465.

Drevets, W., Gadde, K., & Krishnan, K. (2004). Neuroimaging studies of depression. In D. S. Charney, E. Nestler, & B. J. Bunney (Eds.), *The neurobiological foundation of mental illness* (2nd ed., pp. 461–490). New York, NY: Oxford University Press.

Drevets, W., Ongur, D., & Price, J. (1998). Neuroimaging abnormalities in the subgenual prefrontal cortex: Implications for the pathophysiology of familial mood disorders. *Molecular Psychiatry, 3*, 220–226.

Drevets, W., Price, J., Simpson, J., et al. (1997). Subgenual prefrontal cortex abnormalities in mood disorders. *Nature, 386*, 824–827.

Drevets, W., Price, J., Bardgett, M., Reich, T., Todd, R., & Raichle, M. (2002). Glucose metabolism in the amygdala in depression: relationship to diagnostic subtype and plasma cortisol levels. *Pharmacol Biochem Behav., 71*(3), 431–447.

Eslinger, P., Moore, P., Antanib, S., et al. (2012). Apathy in frontotemporal dementia: Behavioral and neuroimaging correlates. *Behavioral Neurology, 25*(2), 127–136.

Filley, C., & Cullum, C. (1993). Early detection of fronto-temporal degeneration by clinical evaluation. *Archives of Clinical Neuropsychology, 8*(4), 359–367.

Floden, D., Alexander, M., Kubu, C., Katz, D., & Stuss, D. (2008). Impulsivity and risk-taking behavior in focal frontal lobe lesions. *Neuropsychologia, 46*, 213–223.

Freeman, W., & Watts, J. W. (1936). Prefrontal lobotomy in agitated depression. Report of a case. *Ann. District of Columbia, 5*, 326.

Freeman, W., & Watts, J. (1939). An interpretation of the functions of the frontal lobe: Based upon observations in forty-eight cases of prefrontal lobotomy. *Yale Journal of Biology and Medicine, 11*(5), 527–539.

Gainotti, G., Azzoni, A., & Marra, C. (1999). Frequency, phenomenology, and anatomical correlates of major post-stroke depression. *British Journal of Psychiatry, 175*, 163–167.

Gerstenbrand, F., Poewe, W., Aichner, F., & Saltuari, L. (1983). Klüver–Bucy syndrome in man: Experiences with posttraumatic cases. *Neuroscience and Biobehavioral Reviews, 7*(3), 413–417.

Greene, K., Marciano, F., Dickman, C., et al. (1995). Anterior communicating artery aneurysm paraparesis syndrome: Clinical manifestations and pathologic correlates. *Neurology, 45*, 45–50.

Hama, S., Yamashita, H., Shigenobu, M., et al. (2007). Post-stroke affective or apathetic depression and lesion location: Left frontal lobe and bilateral basal ganglia. *European Archives of Psychiatry and Clinical Neuroscience, 257*, 149–152.

Hardy, T., & Aldridge, J. (1981). Traumatic transient Klüver–Bucy syndrome. *Surgical Neurology, 15*(5), 338–340.

Huey, E., Zahn, R., Krueger, F., Moll, J., Kapogiannis, D., Wassermann, E., et al. (2008). A psychological and neuroanatomical model of obsessive–compulsive disorder. *Journal of Neuropsychiatry and Clinical Neurosciences, 20*(4), 390–408.

Irle, E., Exner, C., Thielen, K., Weniger, G., & Rüther, E. (1998). Obsessive–compulsive disorder and ventromedial frontal lesions: Clinical and neuropsychological findings. *American Journal of Psychiatry, 155*, 255–263.

Kile, S., Ellis, W., Olichney, J., Farias, S., & DeCarli, C. (2009). Alzheimer abnormalities of the amygdala with Klüver–Bucy syndrome symptoms: An amygdaloid variant of Alzheimer disease. *Archives of Neurology, 66*(1), 125–129.

Kluver, H., & Bucy, P. (1939). Preliminary analysis of functions of the temporal lobe in monkeys. *Archives of Neurology and Psychiatry, 42*, 979–1000.

Knutson, K., Rakowsky, S, Solomon, J., et al. (2013). Injured brain regions associated with anxiety in Vietnam veterans. *Neuropsychologia, 51*, 686–694.

Krueger, C., Laluz, V., Rosen, H., et al. (2011). Double dissociation in the anatomy of socioemotional disinhibition and executive functioning in dementia. *Neuropsychology, 25*(2), 249–259.

Ku, H., Chen, C., Yang, Y., et al. (2013). Association between cerebral lesions and emotional changes in acute ischemic stroke patients. *Journal of Nervous and Mental Disease, 201*, 400–406.

Laplane, D., Levasseur, M., Pillon, B., et al. (1989). Obsessive–compulsive and other behavioural changes with bilateral basal ganglia lesions: A neuropsychological, magnetic resonance imaging and positron tomography study—Part 3. *Brain, 112*, 699–725.

Levy, R., & Dubois, B. (2006). Apathy and the functional anatomy of the prefrontal cortex–basal ganglia circuits. *Cerebral Cortex, 16*, 916–928.

Lindermann, D., Ostendorf, F., Kopp, U., et al. (2013). Subjective cognitive–affective status following thalamic stroke. *Journal of Neurology, 260*, 386–396.

Marin, R. (1991). Apathy: A neuropsychiatric syndrome. *Journal of Neuropsychiatry and Clinical Neurosciences, 3*(3), 243–254.

Marlowe, W., Mancall, E., & Thomas, J. (1975). Complete Klüver–Bucy syndrome in man. *Cortex, 11*(1), 53–59.

Müller, A., Baumgartner, R., Röhrenbach, C., & Regard, M. (1999). Persistent Klüver–Bucy syndrome after bilateral thalamic infarction. *Neuropsychiatry, Neuropsychology, and Behavioral Neurology, 12*(2), 136–139.

Nakada, T., Lee, H., Kwee, I., & Lerner, A. (1984). Epileptic Kluver–Bucy syndrome: Case report. *Journal of Clinical Psychiatry, 45*(2), 87–88.

Narushima, K., Kosier, J., & Robinson, R. (2003). A reappraisal of poststroke depression, intra- and inter-hemispheric lesion location using meta-analysis. *Journal of Neuropsychiatry and Clinical Neurosciences, 15*, 422–430.

Nauta, W., & Domesick, V. (1984). Afferent and efferent relationships of the vassal ganglia. *Ciba Foundation Symposium, 107*, 3–29.

O'Brien, J., Firbank, M., Krishnan, M., et al. (2006). White matter hyperintensities rather than lacunar infarcts are associated with depressive symptoms in older people: The LADIS study. *American Journal of Geriatric Psychiatry, 14*, 834–841.

Oliveira, V., Ferro, J., Foreid, J., Costa, T., & Levy, A. (1989). Kluver–Bucy syndrome in systemic lupus erythematosus. *Journal of Neurology, 236*(1), 55–56.

Ongur, D., Ferry, A., & Price, J. (2003). Architectonic subdivision of the human orbital and medial prefrontal cortex. *Journal of Comparative Neurology, 460*, 425–449.

Ongur, D., & Price, J. (2000). The organization of networks within the orbital and medial prefrontal cortex of rats, monkeys and humans. *Cerebral Cortex, 10*, 206–219.

O'Reilly, R., & Frank, M. (2006). Making working memory work: A computational model of learning in the prefrontal cortex and basal ganglia. *Neural Computation, 18*, 283–328.

Ramsey, L., Xu, M., Wood, N., & Pittenger, C. (2011). Lesions of the dorsomedial striatum disrupt prepulse inhibition. *Neuroscience, 180*, 222–228.

Robinson, R., Kubos, K., Starr, L., Rao, K., & Price, T. (1983). Mood changes in stroke patients: Relationship to lesion location. *Comprehensive Psychiatry, 24*, 555–566.

Robinson, R., Kubos, K., Starr, L., Rao, K., & Price, T. (1984). Mood disorders in stroke patients: Importance of location of lesion. *Brain, 107*, 81–93.

Saleem, K., Kondo, H., & Price, J. (2008). Complementary circuits connecting the orbital and medial prefrontal networks with the temporal, insular, and opercular cortex in the macaque monkey. *Journal of Comparative Neurology, 506*(4), 659–693.

Sandson, T., Lilly, R., & Sodkol, M. (1988). Kluver–Bucy syndrome associated with delayed post-anoxic leukoencephalopathy following carbon monoxide poisoning. *Journal of Neurology, Neurosurgery, and Psychiatry, 51*(1), 156–157.

Santos, M., Kövaria, E., Gold, G., et al. (2009). The neuroanatomical model of post-stroke depression: Towards a change of focus? *Journal of the Neurological Sciences, 283*(1/2), 158–162.

Shimoda, K., & Robinson, R. (1999). The relationship between poststroke depression and lesion location in long-term follow-up. *Biological Psychiatry, 45*, 187–192.

Singh, A., Black, S., Herrmann, N., et al. (2000). Functional and neuroanatomic correlations in poststroke depression: The Sunnybrook Stroke Study. *Stroke, 31*, 637–644.

Starkstein, S., Fedoroff, P., Berthier, M., & Robinson, R. (1991). Manic–depressive and pure manic states after brain lesions. *Biological Psychiatry, 29*, 149–158.

Swedo, S., Leonard, H., Garvey, M., et al. (1998). Pediatric autoimmune neuropsychiatric disorders associated with streptococcal infections: Clinical description of the first 50 cases. *American Journal of Psychiatry, 155*, 264–271.

Terroni, L., Amaro, E., Iosifescu, D., et al. (2011). Stroke lesion in cortical neural circuits and post-stroke incidence of major depressive episode: A 4-month prospective study. *World Journal of Biological Psychiatry, 12*, 539–548.

Terzian, H., & Ore, G. (1955). Syndrome of Klüver and Bucy; Reproduced in man by bilateral removal of the temporal lobes. *Neurology, 5*(6), 373–380.

Vataja, R., Leppavuori, A., Pohjasvaara, T., et al. (2004). Poststroke depression and lesion location revisited. *Journal of Neuropsychiatry and Clinical Neurosciences, 16*, 156–162.

Vuilleumier, P., Ghika-Schmid, F., Bogousslavsky, J., Assal, G., & Regli, F. (1998). Persistent recurrence of hypomania and prosopaffective agnosia in a patient with right thalamic infarct. *Neuropsychiatry, Neuropsychology, and Behavioral Neurology, 11*, 40–44.

Zamboni, G., Huey, E., Krueger, F., Nichelli, P., & Grafman, J. (2008). Apathy and disinhibition in frontotemporal dementia: Insights into their neural correlates. *Neurology, 71*, 736–742.

12

White Matter and Cognition

Throughout several of the previous chapters, there are references to lesions confined to or including white matter regions that result in specific cognitive/behavioral deficits. These examples can represent true disconnection syndromes because white matter lesions result in cortical regions that perform specific functions being disconnected from other cortical regions with which they were receiving/sending information or performing interactive analysis.

References to white matter lesions in the other chapters are sporadic due to the fact that studies of these regions rely on the accumulation of random lesions co-occurring in the same area and resulting in the same common deficit. These lesions were generally uncommon and thus did not lead to a plethora of studies. However, with the advent of diffusion tensor imaging (DTI) to delineate the structural integrity of white matter tracts, tract-based statistical analytic techniques to perform group analyses of white matter tracts, and the development of white matter atlases, it is now possible to study systematically the integrity of white matter tracts vis-à-vis behavioral and cognitive disorders.

Previous chapters mentioned the use of DTI to assess the integrity of white matter pathways. Here, the basic tenets of this indirect neuroimaging measure of assessing white matter are described. DTI does not visualize axons directly but, rather, uses a measure of the trajectory that water diffuses through an axon to derive the trajectory that the axon may be coursing in the brain. In short, as seen in Figure 12.1, vectors can be calculated for the three-dimensional directions that water can diffuse in the brain. Through DTI, these vectors can be computed for each voxel in the DTI image.

The mobility of water molecules in white matter is constrained predominantly by the myelin and axonal membranes. In a normal white matter fiber, the water will diffuse along the long axis of the axon when there is unimpeded diffusion, which is referred to as anisotropic diffusion. Each voxel in a white matter region is characterized by a vector, referred to as a tensor, that reflects the diffusion path of water in that white matter region. It is important to note that these vectors are at the voxel-size level (at best, several cubic millimeters) at which the images were acquired, with each voxel containing thousands of axons.

To calculate the diffusion vectors from DTI, it is typical to acquire images of those regions with six or more imaging acquisitions, each obtained from a different orientation. This provides both a direction and speed of water diffusion for each voxel. The more information used to derive the diffusion measures for each voxel, the more sensitive that measure is to disruption in white matter integrity secondary to damage, and the more stable it will be if the region is intact.

The result of these computations is to construct, in essence, an ellipsoid of what would be the approximate shape of a water molecule in the white matter tract (Figure 12.2). This ellipse has a long (principal) axis, which should best reflect the direction of water diffusion in the white matter tract, as well as measures of the width and depth of the ellipse. The measures of the lengths of these axes are referred to as eigenvalues, which are considered a measure of the diffusivity of water along each of the three axes of an axon. The diffusivity along the longitudinal, principal axis is referred to as axial diffusivity. The diffusivities of the two minor axes are averaged together and referred to as the radial diffusivity. This measures the degree of restriction of diffusivity of the water molecule against the walls of the white matter tract, which reflects factors impeding water diffusion along the long axis of the white matter tract. A third measure of diffusivity used occasionally is mean diffusivity, an overall reflection of total diffusivity that takes the average value of all three of the eigenvalues.

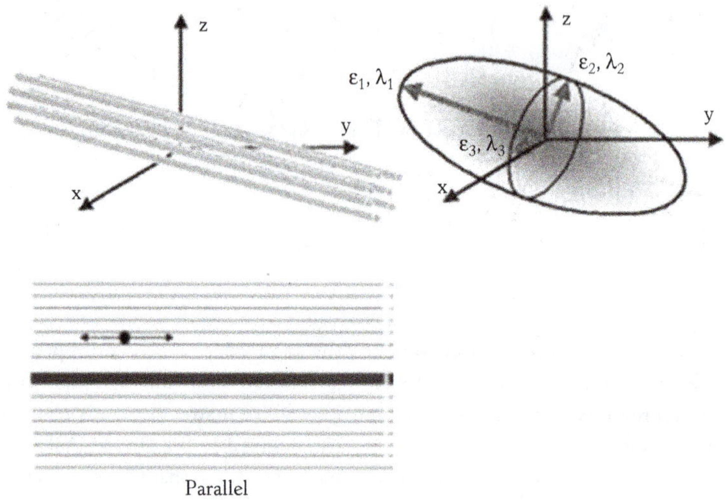

FIGURE 12.1: Schematic drawing of myelinated fibers. On the top left, fibers that represent axons can be measured by the flow of water in terms of a vector represented in the *x, y,* and *z* directions. The ellipsoid next to the fibers shows the representation of the water molecule if it is flowing in the direction of the axon unimpeded. On the bottom is a single fiber, with the arrow showing the other vector that a water molecule can move, which is parallel to fibers. This direction does not cross myelin.

Source: http://www.ajnr.org.

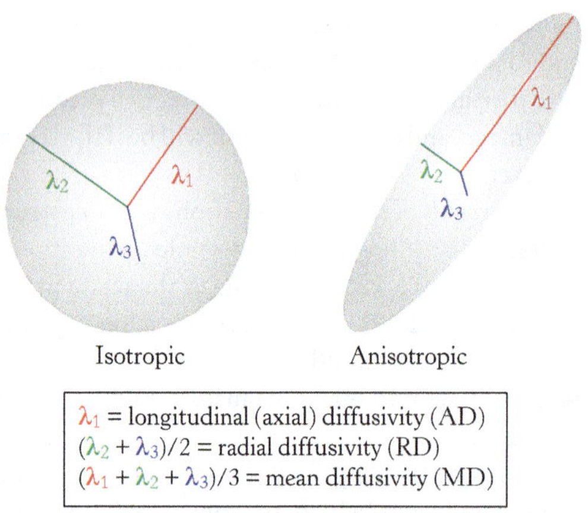

FIGURE 12.2: Representation of a diffusion ellipsoid showing the eigenvectors. Gray matter is predominantly isotropic (sphere-like) and white matter tracts are anisotropic (cigar-shaped) in terms of water diffusion. The measure most commonly used to characterize directional diffusion is fractional anisotropy. This ranges between 0 and 1 to signify the fraction of diffusion in the longitudinal direction. Other measures that can be used are axial diffusivity (AD), radial diffusivity (RD), and mean diffusivity (MD).

Source: http://www.diffusion-imaging.com.

The importance of these diffusivity measures is their use in obtaining a marker of white matter integrity. The mathematically optimized measure of the "square root of the sum of the squares (SRSS) of the diffusivity differences, divided by the SRSS of the diffusivities" is referred to as fractional anisotropy (FA). When the factors impeding diffusion down the long axis of the white matter tract are relatively small and thus diffusion of materials appears to be flowing along the axon in the optimal, intended direction, then the FA is near 1. This optimal diffusion down the intact long axis of the white matter tract is pictured as a strongly linear-looking, cigar-shaped ellipsoid that travels efficiently down the white matter path. When the FA is closer to 0, the ellipsoid is more spherical, diffusion is equal in all directions, and water is not traveling effectively down the white matter tract. This will occur from the FA equation when the radial and mean diffusivities, those values reflecting factors impeding diffusion down the long axis, are large. This would occur with damage to axons or myelin, which would result in the water not diffusing along the long axis of the axon and reflected in a low fractional anisotropy toward 0. Using these measurements of fractional

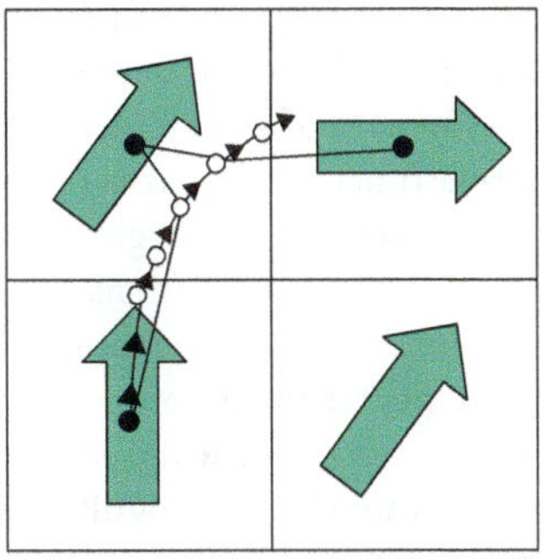

FIGURE 12.3: Interpolating how voxels align for DTI tracking. Large arrows indicate the vector of the largest principal axis for each of the four voxels represented by the boxes The smaller black arrowheads depict how algorithms would line up the voxels to show the orientation of a tract moving up from the bottom and curving to the right.

Source: Mori and van Zijl (2002).

anisotropy of the water diffusion of the voxels in white matter, it is possible to obtain maps of white matter tract integrity.

Another measurement of the structural framework of white matter tracts is the technique of tractography. Tractography is a method by which one can localize where there may be a disruption in a white matter region by reconstructing a framework of a skeleton of the white matter tracts in the brain (Mori et al., 1999). In tractography, algorithms are used to construct the trajectories of white matter tracts by piecing together diffusion signals from contiguous voxels. These tracking algorithms use a set of conditions to test if the effective diffusion vector of a voxel is connected to the next voxel. This is done in the following manner. If the vectors of two contiguous voxels are aligned and the direction of the water diffusion is in the same direction, then the voxels are linked together as part of a tract, reflecting the direction that the water molecules would flow if unimpeded (Figure 12.3). If axonal membranes and/or myelin are disrupted so that the water molecules do not flow in the direction of the tract, then the tract will appear to be disrupted at the damaged spot when constructing it (Figure 12.4).

The figures typically being used in many DTI studies, and particularly tractography studies, illustrate fibers that appear to resemble white matter. It is important to note that these depictions do not represent actual white matter fibers nor do they represent a one-to-one correspondence to white matter fibrils. Thus, the images that are generated from these studies should not be interpreted as an actual quantitative depiction of white matter tracts.

Interpretation of disrupted white matter tracts must be considered in terms of the role the regions that they are connecting play in cognition. A disrupted white matter tract connecting two independent cortical regions can produce varying types of behavior, based on the roles of those cortical regions and the degree and type of white matter disruption. A complete disruption of white matter transmission in this type of system could lead to the performance described in patients with clear disconnection syndromes. If the two cortical regions being connected were more distributed or interactive in their processing roles, as opposed to independent, this leads to more complex behavioral outcomes, again depending on the nature and degree of white matter

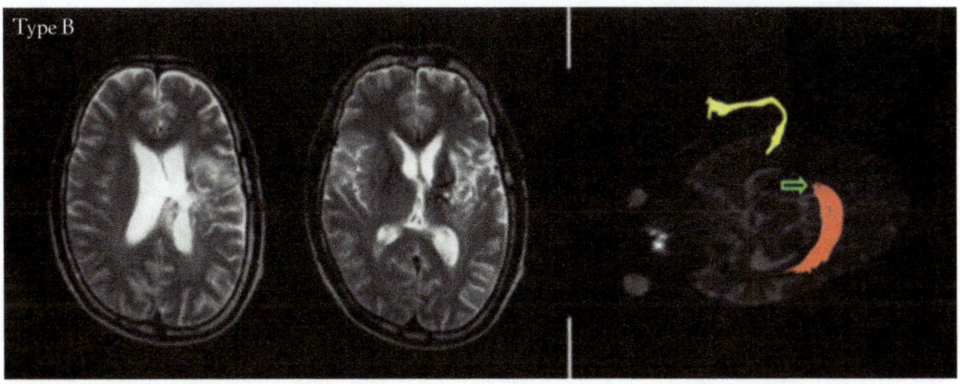

FIGURE 12.4: Disruption of the arcuate fasciculus white matter tracts in aphasic patients. The two images on the left are T2-weighted brain MRIs in a chronic stroke patient with aphasia. The image on the right is diffusion tensor imaging tractography for the arcuate fasciculus (AF). Right AF, yellow; left AF, red; arrow, discontinuation.

Source: Tak and Jang (2014).

disruption. If the white matter connections link multiple geographically distributed cortical and subcortical regions, the behavioral outcomes can be further complicated.

The white matter connections that link regions together may be linking multiple subpopulations of neurons in a cortical region to a variety of other cortical regions dispersed throughout the brain. These dispersed cortical regions may be performing tasks in multiple different networks. Thus, clinical outcomes from a white matter lesion depend on the cortical regions to which white matter is connected, the subpopulation of neurons in those cortical regions, and, most important for this chapter, the connecting axons in the white matter tract that are disrupted.

Given these potential variables that can lead to a variety of behavioral outcomes given a particular white matter lesion, there remains some consistent behaviors that occur after specific white matter lesion. The lack of standardized anatomical localizations and variable image acquisition techniques still provide some limitations so that the development of an extensive white matter tract–cognitive function map is off in the future. However, the presence of regularly occurring white matter–behavior correlations argues for the existence of some consistent relationships existing between white matter function and cognitive performance (see overview of white matter pathways and possible relationships to cognitive systems in Figure 12.5), which are described next.

The following descriptions of white matter lesions associated with cognitive dysfunction have only been described recently with the advent of DTI imaging. Thus, the white matter correlations provided are evolving and do not contain the cognitive delineations and mechanistic accounts of previous chapters. As the maps of white matter tracts across multiple individuals evolve, atlases of white matter tracts will allow for an increase in the

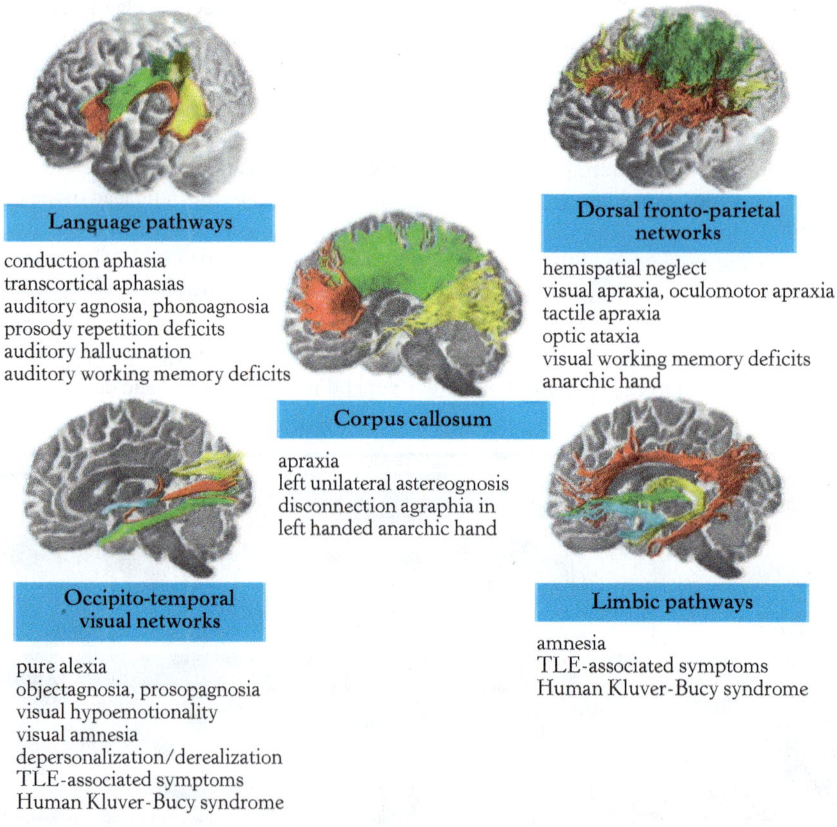

FIGURE 12.5: Representations of large-scale white matter network-supporting cognitive networks that were developed using DTI tractography. Listed below each white matter network are neurological and neuropsychiatric syndromes associated with each network for which a disconnection mechanism has been proposed.

Source: Catani (2006).

number of individuals to assess for both the presence and the absence of a cognitive association and determine if consistent associations exist. The current descriptions provide details of the associations that are beginning to develop between white matter lesions and disruption of cognitive function across multiple cognitive domains. As further studies are performed, the details and consistency of the associations described here will evolve.

CALLOSAL SYNDROMES

Patients with callosal degradation/lesions, in general, have been the most studied individuals with white matter lesions and the resultant impairments in cognition and behavior (Schulte & Müller-Oehring, 2010). The corpus callosum (CC) is anatomically segregated into three regions: (1) an anterior part (referred to as the genu and rostrum) that connects frontal and premotor regions of the two hemispheres; (2) a middle part (the body) that interconnects motor, somatosensory, and parietal areas; and (3) a posterior part of the corpus callosum (the splenium) that interconnects temporal and occipital cortices (Figure 12.6). It is important to note that the CC is not the only white matter connection between the two hemispheres. The other pathways connecting the hemispheres are the anterior and posterior commissures, dorsal and ventral hippocampal commissures, habenular commissure, and intercollicular commissure (Bayard et al., 2004).

The larger number of studies of individuals with CC lesions is due to the history of using corpus callosotomy in the treatment of refractory seizures (surgically splitting the anterior two-thirds of the CC to reduce seizure severity and generalization). The landmark work of Sperry, Gazzaniga, and colleagues, who studied patients with "split-brains," has been detailed extensively in previous publications demonstrating what functions appear to be more lateralized to the right hemisphere compared to the left (Gazzaniga, 2005).

An example of some of the initial key findings from studying callosal resection patients is the lateralization of language functions. This was best exemplified by presenting a patient an image to the right visual field so that only the left hemisphere received the information. Patients were then asked to describe the picture, which they could do perfectly. When the image was presented to the right hemisphere by only projecting it to the left visual field, the patients would respond by saying, "I can't describe it." However, they could make a nonverbal response to the stimulus by pointing to an object in the picture, for example. This demonstrates that the language component required to describe the picture is only present in the left hemisphere. The right hemisphere saw the image and registered it, but due to the callosal resection, it could not get to the left hemisphere language structures needed to provide a description (Devinsky & Laff, 2003).

Occasionally after a callosal resection, a phenomenon referred to as the alien hand sign will spontaneously occur. The patient will find that in attempting to perform a motor task with one hand,

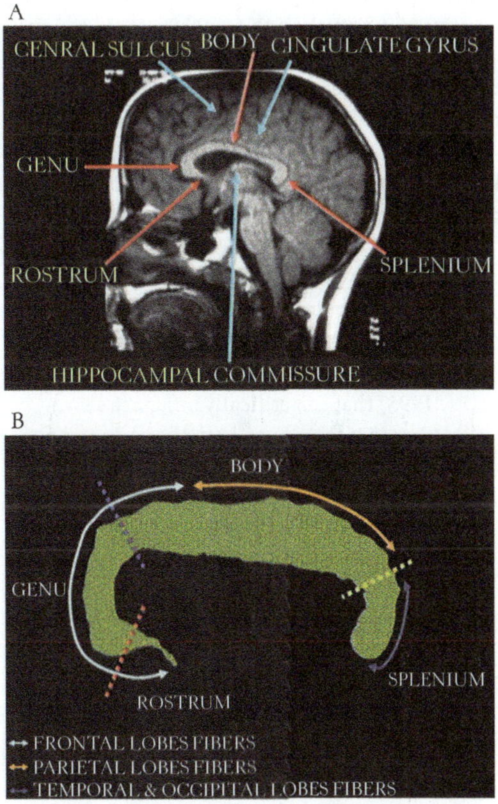

FIGURE 12.6: Sections of the corpus callosum. The top image is a sagittal view of the brain, and the bottom is a schematic of the corpus callosum showing its subdivisions. The splenium is the posterior section connecting parietal and occipital aspects of the two hemispheres. The body is the main portion of the corpus callosum connecting frontal and parietal lobe regions between the hemispheres. The genu is the curvature at the most anterior portion of the corpus callosum. The rostrum is the front end of the corpus callosum.

Source: http://www.pediatricneuro.com.

the other hand will try to perform the same action and ultimately interfere with the hand meant to perform the motor task. This was further described in an interesting manner in a split-brain patient who reported being "surprised" that the unintended (left) hand interfered with task performance of the intended (right) hand. This surprise was attributed to the left hemisphere being unaware of and confused by the actions of the left hand. This typically occurs after anterior callosal lesions (Leiguarda et al., 1989).

In addition to being able to determine that certain functions are lateralized to one hemisphere or the other, callosal resections can help determine which functions require or use interhemispheric transfer of information to complete cognitive operations. The following are key examples from the numerous studies combining lesion (split-brain), functional imaging (e.g., functional magnetic resonance imaging (fMRI)), and DTI to delineate the key types of transfers of information that courses the CC:

1. Transfer of visuomotor information between hemispheres (Iacoboni & Zaidel, 2004; Pollmann & Zaidel, 1998).
2. Shifts in spatial attention (Corbetta et al., 1995) that can critically influence sensorimotor integration, with the premotor and parietal cortex regions being linked through the mid-body and anterior regions of the CC (Iacoboni & Zaidel, 2004).
3. Posterior callosal areas connecting information from visual areas to structures for visuomotor integration.
4. Temporoparietal junction communicates with its homolog in the opposite hemisphere via the CC to mediate coactivation for visuomotor integration and attentional mechanisms (Mooshagian et al., 2008).
5. Posterior callosal splenium area is associated with visual local–global integration (Müller-Oehring et al., 2007).
6. Left pre-supplementary motor area (SMA) region communicates with its homolog on the right for praxis performance (see Chapter 5).

Lesions in these callosal regions result in disconnections between hemispheric communication and disruption of the functions noted to be mediated via that callosal connection.

LANGUAGE

Many theories have been proposed concerning the network of cortical regions supporting language functions; however, there is little that has been explored in terms of the role played by white matter pathways in this collection of cortical regions, except for the arcuate fasciculus—the white matter pathway that connects Wernicke's area to Broca's area. Using the technique of DTI, Catani and ffytche (2005) isolated the direct arcuate fasciculus pathway between Broca's and Wernicke's area. In addition, an indirect pathway was found by DTI connecting Broca's and Wernicke's territory that passed through the inferior parietal lobe (Catani et al., 2005) (Figure 12.7). This indirect pathway contains two segments—a posterior one connecting the temporal and parietal cortices involved in language processing and an anterior segment connecting parietal and frontal cortices. These two connected segments together establish a network of connected regions consisting of the posterior aspects of middle and inferior frontal gyri (Broca's area plus), the angular and supramarginal gyri, and the posterior part of the superior and middle temporal gyri (Wernicke's area plus additional regions).

The three parts of this perisylvian white matter tract (see Figure 12.7) were labeled by Catani et al. as the direct pathway (traditional arcuate

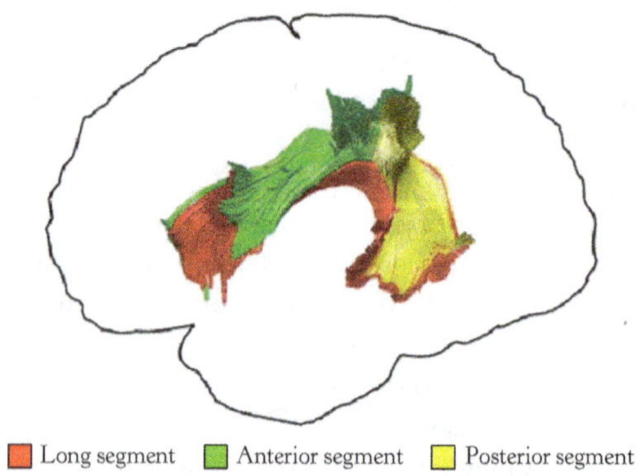

FIGURE 12.7: The perisylvian language network. The figure is a three-dimensional reconstruction of the direct and indirect perisylvian pathways in the left hemisphere. The long segment fibers (red) connect Broca's and Wernicke's area and represent the more traditional arcuate fasciculus. The anterior segment fibers (green) connect Broca's area and the IPL. The posterior segment fibers (yellow) connect the IPL to Wernicke's area.

Source: Catani and ffytche (2005).

fasciculus); the anterior segment or anterior indirect pathway, which is the connection between frontal and inferior parietal cortices; and the posterior segment or posterior indirect pathway connecting the temporal and inferior parietal cortices. These connections have been postulated to be selectively engaged in connecting regions supporting different language operations: (1) the direct pathway with phonological functions, (2) the posterior indirect pathway engaged in lexical–semantic operations (e.g., auditory comprehension), and (3) the anterior indirect segment involved in vocalization of semantic content (Catani et al., 2005). Catani and ffytche (2005) postulated that disruption of white matter in the inferior parietal lobe (IPL) could result in a variety of behavioral variants. If a white matter lesion involves predominantly the arcuate fasciculus, the resultant disorder would resemble conduction aphasia with impaired repetition. If both direct and indirect pathways are lesioned, then global aphasia would be proposed to occur, even with all of the language cortices intact (Naeser et al., 2005). Lesions cortically involving the IPL could result in a variety of deficits depending on what subregion of the IPL was involved and the extent of the underlying white matter connections that are also disrupted. If the lesion was part of the anterior aspects of the IPL, the resultant aphasia would consist of nonfluent spontaneous speech with intact repetition and comprehension (Basso et al., 1985). If both anterior and posterior aspects of the IPL are lesioned, the resultant behavior would be proposed to be a mixed transcortical aphasia, which consists of severe comprehension and verbal output impairments, except the patients have intact repetition. If both anterior and posterior cortices of the IPL are involved as well as the underlying white matter, then global aphasia would be expected to occur. The predictions from this model, when delineated, will allow for future hypothesis testing resulting in empirical determination of model accuracy.

Another region associated with language-related functions is the auditory association cortex, a region proposed to be engaged in auditory word recognition. The auditory association cortex is connected to more posterior visual occipital regions and more anterior temporal areas through the inferior longitudinal fasciculus and U-shaped fibers. Patients with lesions to the previously mentioned connections may show difficulty in using words to name objects (e.g., anomic aphasia).

Semantics

Semantic networks have been outlined in meta-analyses (Binder et al., 2009), but the white matter pathways associated with semantic subsystems have not been fully outlined. The relationship between white matter tracts and semantic deficits was studied in a group of 76 right-handed brain-damaged patients (Han et al., 2013). The percentage of white matter lesion voxels that were part of the patients' lesions detected in structural imaging and the voxels with dysfunctional FA values detected with DTI were compared to both the individual test performance and the average test scores across three semantic tasks (across multiple different modalities). The findings showed that the white matter tracts of the left inferior fronto-occipital fasciculus (IFOF), left anterior thalamic radiation, and left uncinate fasciculus significantly correlated with severity of impairment across all semantic tasks. However, lesion damage on structural MRI and/or reduced FA values associated with these tracts were not correlated with performance on two control tasks of repetition and number processing. This suggests that these tracts are more likely linking semantic-related cortical regions and not language regions in general. The finding of IFOF lesions being associated with semantic tasks that were administered to the patients in two different modalities (auditory and visual) suggests that this tract may be involved in connecting regions involved in multimodality semantic processing, likely between the left posterior middle temporal gyrus and the anterior inferior frontal cortex. The left anterior thalamic radiations that correlated with semantic testing are known to connect the inferior frontal region (engaged in multiple semantic operations) to the thalamus, with the thalamus able to further link this inferior frontal lobe region to numerous other cortical regions. In addition, the thalamus and its white matter connections have also been shown to contribute to lexical–semantic processing (Crosson, 1984, 2013; Crosson et al., 1997) as well as to the semantic binding process (Kraut et al., 2002; Slotnick et al., 2002). The left uncinate connects the anterior temporal lobe, implicated in a variety of semantic processes, to frontal lobe regions engaged in semantic operations as well as domain-general cognitive control functions (Han et al., 2013). Thus, the white matter pathways identified in this group analysis have been shown to independently be connecting regions previously linked to semantic processing, but now with DTI tracking,

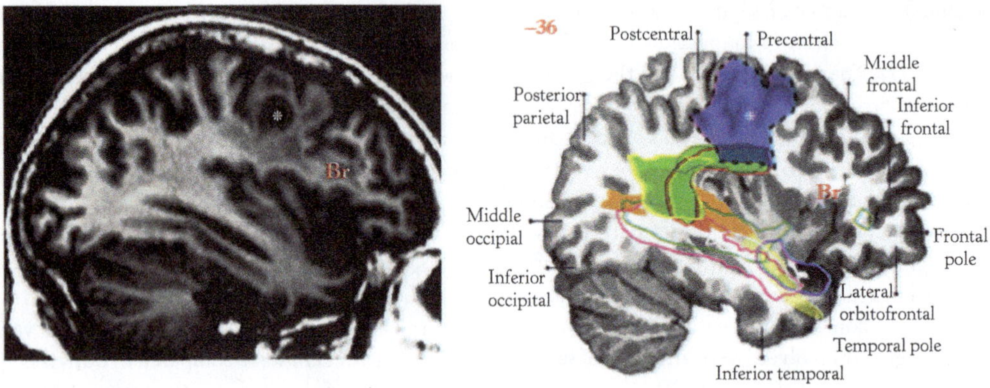

FIGURE 12.8 (Left) MRI of a 72-year-old patient with a language impairment characterized by reduced verbal fluency and repetition deficits that is consistent with a Broca's aphasia; however, Broca's area is intact in this patient. The MRI shows a tumor (asterisk) localized in the precentral gyrus with perilesional edema extending into adjacent parietal and frontal white matter. (Right) The area of the tumor and edema is indicated in blue and overlaid onto the corresponding sagittal image of the atlas, showing the affected white matter tracts (e.g., anterior and long segment of the arcuate fasciculus).

Source: Catani et al. (2012).

a more integrated view of how the semantic regions are connected can be envisioned.

These types of white matter group lesion studies can be performed in degenerative diseases, if the pathology of the degenerative disorder is fairly consistent. In a study of 35 patients with primary progressive aphasia and 29 control subjects, disrupted tractography of the frontal aslant tract and uncinate fasciculus was found to be correlated with performance on specific cognitive tasks. Specifically, damage to the frontal aslant tract correlated with performance in verbal fluency (letter-driven verbal fluency), whereas damage to the uncinate fasciculus is correlated with deficits in semantic processing, which is consistent with results of numerous other studies linking the uncinate fasciculus and its connections between the frontal and temporal lobes with a role in semantic processing (Catani et al., 2013).

A network-based approach in clinico-anatomical correlation studies that includes white matter connections in the model offers the advantage of explaining how symptoms classically attributed to damage of a cortical area (e.g., nonfluent aphasia with lesions to Broca's area) can manifest in patients with lesions outside of that area. For example, studies suggest that 15% of patients with clinical symptoms of Broca's aphasia have lesions that lie outside of Broca's area, often in regions of the parietal lobe that are clearly posterior to the typical frontal lobe Broca's area regions (Basso et al., 2000). This is the case in a patient with a brain tumor (Figure 12.8) in which there is tumor invasion of the anterior aspects of the arcuate fasciculus without direct damage to Broca's area, but the patient presents with symptoms most consistent with Broca's aphasia. In this case, dysfunction in Broca's area can result from a white matter lesion causing Broca's area to be disconnected from posterior parietal and temporal language regions (Catani et al., 2012).

Alexia

Disconnection accounts of alexia without agraphia postulate that left hemisphere regions specialized in visual perceptual processing of letters in words can no longer access regions in which visual language word stores are located. This classic disconnection syndrome has been described when a lesion both causes a right hemianopia (typically from a lesion involving the left primary visual cortices and the corresponding underlying white matter) and also extends into the white matter to interrupt the splenial callosal fibers crossing over from the right occipital lobe where the right primary visual cortices are located that could also process letters at a perceptual level. This same clinical picture can also occur from a subcortical lesion undercutting Wernicke's area, in essence disconnecting visual input to the language comprehension and word store networks (Geschwind, 1965).

Investigators studying the organization of the visual "what" system, which encodes for the visual memory representations, have identified a region that they postulate is involved in the processing of visual letter information to the point that the perceptual information is processed into visual representations of whole words. This region has been referred to as the "visual word form area" (VWFA). It was thus hypothesized that lesions disrupting the connections associated with the VWFA may result in alexia without agraphia. In this respect, a prospective set of language testing and imaging studies were conducted on a patient about to undergo a surgical resection. Prior to and post-surgery, the patient received an fMRI study during identification of letter strings as words or not and also a DTI to assess the white matter surrounding a surgical lesion near the VWFA. Pre-op DTI showed that the VWFA was linked to the occipital cortex through the inferior longitudinal fasciculus (ILF) and to perisylvian language areas (supramarginal gyrus) through the arcuate fasciculus. Surgery disrupted the ILF white matter tract (seen with serial DTI scans), and this surgical lesion was correlated with a post-op decrease in reading abilities, thus establishing the ILF as critical for normal reading, with its disruption being another mechanism to developing alexia (Epelbaum et al., 2008).

PRAXIS

As previously reported, apraxia is an inability to execute learned, purposeful commands even though the subject has the physical capacity to perform the commands. A frontoparietal network associated with the function of praxis has been proposed. The praxis system encodes the representations for tasks related to object manipulation and their associated motor acts as well as the neural mechanisms to carry out these acts. One of the key ways to assess the integrity of this system is to provide a verbal command for a subject to gesture the motor action associated with an object (e.g., "Show me how you would hold and use a hammer"). This task probes the integrity of the connection between the verbal system that processes the command and the praxis system to carry it out.

A major white matter lesion to the corpus callosum that results in apraxia when using the left hand is described in detail in the chapter on apraxia. This corpus callosum lesion demonstrated the disconnection between the left hemisphere system that encodes the spatiotemporal movement representations in the left parietal lobule and the left SMA, which is engaged in translating spatiotemporal motor representations into motor programs being disconnected from the right hemisphere SMA, and the motor system that guides performance of the motor act with the left hand.

DTI studies have allowed for further isolation of the connections between the different brain regions performing functions within the praxis system. These connections include the dorsolateral frontoparietal white matter tracts connecting the dorsal motor and premotor cortex to the parietal lobe, the ventrolateral frontoparietal tracts connecting the ventrolateral motor and premotor cortices to the parietal lobe, and the medial frontoparietal tracts connecting the medial frontal lobe to the medial parietal lobe (Figure 12.9).

Lesions extending into these white matter tracts result in disconnecting the cortical regions performing these praxis functions (Leiguarda & Marsden, 2000). The white matter tracts that are typically affected and result in disconnection apraxias are left hemisphere involvement of the connections of the inferior parietal lobule to the frontal lobes—the superior longitudinal fasciculus, arcuate fasciculus, or callosal fibers (Glickstein & Berlucchi, 2008; Heilman & Watson, 2008; Ramayya et al., 2010).

Ideomotor apraxia, in which patients are impaired in performing a motor action from a verbal command but are better able to pantomime the action, has been most often linked with white matter lesions that affect the anterior two-thirds of the CC (Heilman & Watson, 2008). These patients demonstrate an inability to perform a complex motor act to command with their left hand while still being able to perform the act with their right hand. This demonstrates an inability to transfer movement representations stored in their left hemisphere to their right hemisphere to be performed with their left hand.

Another mechanism by which ideomotor apraxia (typically for both hands) has been proposed to occur is via a lesion in the region of the left supramarginal gyrus that also extends to disrupt the underlying white matter of the arcuate fasciculus (Geschwind, 1965). This purportedly results in disconnection of the supramarginal gyrus (where aspects of movement representations could be encoded) and the premotor area that translates these representations to a motor code. Because they have intact movement representations, these patients are able to discriminate whether a movement performed by the examiner is correct, but they cannot make the movement to verbal command.

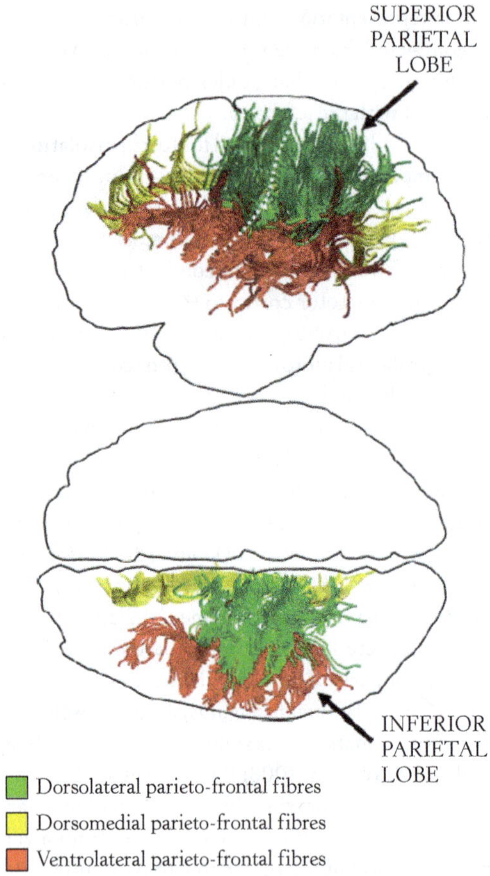

FIGURE 12.9: Praxic frontoparietal circuitry. A three-dimensional reconstruction of the fiber connections between parietal and frontal lobes in the left hemisphere and shown from the left (top) and top of the brain (bottom). The dorsolateral fibers connect the superior parietal lobe and dorsal motor and premotor cortex (green fibers). The ventrolateral fibers connect the inferior parietal lobe and ventrolateral motor and premotor cortex. The dorsomedial fibers connect the medial parietal lobe with the medial frontal lobe. The dotted white line is the central sulcus.

Source: Catani et al. (2002).

Recent DTI studies suggest that the lesion is located in the white matter tract referred to as the ventrolateral frontoparietal tract, which extends from the IPL to the premotor areas (Figure 12.9) (Geschwind, 1965; Schmahmann et al., 2008).

Limb-kinetic apraxia is notable for a loss of dexterity, with patients having unilateral difficulty making precise, coordinated finger movements. This deficit is the result of lesions of the white matter corticospinal tract in the brain stem or the subcortical white matter in the posterior limb of the internal capsule. These lesions disconnect the motor programs to perform motor acts that are encoded in the primary motor cortex from the anterior horn cells in the spinal cord that more directly control the muscles in the hand.

MEMORY

Another set of white matter lesions covered extensively in Chapter 6 and worth repeating here are those lesions resulting in episodic memory disorders. The mamillothalamic tract (MMT) and fornix are two white matter pathways in the Papez circuit with the hippocampus connected to the mammillary bodies by the fornix, and the mammillary bodies are connected to the anterior nucleus of the thalamus via the MMT (Brodal, 1981). Damage to either of these white matter tracts results in notable anterograde and retrograde memory loss via disconnection of key regions of the Papez circuitry required for encoding and retrieving new episodic memories. In addition, there is another white matter pathway providing a link to the memory circuitry, which is an input from the emotion system. The ventral amygdalofugal pathway links the amygdala with the medial part of the dorsomedial nucleus of the thalamus and mediates the attachment of aspects of the emotion of fear to an episodic memory. Damage to this pathway can contribute to the development of both amnesia and emotional dysregulation (Graff-Radford et al., 1990).

VISUAL NETWORK

Visual agnosias have been segregated into more perceptual and more associative disorders. Tractography has helped delineate occipitotemporal white matter tracts (Figure 12.10) that connect higher-order visual processing areas to other associated brain regions. In addition to these white matter tracts, higher-order visual processing information can also be transmitted to other brain areas via short chains of U-fibers connecting cortical to neighboring cortical regions. These U-fibers are short-range white matter connections located immediately under the cortex that pass information from one gyrus to the next neighboring gyrus in a chain-like manner. Unfortunately, this gyrus-to-gyrus transmission of information via U-fibers is slow and theoretically is more likely to result in a loss of information.

The main direct occipitotemporal pathway is the ILF connecting occipital cortices to medial temporal structures (the hippocampus, parahippocampal

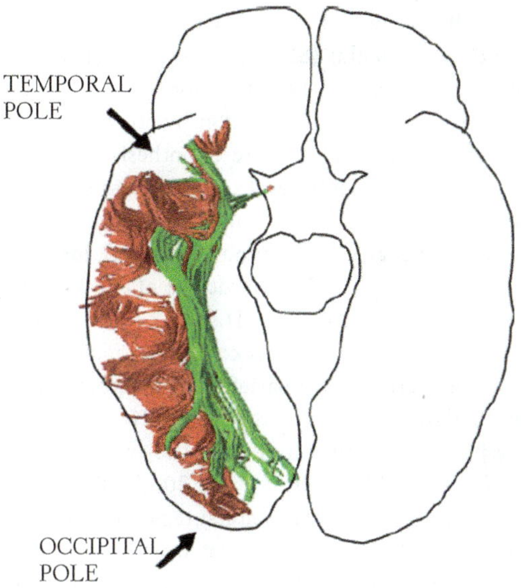

FIGURE 12.10: Occipitotemporal pathways. A three-dimensional reconstruction of fiber connections between right hemispheric occipital and temporal lobes. One consists of a chain of U-shaped fiber connections (red). The other is the inferior longitudinal fasciculus system connecting the occipital to the temporal lobe (green).

Source: Catani et al. (2003).

gyrus, and amygdala) (Catani et al., 2003). A ventral or lateral temporal cortical lesion would lead to specific deficits related to the cortical specializations disrupted. On the other hand, a white matter lesion to the ILF can also lead to disconnecting aspects of one region engaged in higher-order visual processing from other visual processing areas or other cognitive domains.

If the ILF white matter lesion disrupts communication from visual processing areas to other domains such as language, the resultant deficit would be an inability to name an object. If the medial tracts of the ILF are lesioned, there can be a disconnection of the visual processing system to the limbic system, resulting in the phenomena referred to as visual hypoemotionality, in which a patient experiences a deficit in expressing emotional responses to visually presented stimuli that would normally induce an emotional response but also demonstrates preserved emotional responses to the same stimuli if they are presented in a nonvisual domain (Bauer, 1982).

The involvement of long association tracts connecting the occipital lobe to more anterior brain regions can lead to other syndromes that also lead to predominantly visual symptoms. For example, symptoms called "reduplicative phenomena" are thought to relate to a disconnection between visual, affective, and memory regions due to lesions of the ILF and IFOF (ffytche et al., 2010). In disorders in which these reduplicative symptoms are prominent, familiar people, places, and objects are perceived as duplicates that have replaced the real person, place, or object. One of these disorders is referred to as Capgras syndrome, in which the misidentifications involve a person. Other psychiatric symptoms have been accounted for by white matter disconnection, including when a person feels that experiences, particularly visual ones, seem strange or unreal—referred to as derealization, a symptom that appears in a variety of disorders, including schizophrenia, dissociative states, anxiety disorders, bipolar disorder, and epilepsy (Sierra et al., 2002).

Patients with cortical blindness due to extensive occipital lesions can sometime deny their visual impairment, with this denial of blindness referred to as Anton's syndrome (Anton, 1889). Patients with Anton's syndrome may also report visual experiences that traditionally have been interpreted as confabulations—a false memory or false report of visual perceptual experiences. Anton's syndrome with blindness yet denial of this blindness has been conceptualized as a white matter disconnection of the visual cortices from body schema representations in the parietal lobe (ffytche et al., 2010).

In the case of prosopagnosia, impaired face recognition, the inferior longitudinal fasciculus is the white matter pathway that extends posteriorly for connecting regions of the face processing system in the lingual/fusiform gyri to visual processing regions in the occipital lobe and anteriorly to the temporal lobe areas that encode for higher-order semantic and emotional processing associated with faces. Various lesions to the ILF may result in prosopagnosia depending on the location of the lesion, with the deficit occurring in some cases by disconnecting the OFA and FFA from each other or by disconnecting these OFA/FFA regions from the anterior temporal lobe (Catani et al., 2003; Fox et al., 2008).

In some instances, disruption to white matter tracts has been proposed to not result in a loss of connection but, rather, a dysfunctional "overconnection" between regions. This results in what is termed "positive symptoms." The Fregoli syndrome, in which unfamiliar people are perceived as familiar (typically as a person in disguise with threatening intentions), can be interpreted as white matter damage resulting in a hyperconnection between visual, emotional, and memory networks. Similarly, the strong affective and imagery components of "flashbacks" or "re-experiencing" in post-traumatic stress disorder suggest a possible hyperconnection between visual, emotional, and memory regions secondary to white matter dysfunction (ffytche et al., 2010). Further studies are needed to confirm this mechanism and the white matter pathways that result in these types of symptoms or syndromes.

NEGLECT

Unilateral neglect has been described in association with lesions to cortical regions as noted in the visual higher-order deficits (see Chapter 7) and also with white matter damage to the superior longitudinal fasciculus (SLF), ILF, or IFOF (Doricchi et al., 2008) (Figure 12.11). Lesions of the SLF are the most common white matter involvement associated with neglect and are hypothesized to disrupt the linkage between frontal and parietal lobe regions, particularly the connection between the frontal lobe and the temporal–parietal junction (Leibovitch et al., 1998; Verdon et al., 2006). The cases of disruption of the ILF that cause neglect are purported to cause this cognitive deficit due to a disconnection of the parietal and temporal lobes, particularly disrupting the connection between the parahippocampal gyrus and the angular gyrus of the parietal lobe (Bird et al., 2006). The IFOF, connecting the ventral occipital region to the frontal lobe, has also been associated with neglect by impairing the modulation of visual areas from the frontal cortex (Urbanski et al., 2008). It is important to note that not all lesions in these white matter tracts result in neglect; only when the specific white

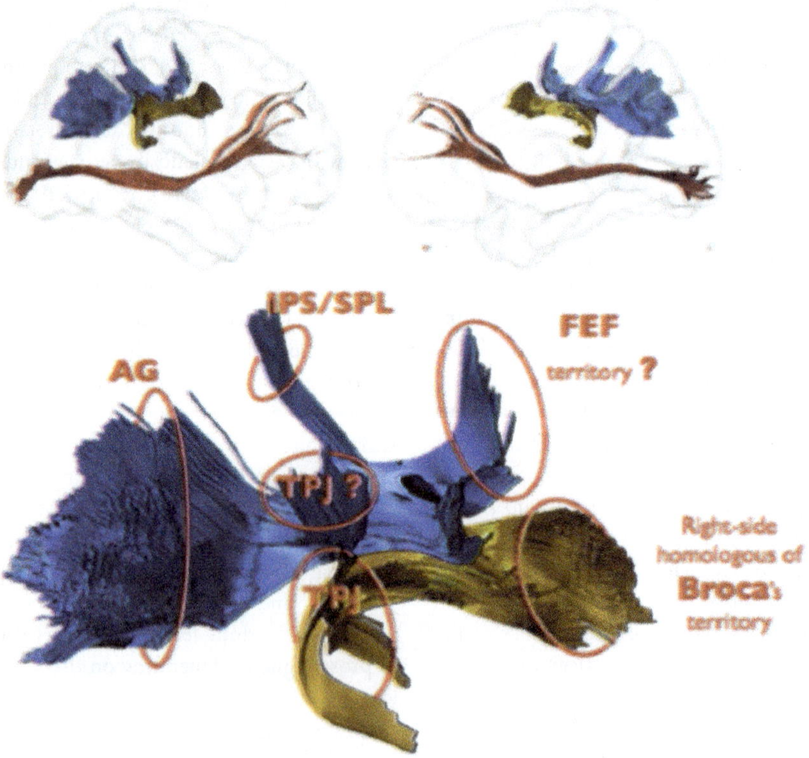

FIGURE 12.11: Three-dimensional reconstruction of the SLF III (gold), SLF II (blue), and IFOF (red). The top left is the lateral view of the right hemisphere, and the top right is the medial view of the right hemisphere. The bottom figure is the frontoparietal connections with cortical projections—angular gyrus, intraparietal sulcus, superior parietal lobule, temporoparietal junction, and frontal eye field.

Source: Doricchi et al. (2008).

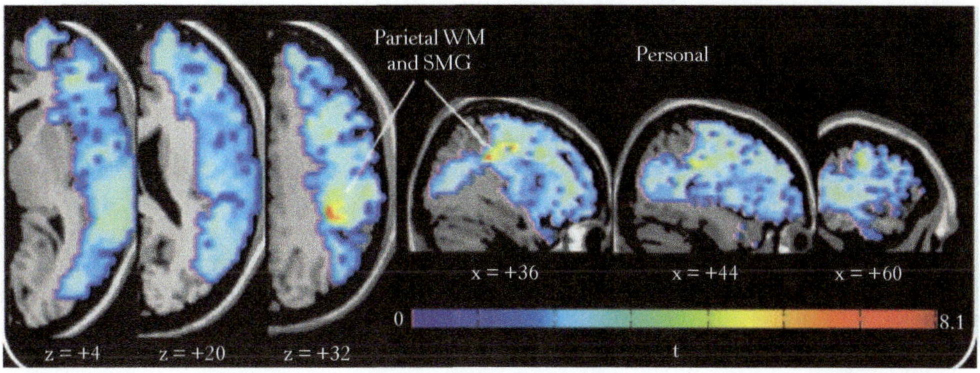

FIGURE 12.12: VBLSM maps for awareness of personal space in right brain-damaged patients. High *t*-scores (red) indicate a significant relationship and low *t*-scores (blue) indicate little relationship to behavior.

Source: Committeri et al. (2007).

matter connections between the cortical regions listed are disconnected may the symptoms occur.

A study assessing a more specific cognitive dysfunction that can result in neglect evaluated 52 patients with strokes, and it was found that awareness of personal space, a key dysfunction purportedly associated with neglect, is rooted in right inferior parietal regions—the supramarginal gyrus, postcentral gyrus, and especially the white matter medial to these two regions. Disruption of personal space awareness seems to be due to a functional disconnection between parietal regions important for coding somatosensory inputs and regions coding more abstract representations of the body in space. This study was essential in demonstrating in a large number of neglect patients that disruption of personal spatial awareness may require that the white matter underlying the parietal region be involved in the lesion (Figure 12.12) (Committeri et al., 2007). Focusing on finer-grained cognitive units such as disruption of awareness of personal space with its associated cortical region and white matter connections is the direction that cognitive neuroscience studies are heading, which provide the clearest account of brain–behavior relationships.

ATTENTION

To ascertain if connections to the attention domain could be isolated, Niogi et al. (2010) examined the correlation of performance on three aspects of attention—alerting, orienting, and conflict processing (assessed with the Attention Network Task)—with white matter tracts as measured by fractional anisotropy. It was found that the three functionally distinct components of attention were each correlated with three distinct white matter tract regions. Structure–function correlations were found between alerting and the anterior limb of the internal capsule, orienting and the splenium of the corpus callosum, and conflict with the anterior corona radiata. (The corona radiata is a white matter sheet that continues ventrally as the internal capsule. This sheet of axons carries nearly all of the communications to and from the cortex to the brain stem and spinal cord; Figure 12.13). A multiple regression/dissociation analysis demonstrated a *triple dissociation* between these three structure–function relationships that provided evidence of three anatomically and functionally separable white matter networks, whose disruption can lead to deficits in selective aspects of attentional processes depending on the specific white matter tracts affected (Niogi et al., 2010).

EXECUTIVE FUNCTION

One key pattern that appears to be emerging in the development of cognitive/behavioral–brain correlations is that cortical lesions with which functions have been associated may not be sufficient to produce a persistent impairment unless the underlying white matter is also involved in the lesion. This was explored in a large study of 516 patients with vascular white matter lesions who were enrolled in the Second Manifestations of ARTerial disease–Magnetic Resonance (SMART-MR) cohort. These patients received neuropsychological testing for the domains of memory, executive functioning, processing speed, and attention (Biesbroek et al., 2013; Geerlings et al., 2009). Using voxel-based lesion–symptom mapping (VBLSM),

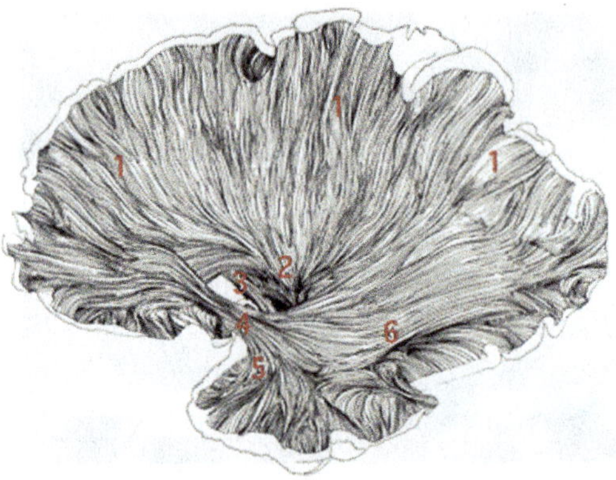

FIGURE 12.13: Depiction of major white matter connections from a sagittal view. 1, Corona radiate; 2, internal capsule; 3, anterior commissure; 4, inferior occipitofrontal fasciculus; 5, uncinate fasciculus; 6, sagittal stratum.

an association was detected between white matter lesions in the superior longitudinal fasciculus and the anterior thalamic radiations with poor executive functioning. These white matter tracts were specifically associated with the executive functions engaged by the tasks of Test of Everyday Attention (executive functions of mental flexibility and shifting attention), Brixton Spatial Anticipation Test (mental inhibition and flexibility), and verbal fluency (lexical search and selection) (Figure 12.14).

Initiative and motivation have long been considered a part of the spectrum of executive functions. A lack of will or initiative has been a major symptom described for disorders of reduced motivation after frontal lobe damage. Akinetic mutism is the term used for the most extreme version of this symptom, which occurs when a patient has a complete lack of initiation and motivation. Apathy is the term typically used for a minor deficit on this spectrum, and abulia refers to a moderate degree of lack of initiative. An abulic patient will have moderate difficulty acting on the external world events presented to him or her and impaired ability to make independent decisions. A white matter lesion has been suggested to be a correlate of developing abulia. The medial prefrontal cortex is connected to the medial parietal, occipital, and temporal lobe

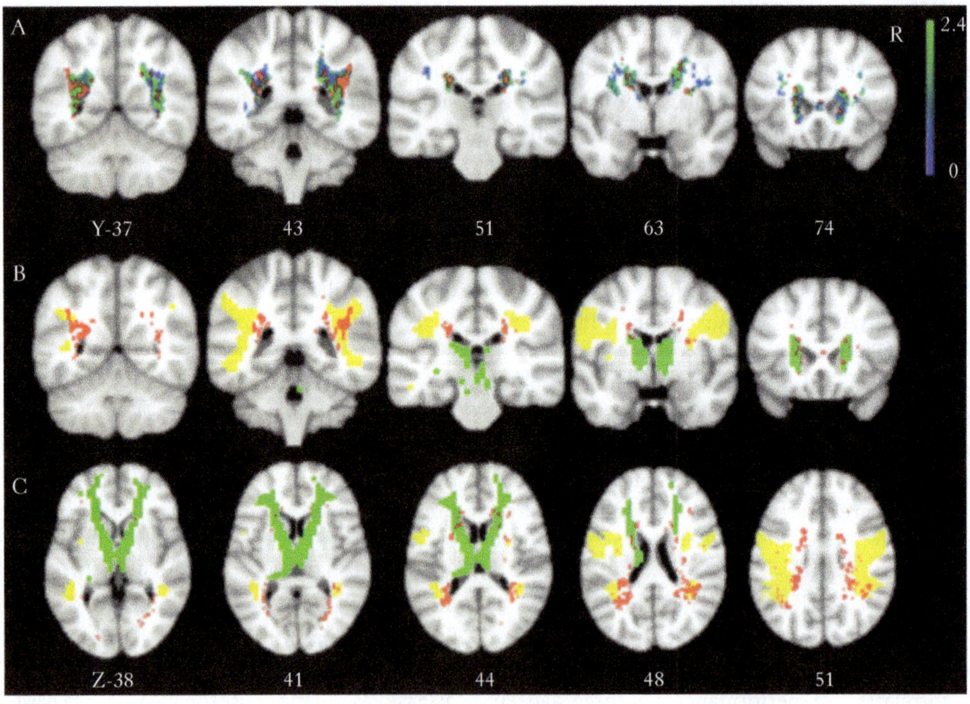

FIGURE 12.14 (A) VBLSM results of the correlation (*t*-statistic) between a lesion in each voxel and executive functioning. Voxels exceeding the false discovery rate are depicted in red, with nonsignificant voxels in a blue to green range. (B and C) The results of the same type of analysis as in row A. Voxels exceeding the false discovery rate threshold overlaid on the superior longitudinal fasciculus (yellow) and anterior thalamic radiation (green) are depicted.

Source: Biesbroek et al. (2013).

by the cingulum. The cingulum is a collection of white matter fibers projecting from the cingulate gyrus to medial temporal lobe structures and is thus a main communication tract between structures in the limbic system. Lesions of the anterior medial frontal lobe and cingulum can result in abulia manifested by apathy, markedly diminished motivation, and inability to make decisions (Mesulam, 2000; Rankin et al., 2006; Zappala et al., 2012). This type of apathy has both the affective and cognitive components of apathy—the affective aspects being blunt affect and the absence of interests, and the cognitive components include decreased engagement with usual activities, lack of interest, inability to initiate things, and reduced ability to sustain effort (Mega et al., 1997).

As with some of the past several studies, other approaches are being developed that allow for making correlations between white matter lesions and behavior. An approach investigating executive functions is to describe patterns of multiple cognitive symptoms that typically occur in varying combinations when a white matter lesion is present. For example, patients with white matter lesions involving the area beneath the dorsolateral frontal lobe have been associated with deficits in altered serial motor sequencing, poor response inhibition, impaired cognitive estimation, and abnormal abstract thinking (Baddeley, 2007; Catani et al., 2012; Thiebaut de Schotten et al., 2012). Executive functions for goal-directed behavior (planning, rule learning, focusing, hierarchical organization, switching, monitoring, etc.) are also affected by these types of lesions (Stuss & Knight, 2002).

LIMITATIONS

Dell'Acqua and Catani (2012) reviewed the use of DTI in clinical applications. The issues that need to be addressed are whether the technique can reliably reproduce normal anatomical pathways, whether there are individual differences that can be both detected and reflect the actual anatomy of individuals, and what are the optimal algorithms/methods that can be reliably applied across brain sites to evaluate patients at different facilities throughout the world. Some studies have confirmed the correlation between tracts detected with DTI and those isolated during postmortem evaluation (Lawes et al., 2008). It has been noted that there are particular tracts that are more reliably reproduced with DTI—the characteristics of optimal tracts to reliably detect are those attached to cortical regions, that do not cross other fibers, and that are without significant curvature (e.g., around the ventricles). Multiple studies of various tracts have demonstrated the presence of interindividual variability for specific tracts, which must be considered when interpreting group data as well as in potential future applications of DTI in the clinical setting (Catani et al., 2007).

The test–retest reliability of DTI has been investigated in 16 older adults using the Tract-Based Spatial Statistics (TBSS) approach. Intraclass correlation (ICC) averaged across the voxels of the TBSS skeleton ranged from 0.524 to 0.798 depending on the specific DTI measure and preprocessing used. The two main preprocessing steps that result in variability and also can be targeted for improvement to enhance the reliability of the technique were using a common individual template and smoothing DTI data using a 1-voxel median filter (Madhyastha et al., 2014). It is clear from the ICC that further enhancements and refinements are indicated, whether in preprocessing methods, analytic tools, degree of specification, image acquisition for DTI, use of other methods to better characterize water molecule displacement, or more direct measures of white matter integrity.

In addition, atlas development continues in this field as the amount of individual variability and longitudinal changes of white matter with age are detected with the use of DTI. New algorithms are being continuously developed that may lead to more reliable tractography at an individual level. As these technological advances are made and more individuals are studied to assess consistency of brain–behavioral correlations, more definitive associations between white matter lesions and cognitive units will be derived, if these exist consistently across individuals.

REFERENCES

Baddeley, A. (2007). *Working memory, thought and action.* Oxford, England: Oxford University Press.

Basso, A., Burgio, F., & Caporali, A. (2000). Acalculia, aphasia and spatial disorders in left and right brain-damaged patients. *Cortex, 36*(2), 265–280.

Basso, A., Lecours, A., Moraschini, S., & Vanier, M. (1985). Anatomoclinical correlations of the aphasias as defined through computerized tomography: Exceptions. *Brain and Language, 26*, 201–229.

Bauer, R. (1982). Visual hypoemotionality as a symptom of visual–limbic disconnection in man. *Archives of Neurology, 39*(11), 702–708.

Bayard, S., Gosselin, N., Robert, M., & Lassonde, M. (2004). Inter- and intra-hemispheric processing of visual event-related potentials in the absence of the corpus callosum. *Journal of Cognitive Neuroscience, 16*, 401–414.

Biesbroek, J., Kuijf, H., van der Graaf, Y., Vincken, K., Postma, A., Mali, W., et al., on behalf of the SMART Study Group. (2013). Association between subcortical vascular lesion location and cognition: A voxel-based and tract-based lesion–symptom mapping study: The SMART-MR study. *PloS One, 8*(4), e60541.

Binder, J., Desai, R., Graves, W., & Conant, L. (2009). Where is the semantic system? A critical review and meta-analysis of 120 functional neuroimaging studies. *Cerebral Cortex, 19*(12), 2767–2796.

Bird, C., Malhotra, P., Parton, A., Coulthard, E., Rushworth, M., & Husain, M. (2006). Visual neglect following right posterior cerebral artery infarction. *Journal of Neurology, Neurosurgery, and Psychiatry, 77*, 1008–1012.

Brodal, A. (1981). *Neurological anatomy in relation to clinical medicine* (3rd ed.). New York, NY: Oxford University Press.

Catani, M. (2006). Diffusion tensor magnetic resonance imaging tractography in cognitive disorders. *Current Opinion in Neurology, 19*, 599–606.

Catani, M., Allin, M., Husain, M., et al. (2007). Symmetries in human brain language pathways correlate with verbal recall. *Proceedings of the National Academy of Sciences of the USA, 104*, 17163–17168.

Catani, M., Dell'Acqua, F., Bizzi, A., Forkel, S., Williams, S., Simmons, A., et al. (2012). Beyond cortical localization in clinico-anatomical correlation. *Cortex, 48*, 1262–1287.

Catani, M., & ffytche, D. (2005). The rises and falls of disconnection syndromes. *Brain, 128*, 2224–2239.

Catani, M., Howard, R., Pajevic, S., & Jones, D. (2002). Virtual in vivo interactive dissection of white matter fasciculi in the human brain. *Neuroimage, 17*(1), 77–94.

Catani, M., Jones, D., Donato, R., & ffytche, D. (2003). Occipito-temporal connections in the human brain. *Brain, 126*, 2093–2107.

Catani, M., Jones, D., & ffytche, D. (2005). Perisylvian language networks of the human brain. *Annals of Neurology, 57*, 8–16.

Catani, M., Mesulam, M., Jakobsen, E., Malik, F., Martersteck, A., Wieneke, C., et al. (2013). A novel frontal pathway underlies verbal fluency in primary progressive aphasia. *Brain, 136*, 2619–2628.

Committeri, G., Pitzalis, S., Galati, G., Patria, F., Pelle, G., Sabatini, U., et al. (2007). Neural bases of personal and extrapersonal neglect in humans. *Brain, 130*, 431–441.

Corbetta, M. (2012). Functional connectivity and neurological recovery. *Developmental Psychobiology, 54*, 239–253.

Corbetta, M., Shulman, G. L., Miezin, F. M., & Petersen, S. E. (1995). Superior parietal cortex activation during spatial attention shifts and visual feature conjunction. *Science, 270*(5237), 802–805.

Crosson, B. (1984). Role of the dominant thalamus in language: A review. *Psychological Bulletin, 96*, 491–517.

Crosson, B. (2013). Thalamic mechanisms in language: A reconsideration based on recent findings and concepts. *Brain and Language, 126*, 73–88.

Crosson, B., Moberg, P., Boone, J., Rothi, L., & Raymer, A. (1997). Category-specific naming deficit for medical terms after dominant thalamic/capsular hemorrhage. *Brain and Language, 60*, 407–442.

Dell'Acqua, F., & Catani, M. (2012). Structural human brain networks: Hot topics in diffusion tractography. *Current Opinion in Neurology, 25*, 375–383.

Devinsky, O., & Laff, R. (2003). Callosal lesions and behavior: History and modern concepts. *Epilepsy and Behavior, 4*, 607–617.

Doricchi, F., Thiebaut de Schotten, M., Tomaiuolo, F., & Bartolomeo, P. (2008). White matter (dis)connections and gray matter (dys)functions in visual neglect: Gaining insights into the brain networks of spatial awareness. *Cortex, 44*(8), 983–995.

Epelbaum, S., Pinel, P., Gaillard, R., Delmaireb, C., Perrin, M., Dupont, S., et al. (2008). Pure alexia as a disconnection syndrome: New diffusion imaging evidence for an old concept. *Cortex, 44*, 962–974.

ffytche, D., Blom, J., & Catani, M. (2010). Disorders of visual perception. *Journal of Neurology, Neurosurgery, and Psychiatry, 81*(11), 1280–1287.

Fox, C., Iaria, G., & Barton, J. (2008). Disconnection in prosopagnosia and face processing. *Cortex, 44*, 996–1009.

Gazzaniga, M. (2005). Forty-five years of split-brain research and still going strong. *Nature Reviews Neuroscience, 6*, 653–659.

Geerlings, M., Appelman, A., Vincken, K., Mali, W., van der Graaf, Y., for the SMART Study Group. (2009). Association of white matter lesions and lacunar infarcts with executive functioning: The SMART-MR Study. *American Journal of Epidemiology, 170*(9), 1147–1155.

Geschwind, N. (1965). Disconnection syndromes in animals and human. *Brain, 88*(3), 585–644.

Glickstein, M., & Berlucchi, G. (2008). Classical disconnection studies of the corpus callosum. *Cortex, 44*(8), 914–927.

Graff-Radford, N., Tranel, D., Van Hoesen, G., & Brandt, J. (1990). Diencephalic amnesia. *Brain, 113*, 1–25.

Han, Z., Ma, Y., Gong, G., He, Y., Caramazza, A., & Bi, Y. (2013). White matter structural connectivity underlying semantic processing: Evidence from brain damaged patients. *Brain, 136*(Pt. 10), 2952–2965.

Heilman, K., & Watson, R. (2008). The disconnection apraxias. *Cortex, 44*(8), 975–982.

Iacoboni, M., & Zaidel, E. (2004). Interhemispheric visuo-motor integration in humans: The role of the superior parietal cortex. *Neuropsychologia, 42*, 419–425.

Kraut, M., Kremen, S., Segal, J., Calhoun, V., Moo, L., & Hart, J. (2002). Object activation from features in the semantic system. *Journal of Cognitive Neuroscience, 14*, 24–36.

Lawes, I., Barrick, T., Murugam, V., et al. (2008). Atlas-based segmentation of white matter tracts of the human brain using diffusion tensor tractography and comparison with classical dissection. *Neuroimage, 39*, 62–79.

Leibovitch, F., Black, S., Caldwell, C., McIntosh, A., Ehrlich, L., & Szalai, J. (1998). Brain–behavior correlations in hemispatial neglect using CT and SPECT: The Sunnybrook Stroke Study. *Neurology, 50*, 901–908.

Leiguarda, R., & Marsden, C. (2000). Limb apraxias: Higher-order disorders of sensorimotor integration. *Brain, 123*(Pt. 5), 860–879.

Leiguarda, R., Starkstein, S., & Berthier, M. (1989). Anterior callosal haemorrhage: Partial interhemispheric disconnection syndrome. *Brain, 112*, 1019–1037.

Madhyastha, T., Mérillat, S., Hirsiger, S., Bezzola, L., Liem, F., Grabowski, T., & Jäncke L. (2014). Longitudinal reliability of tract-based spatial statistics in diffusion tensor imaging. *Human Brain Mapping, 35*(9), 4544–4555.

Mega, M., Cummings, J., Salloway, S., & Malloy, P. (1997). The limbic system: an anatomic, phylogenetic, and clinical perspective. *Journal of Neuropsychiatry Clinical Neuroscience, 9*(3), 315–330.

Mesulam, M. (2000). Principles of behavioral and cognitive neurology. Oxford University Press.

Mooshagian, E., Kaplan, J., Zaidel, E., & Iacoboni, M. (2008). Fast visuomotor processing of redundant targets: The role of the right temporo-parietal junction. *PLoS ONE, 3*, e2348.

Mori, S., Crain, B., Chacko, V., & van Zijl, P. (1999). Three-dimensional tracking of axonal projections in the brain by magnetic resonance imaging. *Annals of Neurology, 45*(2), 265–269.

Mori, S., & van Zijl, P. (2002). Fiber tracking: Principles and strategies—A technical review. *NMR in Biomedicine, 15*, 468–480.

Müller-Oehring, E., Schulte, T., Raassi, C., Pfefferbaum, A., & Sullivan, E. (2007). Local–global interference is modulated by age, sex and anterior corpus callosum size. *Brain Research, 1142*, 189–205.

Naeser, M., Martin, P., Nicholas, M., Baker, E., Seekins, H., Helm-Estabrooks, N., et al. (2005). Improved naming after TMS treatments in a chronic, global aphasia patient—Case report. *Neurocase, 11*, 182–193.

Niogi, S., Mukherjee, P., Ghajar, J., & McCandliss, B. (2010). Individual differences in distinct components of attention are linked to anatomical variations in distinct white matter tracts. *Frontiers in Neuroanatomy*, 4(2). doi: 10.3389/neuro.05.002.2010

Pollmann, S., & Zaidel, E. (1998). The role of the corpus callosum in visual orienting: Importance of interhemispheric visual transfer. *Neuropsychologia, 36*, 763–774.

Ramayya, A., Glasser, M., & Rilling, J. (2010). A DTI investigation of neural substrates supporting tool use. *Cerebral Cortex, 20*(3), 507–516.

Rankin, K., Gorno-Tempini, M., Allison, S., Stanley, C., Glenn, S., Weiner, M., et al. (2006). Structural anatomy of empathy in neurodegenerative disease. *Brain, 129*(11), 2945–2956.

Schmahmann, J., Smith, E., Eichler, F., & Filley, C. (2008). Cerebral white matter: Neuroanatomy, clinical neurology, and neurobehavioral correlates. *Annals of the New York Academy of Sciences, 1142*, 266–309.

Schulte, T., & Müller-Oehring, E. (2010). Contribution of callosal connections to the interhemispheric integration of visuomotor and cognitive processes. *Neuropsychology Review, 20*, 174–190.

Sierra, M., Lopera, F., Lambert, M., Phillips, M., & David, A. (2002). Separating depersonalisation and derealisation: The relevance of the "lesion method." *Journal of Neurology, Neurosurgery, and Psychiatry, 72*(4), 530–532.

Slotnick, S., Moo, L., Kraut, M., Lesser, R., & Hart, J. (2002). Thalamic modulation of cortical rhythms during semantic memory recall in humans. *Proceedings of the National Academy of Sciences of the USA, 99*(9), 6440–6443.

Stuss, D., & Knight, R. (2002). *Principles of frontal lobe function*. Oxford, England: Oxford University Press.

Tak, H., & Jang, S. (2014). Relation between aphasia and arcuate fasciculus in chronic stroke patients. *BMC Neurology, 14*, 46.

Thiebaut de Schotten, M., Dell'Acqua, F., Valabregue, R., & Catani, M. (2012). Monkey to human comparative anatomy of the frontal lobe association tracts. *Cortex, 48*(1), 82–96.

Urbanski, M., Thiebaut de Schotten, M., Rodrigo, S., Catani, M., Oppenheim, C., Touze, E., et al. (2008). Brain networks of spatial awareness: Evidence from diffusion tensor imaging tractography. *Journal of Neurology, Neurosurgery, and Psychiatry, 79*, 598–601.

Verdon, V., Lovblad, K.-O., Hauert, C.-A., & Vuilleumier, P. (2006). *Neuroanatomical basis of hemispatial neglect components using voxel-based lesion symptom mapping.* Paper presented at the second meeting of the European Societies of Neuropsychology, Toulouse, France, October 18–20, 2006.

Zappala, G., Thiebaut de Schotten, M., & Eslinger, P. (2012). What can we gain with diffusion tensor imaging. *Cortex, 48*(2), 156–165.

13

Network Models

Throughout this book, the focus has been on single brain regions that support cognitive units, with the evidence for these associations supported by functional imaging and lesion studies. This is encompassed under the theory of modularity, which proposes that there are functionally specialized regions in the brain encoding for aspects of cognition and behavior (Fodor, 1983). As noted in the introduction, there are other cognitive units that are not supported by isolated regions but are nodes in a network involved in performing the function (e.g., distributed—encoding the process across multiple anatomic nodes of a network).

To clarify these brain–behavior distinctions, it is important to delineate a set of working definitions that are helpful in further framing localizations and functions. To reiterate some of the concepts defined in Chapter 1, a task refers to performing an act or behavior that typically engages several cognitive units. Anatomic units detectable by available neuroimaging techniques were assessed to determine the brain regions supporting these cognitive units (acknowledging that there are also neurophysiological and non-anatomically localizable groups of neurons that support cognitive units). There may well be one or multiple independent brain regions or an integrated network of regions that support each unit. The localizations reported in this book thus far are typically identified when a lesion in a specific location results in a consistent dysfunction of a cognitive unit, referred to as a cognitive–anatomic unit (CAU). Regions that are active during functional imaging studies but not identified as CAUs after assessing lesion studies typically are those whose lesioning does not produce a consistent cognitive deficit, produces no deficit, is engaged by the task in some manner but is not involved in the cognitive process of interest assessed by the lesion data, or is part of a network of anatomic regions working together sharing support for the same cognitive unit and does not result in a consistent deficit. These regions may support a cognitive unit or several cognitive units.

As an example, a task consists of two cognitive units. One cognitive unit is associated with only one region, forming a CAU. The other cognitive unit is associated with four brain regions, with lesioning in any one region not resulting in loss of the functions of the cognitive unit but inconsistent mild dysfunction, suggesting that it is supported by a network of these four regions. Thus, this task consists of a combination of two cognitive–brain systems with the localization of a lesion in one region consistently severely disrupting one cognitive function and lesions to one of the four regions that support the other cognitive function not severely disrupting it but resulting in some decrement in its outcome that is not consistent. (For other network descriptions that will not be repeated here, see Chapter 1.)

Even if a circumscribed lesion results in a consistent cognitive deficit, the question arises whether that region supports that function entirely or whether it is just a node in a set of cooperative nodes in a network in which all the nodes together perform a function but lesioning that particular node does result in a consistent deficit. It could be that this particular brain region represents a hierarchical node in a network such that lesioning it results in disruption of the entire network of regions. This type of network architecture should be considered before assuming a single brain region is responsible, and this shows the value of having an activation study to show all regions involved when interpreting a lesion study.

Also after lesioning of a node, a network may adjust and perform the function that it typically performs but less efficiently. Alternatively, reorganization can occur in the nodes after an injury in a variety of ways, ranging from a consistent anatomic reorganization leading to a consistent output to many different plausible network organizations and outputs or the network functioning inconsistently after a lesion occurs in a particular node in the network.

Networks can thus be complicated in their overall function and even more complicated when a lesion occurs. Irrespective of the complexity of a network, there should be a lesion to a specific location resulting in a consistent deficit for clear inferences to be made at this point about brain–behavior correlations (but see Other Network Approaches later in this chapter).

In many cases in the past, it was unknown whether the lesioned area was performing an isolated function or the deficit was the result of disrupting a network. With the advent of functional imaging, most notably functional magnetic resonance imaging (fMRI) and functional connectivity MRI (fcMRI), networks of regions contributing to a function or a task can now be identified. During fMRI, investigators can have subjects perform a task while in the MRI scanner and image their blood oxygen level-dependent (BOLD) response in the whole brain related to performance of the task. BOLD signal depends on the changes in the magnetic properties of oxygenated/deoxygenated hemoglobin, and it represents an index of oxygen- and blood flow-dependent neural and glial activity. In analyzing fMRI studies to determine which brain regions are associated with cognitive operations, the BOLD response of a brain region while performing a task is compared to the BOLD signal for another "baseline" task for each small volume in the brain referred to as voxels. Voxels with significantly higher BOLD signal during the task than the baseline are considered differentially engaged in task performance. The single brain region or network of brain regions that may be differentially engaged in the task will be isolated using these types of fMRI studies.

fcMRI is typically performed while a subject is lying in the MRI scanner but is not performing a task. BOLD signal is acquired for each voxel in the brain while subjects are performing no specific task, referred to as rest state. The temporal correlation of the spontaneous fluctuations in the BOLD response is then calculated between each voxel and all of the other voxels in the brain (one pair of voxels at a time). Those regions whose resting BOLD signal fluctuations correlate significantly with each other form functional brain networks. It is of note that these "background" fluctuations can also be computed during the performance of a given task to assess for networks that may be engaged by that task. The use of these techniques has established the presence of a variety of networks in the brain that are functionally related. There are multiple resting state networks that have consistently been detected across individuals, establishing these functional networks for further analyses in normal and patient populations. It has been proposed that these networks originate in part from spontaneous neuronal firing so that temporal correlations of the time series of BOLD signal fluctuations between different regions reflect an ongoing connectivity between the nodes detected in these networks, independent of any particular task being performed.

With these fMRI and fcMRI networks, hypotheses can be generated concerning the function and neuroanatomic correlates of these proposed networks and how lesions may affect them. These networks take on various roles in different cognitive operations and behavior. It is speculated that multiple resting state fcMRI networks do not function directly in tasks or processing stimuli (Corbetta, 2012), but they likely play supporting roles such as maintaining a level of engagement, monitoring, and/or intrinsic operations during tasks. This is due to fcMRI networks being imaged only during the regions' spontaneous activity at rest. Once the subject is no longer at rest and is engaged in a task, the network's characteristics change rapidly.

The most consistently detected resting state networks are default mode network (DMN), sensorimotor network (SMN), visual resting state network (VRSN), auditory resting state network (ARSN), executive control network (ECN), lateralized frontoparietal network (FPN), temporoparietal network (TPN), and salience network (Figure 13.1). The sensorimotor, visual, and auditory networks involve areas that when active are normally engaged in primary and secondary perceptual processing in those modalities. The default mode, executive control, frontoparietal, temporoparietal, and salience networks involve regions that when active are most commonly associated with cognition and behavior (Figure 13.2).

These resting state and task-derived networks have been proposed to better represent the neural substrate of cognition and behavior, or deficits after lesions, than a modular organization. The evidence suggests that cognition and behavior are best accounted for by a combination of both types of brain organizational schema—modular and network systems.

This chapter is organized by the network and functions of the network. Because not all of the networks that have been delineated with neuroimaging have been associated with cognitive functions, not all of the networks are discussed. The discussion

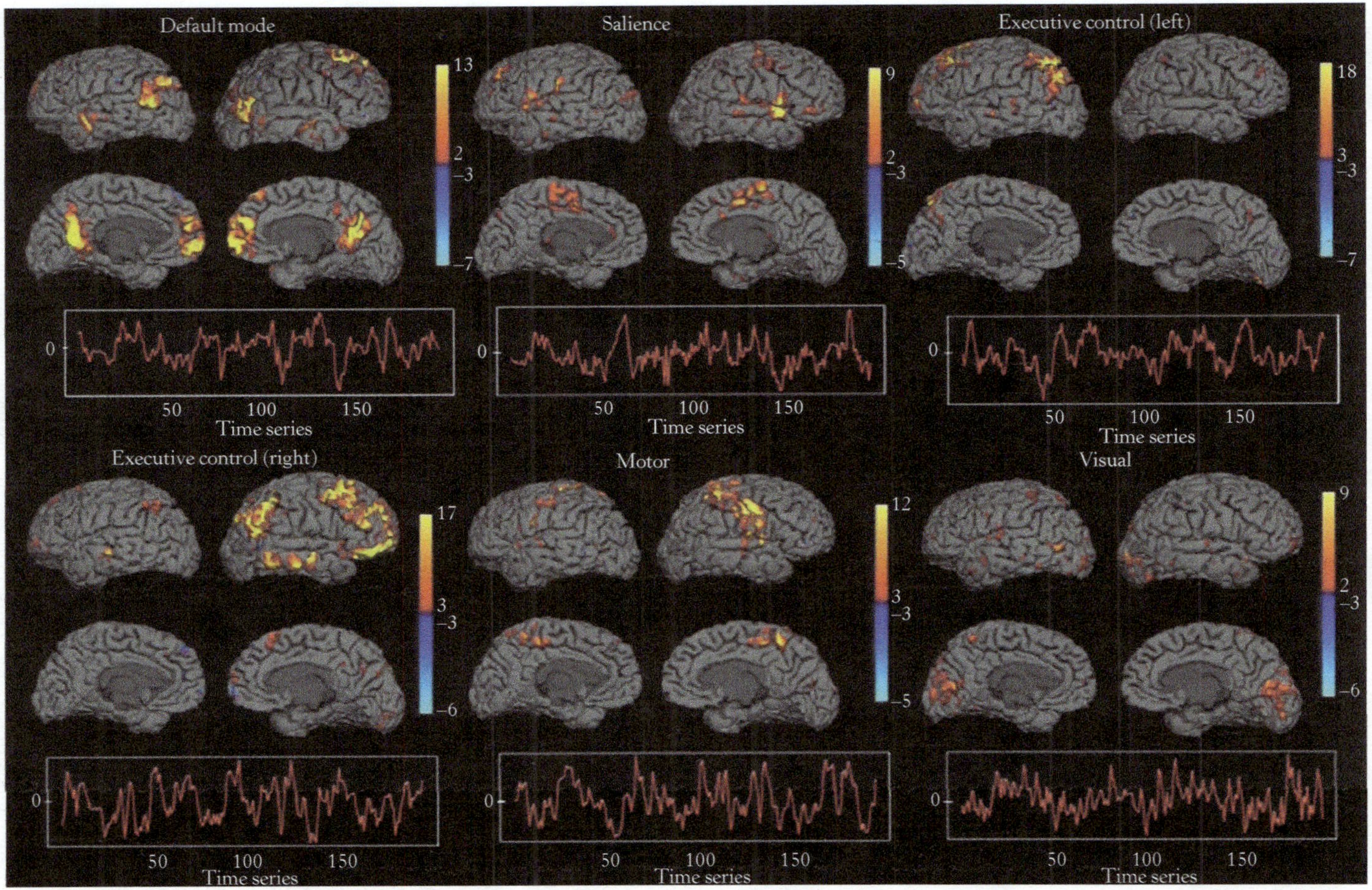

FIGURE 13.1: Functional connectivity from resting state fcMRI in healthy subjects. ICA-derived resting state fMRI networks (DMN, salience, left and right executive control, and visual and motor networks) are depicted with red-to-yellow colors indicating the strength of each voxel's connectivity. The graphs with the red lines show the correlated activity in the baseline fluctuations of BOLD during rest between regions in the networks.

Source: Pievani et al. (2011).

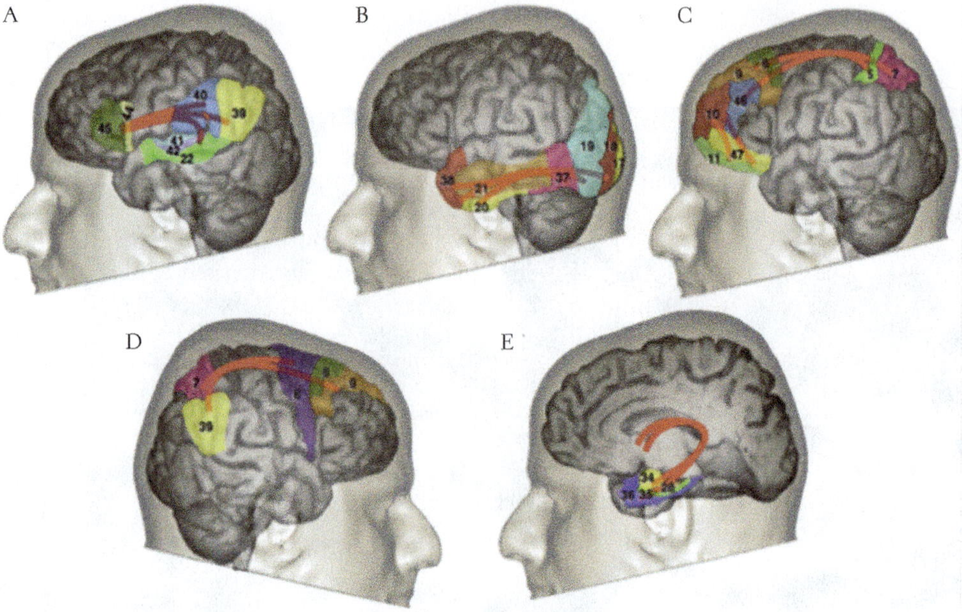

FIGURE 13.2: Several key networks in cognition. (A) A language-related network with anchors at Broca's and Wernicke's areas. (B) The components of a face–object identification network. (C) An executive function network with key regions in the lateral prefrontal, orbitofrontal, and posterior parietal cortices. (D) A proposed spatial attention network from a right lateral view, including posterior parietal cortex, cingulate gyrus, and frontal eye fields. (E) A memory and emotion network including the hippocampal and amygdala regions.

Source: Adapted from Catani et al. (2012).

begins with one well-described network that has been found to be useful in accounting for certain disease states—the default mode network.

DEFAULT MODE NETWORK AND DISEASE STATES

The precuneus is a cortical region that typically has attracted little notice due to its deep location and lack of damage secondary to lesions, either by vascular disease or by other disorders. However, fMRI studies have implicated the precuneus as playing a role in episodic memory (Henson et al., 1999), controlling spatial aspects of motor behavior (Grefkes et al., 2004), shifting attention for visual stimuli (Le et al., 1998), mental imagery and navigation (Knauff et al., 2003), and self-relevant information processing (Kircher et al., 2000). More importantly, the precuneus has been implicated as a key region in the DMN detected during resting fcMRI (Greicius et al., 2003; Gusnard et al., 2001). This network consists of the brain regions of the precuneus, medial temporal, ventromedial prefrontal, dorsolateral prefrontal, posterior medial parietal, and lateral parietal cortices (Figure 13.3).

Originally, the DMN was reported by Raichle and colleagues (see Gusnard & Raichle, 2001 for review) as a group of regions that demonstrated correlated deactivation during task performance across multiple tasks using either fMRI or PET. From this point forward, the DMN will be referenced from here onward as acquired from resting state fcMRI. This set of brain regions' correlated BOLD signal fluctuations are high when an individual is not engaged in specific behavioral tasks and low during focused attention on the external environment. This network, besides consuming a notable amount of energy (Gusnard & Raichle, 2001), has been imputed to represent a variety of cognitive states, including self-consciousness/self-reference (self-referential thought refers to functions such as internal mentation or thinking), spontaneous mental processing, being awake and alert, lack of engagement in a cognitive task, and/or information monitoring. Because these functions do not lend themselves to being easily distinguished from each other, the exact role of the DMN has not been clearly identified. This set of functions on the surface appears to be in contrast to externally oriented goal-directed thought,

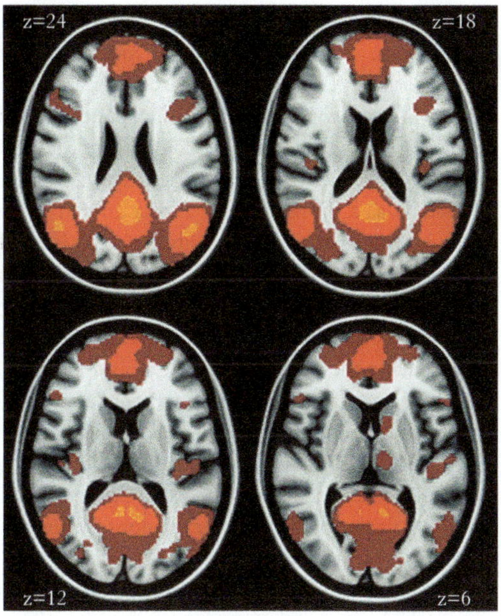

FIGURE 13.3: Group ICA map of the default-mode network from resting state fcMRI scans.

Source: http://oxfordjournals.org.

which makes intuitive sense because the DMN is detected when the subject is not engaged in a task but is at "rest." Overall, however, from this list of possible roles, there is no clear "function" known for the DMN. It appears to be evident that DMN activity could conflict with functions necessary for processes that orient an individual to performing tasks in the world and not just introspecting (Smith et al., 2012) and that suppression of the DMN is necessary for the successful performance of certain types of goal-directed cognitive processes (Spreng, 2012).

Given that the fcMRI networks described here exist at rest and cannot be easily explored experimentally because that would remove the individual from being "at rest," the role that fcMRI rest networks play in cognition is unclear. However, it has been shown that atypical DMNs recorded while a subject is at rest are associated with several neuropsychiatric disease states. The disruption of DMN functional connectivity networks and the role that these networks may play as potential diagnostic markers of neuropsychiatric diseases show considerable promise and are detailed here.

Alzheimer's Disease

DMN dysfunction has most prominently been used in diagnostic implications of dementing illnesses (Zhou & Seeley, 2014). Alzheimer's disease (AD) is associated with hypometabolism/decreased connectivity in the hippocampus, cingulate, temporal, and parietal regions when measured as part of the DMN during rest (Grecius et al., 2003). With AD, decreased resting state activity in the posterior cingulate and hippocampus suggests that disrupted connectivity between these two regions accounts for the posterior cingulate hypometabolism commonly detected in positron emission tomography (PET) studies of early AD patients (Greicius et al., 2004).

This finding of decreased connectivity in the DMN was proposed as an early marker of AD. A meta-analysis of multiple studies totaling 1196 patients and 1255 controls showed that patients with AD have less connectivity in the DMN than controls, notably in the left precuneus, right parahippocampal gyrus, left thalamus, and right postcentral gyrus. These findings were highly replicable across numerous studies (Jacobs, Radua, Lückmann, & Sack, 2013).

It has been proposed that the disruption of the DMN at rest leads to the network not being able to deactivate effectively during task performance; this deactivation from the default mode at rest is needed for successful externally directed task performance (Jacobs, Radua, Lückmann, & Sack, 2013). The imbalance between the inadequate disengagement from the default mode to an active task-related brain has been proposed to result in poor or inefficient task performance. Further studies show that there is a progressive loss of DMN connectivity as disease progression occurs in AD, providing a potential marker of progressive cognitive decline as connectivity decreases or, at some point when treatment options become available, a potential marker of treatment effect.

One of the key correlative findings supporting DMN as a marker of AD is the study that integrated fcMRI findings with PET isotopes of AD pathology. In an investigation of patients developing AD, spatial overlap was found between (1) the DMN regions that demonstrated decreased functional connectivity and (2) regions showing deposition of Pittsburgh compound-B PET (PIB-PET), which is a PET neuroimaging marker of amyloid plaque deposition. Radioactive amyloid plaque markers have been correlated with Alzheimer's pathology, providing a link between disease, pathology, and the PET amyloid imaging marker. The correlation of decreased connectivity of resting state DMN in suspected AD patients with PET amyloid plaque marker detection suggests that resting state fcMRI may one day be able to serve as a clinically diagnostic marker for the development of AD (Mormino et al., 2011).

Frontotemporal Dementia

Patients with the behavioral variant of frontotemporal dementia (BvFTD), in contrast to those with AD, have shown decreased connectivity in the anterior insula, anterior cingulate cortex, medial/orbital prefrontal cortex, striatum, thalamus, and amygdala during fcMRI compared to the connectivity measured in normal, age-matched controls. These hypo-connected regions are part of the salience network, a region identified by resting state fcMRI, with the brain regions of this network proposed to be engaged in social and emotional processing when not in the rest state (Rosen et al., 2002). Whereas AD patients have disrupted DMN connectivity but enhanced salience network connectivity, BvFTD patients show reduced salience network connectivity. In addition, BvFTD patients show enhanced DMN connectivity, opposite to the pattern seen in AD patients. Thus, these networks show potential for use in differentiating these two dementing illnesses from normal controls and potentially from each other.

Traumatic Brain Injury

The relationship of dysfunction in the DMN with traumatic brain injury (TBI) is less consistent than with dementia. Some studies have shown increased DMN connectivity correlated with post-concussive symptoms (Stevens et al., 2012), whereas other studies have shown decreased connectivity (Mayer et al., 2011). This heterogeneity of DMN findings makes intuitive sense because there is considerable variability in the type, location, and extent of damage associated with traumatic injuries. Although this heterogeneity may preclude using DMN status to characterize TBI disease states, ongoing studies are assessing the potential use of DMN connectivity as a marker of prognosis in TBI, with the success likely dependent on how well individual study findings are stable across studies and how networks consistently change with disease progression.

Temporal Lobe Epilepsy

A key region of the DMN is the medial temporal lobe region, which is often implicated in the pathology of patients with temporal lobe epilepsy (TLE). Abnormal neural firing in a brain region can be detected with electroencephalography recording of brain waves from electrodes placed on a person's scalp. The abnormal neural firing associated with seizures is a sharp, spikey wave referred to as a "spike." The neurons abnormally firing to create this spike can recruit other nearby neurons to fire in a similar pattern, which is referred to as spike propagation. If this rhythmical firing continues and remains locally, then this is referred to as a partial seizure and is limited to the region in which the seizure is contained. This is manifested clinically as atypical functioning of the region where the spikes are firing. For example, in the case of the motor region, there will be abnormal motor movements during the partial seizure (e.g., limb jerking). This abnormal neuronal firing can spread because the other neurons to which the spiking neurons are connected will receive a signal through their joining synapse to fire in the same abnormal pattern. If this abnormal firing spreads to other regions throughout the brain, it can lead to a generalized seizure.

In the case of TLE, the seizures are limited to the temporal lobe region and can manifest with a variety of behavioral symptoms. The most typical area where the abnormal spiking originates in TLE is the hippocampal region. However, the area of reduced activation of the DMN in TLE patients, while not having seizures, is the prefrontal cortex (Zhang et al., 2010; see also Liao et al., 2011). It has been proposed that the most typical disruption of DMN in TLE is loss of functional connectivity between the prefrontal cortex and the precuneus (Figure 13.4) (Cataldi et al., 2013; Haneef et al., 2012). Because there is not a direct correlation between the regions where the electrophysiological abnormalities occur and the regions of altered connectivity shown with fcMRI in these patients, further studies are indicated. Further analyses may well find that this prefrontal–precuneus loss of connectivity is a clear and consistent reflection of the temporal lobe electrophysiological dysfunction.

Multiple Sclerosis

Multiple sclerosis (MS) is a disease that primarily disrupts central nervous system white matter by causing its loss of myelin (demyelination), which results predominantly in disruption of the white matter connections between gray matter regions. In addition, to a lesser degree, there is disruption of the gray matter with cortical MS lesions. This disease has long been conceptualized by the white matter pathology causing deficits via disruption of multiple brain networks by which gray matter communicates. Consequently, the deficits resulting from MS lend themselves to best being accounted for by models that focus on the disruption of brain networks. One

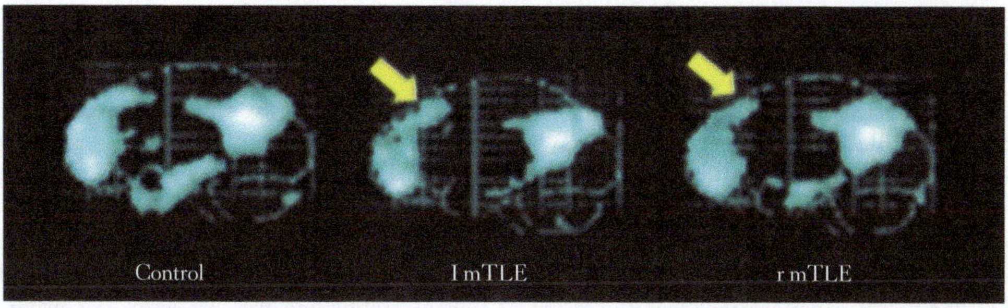

FIGURE 13.4: Temporal lobe epilepsy affects activity and connectivity of the default mode network (DMN). The images show a comparison of the DMN in control subjects and right and left TLE patients. The images represent the averages of DMN signals. Note the significantly smaller areas of correlation in the dorsal medial prefrontal cortex and the mesial and inferior temporal lobe in TLE patients in comparison with controls.

Source: Zhang et al. (2010).

of the emerging chronic deficits in MS is cognitive impairment, which has not easily been accounted for with standard structural brain imaging. Disruption of the resting state networks in MS has showed promise in accounting for deficits, particularly the DMN and its relationship to cognition (Sacco et al., 2013).

Changes in resting state networks, including DMN, do not correlate with gray matter lesions in MS (Gallo et al., 2012; Rocca et al., 2010), suggesting that the disruptions in resting state networks are more likely associated with the prominent white matter pathology of MS. Studies of healthy controls and MS patients, including those with and without a cognitive deficit, showed reduced connectivity in the DMN in MS compared to controls (Rocca et al., 2010). In another study of 36 MS patients, 18 with cognitive deficits and 18 without, the entire MS group showed a reduction in connectivity within the DMN, particularly in the anterior cingulate region of the DMN, and also reported an increase in connectivity at the posterior cingulate region of the DMN compared to controls. Of significance is that the increase in connectivity in the posterior cingulate was in those patients who did not have a cognitive impairment. This provides a potential method to monitor cognitive function in MS patients for both the presence of deficits and response to treatment (Leavitt et al., 2014; Rocca et al., 2010) after the findings reported are confirmed by studies of larger numbers of MS patients.

Attention Deficit Hyperactivity Disorder

Another disease state associated with DMN is attention deficit hyperactivity disorder (ADHD). Decreased connectivity in a set of nodes—the dorsal nodes—of the DMN was found to be associated with a subtype of ADHD in which the most prominent symptom is attention deficit (Anderson et al., 2014). In addition, the more ventral nodes of the DMN show increased connectivity in this inattentive subtype of ADHD. This suggests that in the future, further analysis of nodes within a network may provide more fine-grained distinctions to distinguish between disease states and will need to be systematically explored in investigating disease states.

Psychiatric Conditions

In terms of behavioral disorders, it has been proposed that an inability to suppress the DMN when task engagement is to occur represents a mechanism by which cognitive deficits and/or behavioral symptoms may develop in psychiatric illness. The DMN interacts with other cognitive networks as an individual shifts between resting state to performing tasks in the world. As a task is to be performed, the task-associated networks become activated and the DMN becomes suppressed. The dynamic between activating one network and deactivating another is not clearly known. Whether it is from the inability to suppress the DMN when a task needs to be performed or dysfunction in activating the other networks necessary to perform a task, psychiatric conditions or cognitive impairments in those with psychiatric illnesses have been proposed to be associated with either of these two dysfunctions. A clear example of this is in schizophrenic patients, in whom DMN suppression is impaired during performance of cognitively demanding tasks (Anticevic et al., 2011).

DMN suppression may represent a manner in which the brain suppresses internal activity such as mind wandering or rumination (Anticevic et al.,

2012). In fact, failure to suppress the DMN has been proposed as a possible mechanism to the rumination on negative internal thoughts that occurs in a subset of patients with significant depression (Perrin et al., 2012; Sheline et al., 2009). It has been further hypothesized that in depressed patients, this increased activity in the DMN, particularly the medial prefrontal network nodes, may contribute to both the increased ruminations in these patients and impaired frontal lobe-related cognitive performance that is occasionally exhibited in this group (Nejad et al., 2013).

Recent investigations have also focused on using pharmacologic manipulation of these networks to determine possible underlying dysfunction of network enhancement and/or suppression. The pro-stimulant modafinil has been found to enhance DMN suppression during performance of a working memory task. Modafinil has multiple mechanisms of action, but the most relevant to cognition is its role in increasing dopamine in the brain. It has thus been suggested that the dopamine system is involved in suppressing the DMN based on these working memory findings (Minzenberg et al., 2011). The psychedelic hallucinogen psilocybin was also found to increase DMN suppression at rest, providing further support for a role of the dopamine circuit in modulating DMN suppression (Carhart-Harris et al., 2012).

Overall, dysfunction in the DMN does appear to correlate with certain cognitive and behavioral disorders, even though it is unclear what the DMN itself represents. As further investigations and analyses evolve, the role for the DMN in diagnostic, prognostic, and treatment monitoring may continue to advance. In addition, further studies may better elucidate what the network actually signifies and how it interacts with other networks.

OTHER REST STATE NETWORKS AND DISEASES

Distinguishing other disease states from normal has been pursued using rest state networks other than the DMN or by using seed regions and assessing functional connectivity to those particular seed regions. A seed region in rest state fcMRI analysis refers to a particular voxel or group of voxels that are chosen to find the temporal correlations of the spontaneous fluctuations in the BOLD response of that seed region with every other voxel in the brain, which is the measure of connectivity used with fcMRI. These correlations to the seed region in a patient with a disease can be compared to those of normal controls to determine if there are dysfunctional rest state connections for that region in the patient. One disease examined in this manner was progressive supranuclear palsy (PSP), which clinically presents with gaze paralysis, axial rigidity, gait instability, and a behavioral deficit that is marked by disruption in executive functions and psychomotor speed, apathy, and compulsions. Using fcMRI, connectivity was measured in two control groups and patients with PSP using the dorsal midbrain tegmentum as a seed region. The fcMRI seed analysis showed that PSP patients had disruption of the connectivity of the dorsal midbrain tegmentum to voxels in the brain stem, cerebellum, and basal ganglia. This finding correlates with autopsy findings in PSP patients showing this region to demonstrate focal atrophy and cell loss (Gardner et al., 2013).

Seeley et al. (2009) studied rest state fcMRI in patients with one of five of the following neurodegenerative diseases: AD (n = 24), behavioral variant frontotemporal dementia (BvFTD; n = 24), semantic dementia (SD; n = 24), progressive nonfluent aphasia (PNFA; n = 13), or corticobasal syndrome (CBS; n = 17). The patterns of functional connectivity were assessed using seed regions that were based on brain areas that were characteristically disrupted and/or atrophic for each disease. AD patients had disruption to the DMN, as noted previously (Buckner et al., 2005). BvFTD was again linked to changes in the emotional salience processing network. SD was related to changes in connectivity in the temporal pole–subgenual cingulate–ventral striatum–amygdala network. The PNFA-targeted seed network of brain–behavior correlations included the frontal operculum, primary and supplementary motor cortices, and inferior parietal lobule bilaterally because these regions link the language and motor systems that enable speech. In PNFA in which there is left sided degeneration of the brain, this is reflected in disrupted connectivity on the left side of that network. Corticobasal syndrome, characterized by motor and oculomotor abnormalities on clinical presentation, was found to be associated with disruption of the dorsal sensorimotor association network (Seeley et al., 2009; see also Pievani et al., 2011; Zhou et al., 2012). Further studies are ongoing with more advanced analytic methods to explore how aberrations in network connectivity can be used for diagnostic, prognostic, and therapeutic monitoring purposes. A key advance that could greatly support the use of these resting state connectivity networks for diagnostic purposes is the ability to reliably analyze and apply the results for a single subject because all of the previously mentioned studies have been group studies.

LESIONING OF NETWORKS

A method to determine the localization of the functions of a network or its nodes is to observe how individuals function after a lesion to the network occurs. In the past, this would have proceeded from studying a collection of patients with randomly occurring and variable-sized lesions to find a homogeneous cohort of patients with a consistent-sized lesion located in the same place. As one may imagine, collecting these groups of individuals is logistically difficult. Now with recent advances in neuroinvestigative techniques, there are other opportunities to produce systematic, consistent, reversible lesions in normal individuals to investigate networks. These new techniques allow for probing to seek the causal role of particular brain areas within networks that include several regions by measuring the effects of manipulations for a targeted area on the function of the network. These techniques have also been used to investigate independent anatomic regions performing consistent cognitive operations, but here the focus is on studies using the results of lesions to infer the function of a network and/or the nodes within a network.

One particular technique is repetitive transcranial magnetic stimulation (rTMS). rTMS was introduced in approximately 1985 as a brain stimulation technique. The principle of how rTMS works is based on Faraday's law of induction for time-varying currents. In the case of rTMS, a time-varying alternating pole magnetic field is generated through a stimulator coil (Figure 13.5). This rapidly changing external magnetic field induces an electric current. When this coil is placed over the scalp, the rise and fall of the alternating magnetic field induces a flow of current to the underlying brain tissue that results in a subsequent change in neuron firing. The diameter of the induced field depends on the shape of the coil but is typically approximately 2 or 3 cm. The depth of the effect is also approximately 2 or 3 cm.

The effect of the stimulation on the underlying cortex depends on the frequency of the stimulation parameters. A stimulation frequency of 1 Hz is generally thought to be inhibiting to the underlying cortical regions beneath the coil (e.g., reduce cortical excitability of the neurons underneath the stimulation area of the coil), whereas frequencies of 5 Hz or higher are considered to be excitatory. The effects of these frequency parameters were indirectly determined by studies showing increased blood flow in regions underlying 10 Hz rTMS, with decreased blood flow in regions affected by 1 Hz rTMS.

rTMS application is calibrated and conducted in the following manner. The intensity of the rTMS

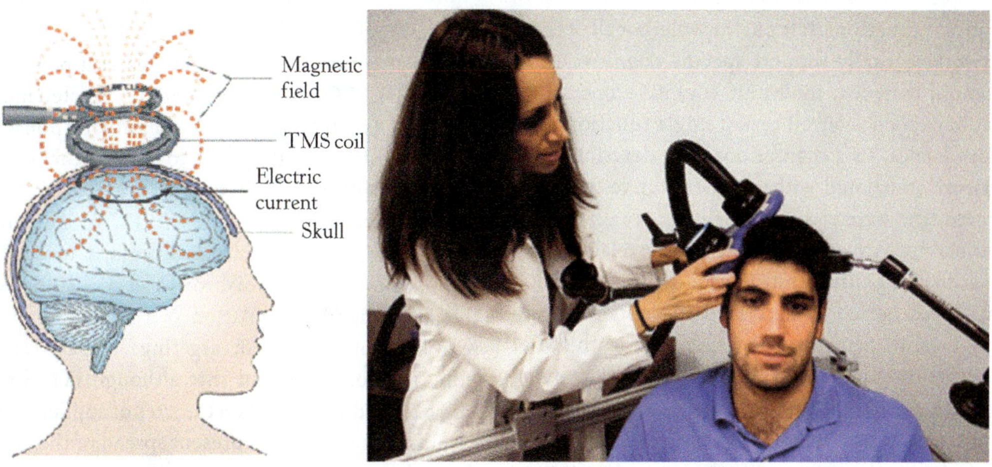

FIGURE 13.5 (Left) Schematic of an rTMS coil that when the polarity of the coil is alternated, an electrical field is induced that affects the underlying cortex. (Right) The coil is placed on the scalp with the electrical field transmitting through the scalp and skull to the underlying cortex.

Source: http://www.brainclinics.com.

to be used is established by determining the threshold required to produce movement of the thumb or fingers when stimulating over the individual's motor cortex (motor threshold). The intensity of stimulation used for rTMS throughout the brain is calculated as a percentage (typically 120%) of the individual motor threshold. To then perform rTMS over a given brain region, the plastic-enclosed electromagnetic coil is held next to the scalp and skull over the targeted brain region. The magnetic field passes through the skin and skull, inducing a directed current in the brain that activates or deactivates nearby neurons, depending on the frequency of stimulation. The path of the current is difficult to model because of the nonuniform shape of the brain and lack of uniform conductance of electromagnetic impulses through the tissues of skin, fat, bone, meninges, and cerebrospinal fluid.

The effects of rTMS are typically temporary and reversible. Occasionally, rTMS produces longer-lasting effects that persist past the initial period of stimulation. The mechanism of these effects is not clear, although it is widely believed to be related to changes in synaptic architecture. This effect has been taken advantage of in some clinical settings to produce long-lasting effects in treating diseases such as depression.

The rTMS technique can be used by applying it consistently to a particular region that is considered part of a network to temporarily produce a virtual lesion and determine if that disruption results in a consistent impairment in cognitive performance. Multiple networks have been proposed for a host of cognitive functions. It is unclear whether all of these networks actually support specific cognitive units or more complex, multiunit cognitive operations that have been referred to as a single function. As a consequence, this chapter does not describe every network associated with every cognitive function. Because the stated goal is to delineate brain regions that can be shown to consistently correlate with a described cognitive unit, the following discussion introduces networks described to support cognition, most of which have been defined with fMRI (not resting state fcMRI unless specified) as being associated with task performance while a subject is in the MRI and that have been investigated with multiple investigative approaches including lesioning techniques or delineated in some manner to provide definitive, consistent roles of the network and nodes.

TASK-RELATED NETWORKS

The following sections delineate networks described to support cognition.

Attentional Networks

Many studies investigating attentional selection have used neuroimaging studies to identify specific cortical networks relating to spatial-based attention (Corbetta & Shulman, 2002; Coull & Nobre, 1998; Steinmetz & Constantinidis, 1995), with a bilateral dorsal frontoparietal network identified that is engaged in voluntary shifts of spatial attention. fMRI studies have further identified one region, the lateral prefrontal cortex, as playing a crucial role in these networks for shifting attention, particularly related to selecting task-relevant information (Brass & von Cramon, 2004). In addition, the right posterior parietal cortex (parietal lobe posterior to the somatosensory cortex, Brodmann area (BA) 5 and 7) has been shown in lesion studies to be associated with deficits in directed spatial attention and unilateral neglect (Mesulam, 1981). Neglect patients have difficulties attending to information in the contralateral visual field to the side of the parietal lobe lesion.

Given that these key regions have been found to be integral in attentional processes, one study investigated the role of this frontoparietal network in the control of motor attention versus spatial attention using rTMS to induce lesions in the network during task performance (Rounis et al., 2007). High-frequency (5-Hz) rTMS was applied to create virtual lesions in the right and left frontal and parietal regions during performance of motor and spatial attention tasks. Left dorsolateral prefrontal cortex (DLPFC) rTMS differentially affected motor attention (switching from one motor response to another), showing this area to be critical to that function within this network. Previously, other studies have shown the left DLPFC to work in a network with the left parietal regions to control response switching (Rushworth et al., 2001). On the other hand, stimulation of the right parietal region disrupted the task targeting left spatial attention. The authors noted that although rTMS may well exert a direct effect on the sites of application as assumed, these could represent spread of the rTMS throughout the network, leading to activity changes through the entire functional network. One way to argue against this type of account is to record fMRI following rTMS to localize the region affected by rTMS and show the extent of disruption. Future approaches such as this recommended one may lead to more definitive localizations.

In another study of stroke patients and attention performance, resting state functional connectivity was assessed for coherence of spontaneous activity in the attention and somatomotor networks (Carter et al., 2010). Correlating performance with functional connectivity in 23 stroke patients and 12 controls, the study showed that abnormal stimulus detection was correlated with disrupted functional connectivity in the resting attention network. Somatomotor network disrupted connectivity was correlated with degree of upper extremity impairment. Importantly, there was no correlation of impaired performance in the motor task with the attention network or attention task with the somatomotor network. These results were interpreted as demonstrating that a loss of coherence in spontaneous BOLD fluctuations in different functional networks at rest can predict clinical outcomes—a loss of functional connectivity in the dorsal attention network correlated with neglect and loss of connectivity in the somatomotor network correlated with measures of a loss of extremity function.

Capotosto et al. (2013) used rTMS to stimulate regions over the intraparietal sulcus (IPS) that were found on fMRI studies to be intimately involved in attentional mechanisms. Inactivation of the right ventral IPS disrupted the ability to discriminate a target that a subject is supposed to attend to in the contralateral visual field. These medial parietal structures of the IPS appear to subsume a detection function in the visual attention system, with each visual field lateralized to the contralateral hemisphere. Repetitive TMS over the medial superior parietal lobule (mSPL) disrupts target detection after shifts of attention in either direction, either shifting left to right or right to left, irrespective of the object's spatial location. The role in this attentional network of the mSPL in shifting attention between locations in both hemifields is consistent with the lesion location seen as part of Balint's syndrome, in which patients present with bilateral damage of the occipitoparietal cortex extending into the mSPL. Because patients with Balint's syndrome present with simultagnosia (being able to see only one object at the time), this symptom can now be explained by impairment in shifting attention, irrespective of the direction of the shift.

Another theoretical framework for attention proposes the existence of three separable attention networks—alerting, orienting, and conflict resolution (Petersen & Posner, 2012)—with imaging support provided for each of these three networks (Westlye et al., 2011). Rinne et al. (2013) studied 110 stroke patients using the Attention Network Test, which delineates deficits in any of these three domains. Deficits were identified in each domain, and voxel-based lesion–symptom mapping (VBLSM) was used to determine the regions associated with each network. The networks were delineated as follows: conflict resolution with bilateral prefrontal and premotor areas, orienting with right pulvinar and temporoparietal regions, and alerting with anteromedial bithalamic nuclei and upper brain stem regions. These anatomical correlates for alerting follow the projections of the locus ceruleus and reticular thalamic nuclei to the cerebral hemispheres, which are consistent with the ascending norepinephrine activation system. These results also showed dependence among the attention networks and their neural substrates. Lesions of the premotor area resulted in an inability to choose between conflicting choices. This area is an uncommon location for strokes and thus has not been seen often clinically. It was also noted that conflict processing was impaired most strongly with lesions to prefrontal–premotor white matter projections, demonstrating the key role of white matter connections in these circuits. Lesions to the right temporoparietal junction and pulvinar interfered most strongly with orientation and thus are consistent with lesions associated with hemispatial neglect, the clinical syndrome that most closely parallels this function.

In contrast, Murakami et al. (2014) studied 115 post-stroke patients who were assessed for attention deficits using the Clinical Assessment for Attention, which included multiple assessments of differing aspects of attention, in addition to structural imaging studies. These tests included measures of working memory, sustained/divided attention, neglect, and processing speed. A lesion overlapping analysis technique was used, which showed that right hemisphere abnormalities were associated with poor visual cancellation test performance but that performance on all other attention tests was associated with left hemisphere dysfunction. A key finding from this study is that whereas cortical lesions differed across various task domains, lesions from the thalamus and basal ganglia in the dominant hemisphere overlapped across all attention tests studied, suggesting that these regions anchor a large, multimodal attentional network. Although it appears that these findings may contradict those of Rinne et al. (2013), the differences in network descriptions can result from the different tasks used and the fact that the image–symptom correlation techniques differ, with the Murakami et al. study using an approach that does not result in focused localizations. It is of key interest, however, that the thalamus and basal ganglia play such a prominent role in attentional networks, irrespective of tasks and lesion analysis techniques used.

The studies of attention networks have also been informed from investigations of patients with attentional deficits. The most obvious disorder associated with inattention is the syndrome of neglect. Functional imaging studies of spatial attention suggest that the IPS and dorsal premotor cortex are key regions required for shifting attention, with this operation being an essential attentional component required to avoid neglect. One study analyzed 29 right hemisphere stroke patients based on performance on a cuing task to measure spatial attention (Ptak & Schnider, 2011). Using a region of interest (ROI) analysis of eight areas hypothesized to be key regions involved in cuing tasks, a direct comparison between neglect patients and control subjects was made. Those with neglect had damage to the TPJ, the middle frontal gyrus, and the posterior IPS. In addition, damage to the frontal eye fields (FEF) and posterior IPS was correlated with neglect patients' difficulties in orienting attention. Overall, this study supported the approach for a network account of spatial attention and neglect, with attentional selection of stimuli involving the reorienting of attention, via nodes of a distributed network comprising the TPJ, the IPS, and the dorsal premotor cortex including the FEF and middle frontal gyrus (MFG). Of course, this network also includes the white matter connections of these regions. The IPS has projections to the FEF and adjacent premotor cortex (BA 6 and 8), the FEF projects to the TPJ region via the superior longitudinal fasciculus, the dorsal premotor cortex is connected with the IPS, and the inferior and superior parietal lobe have local interconnections with each other.

When attentional networks are disrupted, the symptoms of neglect can develop. Disruption of the inferior parietal lobule (IPL) could result in an inability to access representations of items in the contralateral visual field. Damage in the mid-IPS might impair the ability to maintain representations of task-relevant locations; whereas, extension to more posterior IPS might abolish the representation of visual locations. Disruption of bilateral dorsal premotor regions would disrupt the ability to bias the selection of external stimuli in contralateral visual fields. Lesions to the right pulvinar or temporoparietal regions would impair orienting to the contralateral visual field (Vuilleumier, 2013).

In summary, although these multiple platforms of investigation are still evolving and are the product of the use of different cognitive tests and analytic techniques across studies, there are distinct patterns emerging from these studies that are outlining the network engaged in attention. A collection of derived operations for nodes in the network (Figure 13.6) includes the following:

1. A key role of the TPJ in the detection of unexpected but relevant events as well as reorienting toward task-relevant novelty information (Singh-Curry & Husain, 2009).
2. The IPL forms the token representation of the target in a visual field by integrating inputs from both the dorsal (occipitoparietal) and the ventral (occipitotemporal) visual object processing streams and processing information about object location and linking them together. Other functions that may be subserved by subsets of this region include the supramarginal gyrus, whose function is to respond to novel information, and the angular gyrus, having a role in attention reorienting.
3. Anterior regions around the IPS are involved in coding spatial locations for eye and limb movements.
4. Middle IPS plays a role in controlling selective attention to contralateral locations in the presence of competing inputs (for anatomy of IPS, see Figure 13.7).
5. Bilateral prefrontal areas resolve conflict resolution.
6. Dorsal premotor regions function to bias the selection of external stimuli in keeping with tasks and goals.
7. Right pulvinar and temporoparietal regions aid in orienting.
8. Anteromedial bithalamic nuclei and upper brain stem regions function in alerting.

These associations between brain regions and cognitive units engaged in the attention domain are an evolving process leading to greater specification over time.

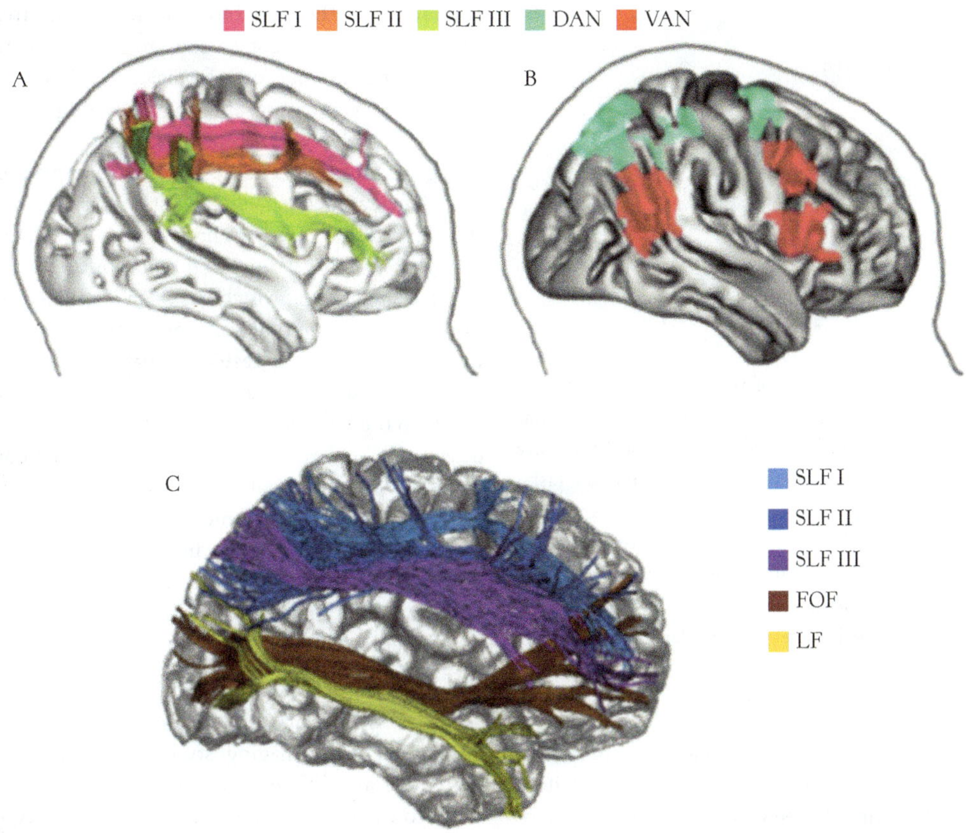

FIGURE 13.6: Frontoparietal networks controlling spatial attention. (A) The parietal and frontal cortices in the dorsal attention network are connected by three white matter pathways in the superior longitudinal fasciculus (SLF). (B) The projection cortically of the network. (C) The SLF in comparison to the inferior longitudinal fasciculus (ILF) and the inferior fronto-occipital fascicle (IFOF).

Source: Vuilleumier (2013).

This includes clarifying the cognitive units of attention and determining if one or several regions support each of these units. It is clear, however, that the framework of an attentional system is beginning to form.

Sustained Attention/Vigilance Network

The ability to maintain attention for an extended period of time is referred to as vigilance. Neuroimaging during vigilance tasks has demonstrated changes in cerebral blood flow and glucose metabolism in the ventral frontal cortex and IPL (Demeter et al., 2010; Tana et al., 2010). Patients with hemineglect are also impaired on sustained attention and vigilance tasks when their lesions include the right IPL and ventral frontal cortex (Samuelsson et al., 1998).

Studies of individuals with lesions of the right IPL showed deficits in spatial but not nonspatial vigilance tasks (Malhotra et al., 2009). A study using rTMS over the left and right parietal lobe while subjects performed spatial and nonspatial visual sustained attention tasks showed a decrement in performance over time on the spatial task when either the right or the left IPL was disrupted. There were no changes in performance when the SPL was stimulated on either side for the nonspatial task. These findings indicate that the left IPL plays a role in the maintenance of sustained attention with spatial information (Lee et al., 2013). Taken together, the IPLs and ventral frontal cortex form a network for at least sustained visual attention and vigilance, and possibly other attention-related functions.

Visuomotor Network

The visual system has been proposed to consist of two processing streams—the dorsal stream, which

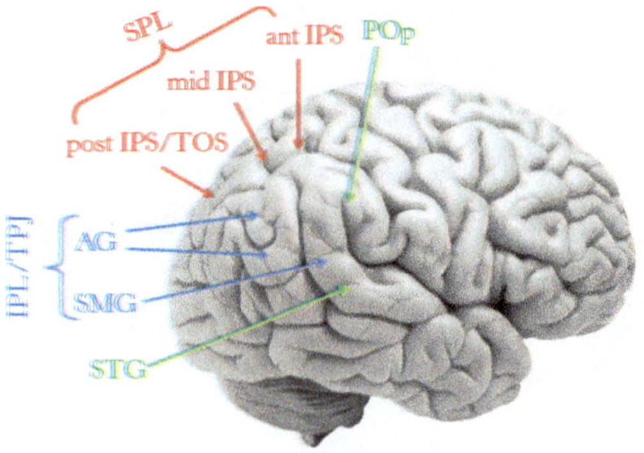

FIGURE 13.7: Regions of the parietal lobe engaged in attention. The intraparietal sulcus (IPS; red) contains distinct subareas (anterior, mid, and posterior) that have been shown to have different roles in attention tasks. The inferior parietal lobule (blue) includes the angular gyrus (AG), which is engaged in re-orienting, and the supramarginal gyrus (SMG). The parietal operculum (POp) and posterior superior temporal gyrus (STG) are purportedly involved in interpreting balance information.
Source: Vuilleumier (2013).

processes "where" an item is located in space, and the ventral system, which identifies "what" an item is (for further details, see Chapter 7). Disruption of the "what" system is associated with visual agnosia as described in Chapter 7. The "where" system is typically not associated with isolated "where" system lesions and primary "where" deficits. One syndrome that is associated with the "where" system, optic ataxia, is associated more with the networks that engage both the "where" system and visuomotor networks. Optic ataxia is characterized by an inability to coordinate a motor response of grasping for an object based on visual location information, with this action appearing to require engagement of the "where" system with motor function. Pisella et al. (2006) proposed several network pathways to account for visuomotor functions, with distinct lesions disrupting them. A dorso-dorsal pathway for visuomotor processes was proposed involving the projections from the superior parietal lobule, the intraparietal sulcus, and occipitoparietal sulcus connected to the premotor and prefrontal regions. This pathway is dedicated to mediate visuomotor control functions. Optic ataxia patients engage this network because the task of grabbing an object requires the most direct route to perform the visuomotor transformations needed for grasping. A second network pathway, the ventrodorsal pathway, involves the IPL connected to the premotor and prefrontal areas. This circuit is thought to support advanced processing of sensorimotor information such as complex planning and programming and is proposed to rely on complex visual representational levels and engages a more bilateral hemispheric organization. One deficit associated with this stream is a lesion of the left IPL that results in limb apraxia. A lesion to this region results in impaired imitation and pantomime of object use, which has been attributed to a loss of spatial-temporal movement representations. Lesions of right IPL result in spatial neglect, an inability to attend to and make intentional movements to the left side of space. Although many have described the mechanism for the attentional component, the intentional (e.g., an agent performing an action in the environment) aspect is proposed to result from difficulty in initiating and guiding movements toward the left space, which is based on lesions affecting spatiotemporal organization of mental representations in the right IPL.

Spatial Relations Network

Functional neuroimaging studies have suggested that there are different networks of regions dedicated to categorical spatial relations (e.g., categorical decisions are the type in which a judgment of a yes/no spatial decision is made—to decide whether an item is on the right or the left of the center spot) between objects as opposed to object identification. A study comparing spatial relations of objects to the identity of objects detected increased activity in bilateral superior and inferior parietal cortices and bilateral posterior middle frontal cortices for spatial relations (Amorapanth et al., 2010). In a companion lesion study, VBLSM analysis of 34 patients with unilateral hemispheric lesions was performed assessing categorical and coordinate spatial matching tasks. VBLSM analysis revealed that damage to the left supramarginal and angular gyri, the posterior middle and inferior frontal gyri, and the white matter undercutting the superior temporal gyrus was associated with deficits in categorical spatial judgments. Damage to the same regions on the right also results in a deficit, but a less severe one. VBLSM analysis also revealed that damage to the right middle temporal gyrus produced deficits in coordinate spatial processing, whereas damage to the left angular gyrus and inferior frontal gyrus produced milder deficits in coordinate spatial processing (e.g., to decide whether or not an item is more than 2 inches from the center spot). Thus, damage to the left angular gyrus and inferior frontal gyrus produced deficits in both coordinate (metric of how far apart things are) and categorical spatial processing (qualitative terms of location—next to, right, left, on top of, etc.). The conclusion was that the left angular and inferior frontal gyri process coordinate spatial information over and above the categorical processing. These results demonstrated two overlapping networks with differential contributions from the nodes involved (Amorapanth et al., 2010).

Symptom of Simultanagnosia

Humans process a scene with all of its components by allocating attention to the background of the scene and all of the objects in it. However, individuals have a limited attentional capacity that can only process the number of objects up to their capacity. The clearest example of a deficit in this capacity is the condition of simultanagnosia (in general, not by the subtypes described in Chapter 7), which is characterized by impaired spatial attention to more than one object at a given point in time. In a study of lesioned patients with visuospatial deficits (Chechlacz et al., 2012), the loci of anatomic lesions for those with simultanagnosia were compared to those of patients with neglect and those with posterior hemispheric lesions but without visuospatial deficits. It was found that bilateral parieto-occipital white matter lesions that produced disconnections are necessary, but not sufficient, to create the symptoms of simultanagnosia. In addition, damage to the middle frontal area (BA 46), cuneus, calacarine, and parieto-occipital fissure as well as right hemisphere parietal lesions within the intraparietal and postcentral gyri were associated with simultanagnosia. Another set of analyses showed that disruption of the bilateral white matter pathways (superior longitudinal fasciculus and inferior longitudinal fasciculus) of the visuospatial attention network results in simultanagnosia. Overall, damage to the parieto-occipital regions and the intraparietal sulcus, together with bilateral white matter disconnections within the visuospatial attention network, contributes to poor visual attention for multiple objects in a scene (Chechlacz et al., 2012).

Motion Perception Network

Recognizing that objects are in motion is a skill in which humans and animals are highly competent. Multiple studies have demonstrated that irrespective of the item in motion (e.g., using only points of light attached to the appendages of an undetectable object), a network of regions associated with motion perception is engaged, including the posterior superior temporal gyrus (pSTG) and sulcus (pSTS), posterior middle temporal gyrus, ventral temporal cortex, and parietal cortex (Beauchamp et al., 2002; Saygin et al., 2004; Vaina et al., 2001). The most reliably engaged anatomic region across studies has been the pSTG/STS. Other fMRI studies have also demonstrated the importance of the premotor and inferior frontal regions, showing a role for the motor system in motion detection, particularly regions involved in action planning (Saygin et al., 2004).

To better clarify the regions involved, in a large group study of 60 unilateral stroke patients, including both right and left hemisphere strokes, motion detection was assessed as well as lesion location and size (Saygin, 2007). VBLSM analysis demonstrated that lesions in the superior temporal and premotor frontal areas had the largest influence on motion perception, with each region's response being independent of the other. These findings provided further support for these areas playing an integral role in the motion detection network and indicated that lesioning of these two regions resulted in a detectable motion detection deficit. However, the cognitive role of each region could not be clearly identified from this study, and further investigations are ongoing to delineate the cognitive operations supported by each region.

Gesturing Object Use

The left IPL has been implicated in gesturing the use of an object; however, lesions in this region do not consistently lead to an impairment. In addition, the possible network of regions involved in this function has not been established. One study attempting to determine if a network was involved took a novel, two-stage approach to the analysis of lesion data (Price et al., 2010). First, lesion overlap maps were used to identify the most consistent network of regions that were involved in patients with gesturing deficits. This was followed by a voxel-based morphometry analysis to identify where the lesion sites in patients with gesturing difficulties differed from the lesion sites in patients who had difficulty naming actions and repeating words but no difficulty gesturing object use. The investigators identified 5 lesioned patients with difficulty gesturing object use. All patients had damage to the white matter underlying the left ventral supramarginal gyrus, extending to the midline and into the temporal lobe. Forty percent of the patients had involvement to the left posterior middle temporal cortex, and 60% had damage to the left dorsal supramarginal gyrus and left premotor cortex. These regions were deemed to be part of the network of regions engaged in object gesturing. The second aspect of the study consisted of searching a database of 157 patients with lesions in these regions to determine which areas are the best predictors of developing a gesturing deficit. The results indicated that combinations of regions are better predictors of a deficit than any one single region. The best predictor of a deficit was found when there was damage to the left posterior middle temporal gyrus or the left dorsal supramarginal gyrus in addition to damage to parietal lobe white matter tracts. There were numerous other probabilities of having a deficit with other combinations of lesions in various anatomical regions. This type of innovative approach to determining how lesions affect networks will lead to a clearer understanding of the interaction between nodes in a network and further clarify the roles each node plays in a cognitive unit or task.

Sound Network

Neuroimaging studies suggest that sound recognition and sound localization are processed in anatomically distinct cortical networks. Sound stimuli conveying the *identity* of the sound were proposed to engage a network that involves bilaterally the temporal convexity as well as a part of the left inferior frontal gyrus. Sound *localization* was proposed to engage a bilateral network including the posterior parietal and prefrontal cortices. A study of 15 right hemisphere lesioned patients and 15 with left hemisphere lesions (Adriani et al., 2003) assessed the capacity of patients to recognize environmental sounds, to localize sounds in space, and to perceive if the object making a sound is moving and in what direction. Patients had a variety of combination or isolated deficits, leading to several insights on the network of regions outlined previously. Impaired performance in sound recognition, sound localization, and/or sound motion perception was always associated with a lesion that involved the networks outlined. Normal performance, however, could be associated with lesions in or outside the networks. The conclusion from the study was that lesions to regions in these networks are necessary, but not sufficient, for a deficit to occur. In addition, deficits to the aspects of sound processing assessed in this study were not associated predominantly with lesions of the proposed networks (Adriani et al., 2003). Currently, the networks for nonverbal sound processing are poorly understood and will likely require studies with considerably larger numbers of subjects or different analytic techniques to determine if and what type of network processing is involved.

Language Networks

Language processing, in addition to the two network models proposed in Chapters 3 and 4, can be instantiated as an interconnected cortical network of distributed brain areas consisting of the bilateral temporal lobes, left IPL, the left-hemispheric posterior inferior frontal gyrus (pIFG, overlapping with Broca's area), and the left hemisphere dorsolateral premotor area (Hickok & Poeppel, 2007; Murakami et al., 2012).

In further elucidating the connectivity in the language network, an fcMRI study of 970 healthy subjects used Broca's and Wernicke's areas as seed regions to determine the network of associated regions to these two areas at rest. The study found high connectivity to the prefrontal, temporal, and parietal regions but also to the bilateral caudate and left putamen/globus pallidus and subthalamic nuclei. The connections in the network are typically short range in distance except for those from Wernicke's area, which are long-range connections (Tomasi & Volkow, 2012).

Some have suggested that there are two language tracts. One is a dorsal stream that connects the temporoparietal with frontal premotor regions through the superior longitudinal and arcuate fasciculus and integrates sensorimotor language processing (e.g., repetition). The other is a ventral stream that connects temporal and prefrontal regions via the extreme capsule and mediates meaning (e.g., semantics/comprehension). To test this organization, 100 aphasic stroke patients were administered repetition and comprehension tests with lesions correlated by VBLSM, and white matter fiber tract involvement was also assessed as determined by probabilistic fiber tracking. Repetition deficits were associated with lesions of the posterior temporoparietal region and dorsal superior longitudinal and arcuate fasciculi. Comprehension deficits were associated with lesions of the temporo-prefrontal region, insular cortex, putamen, and extreme capsule (Kummerer et al., 2013). This large-scale study supports the notion of these two major language networks; however, these were based on the two tasks, repetition and comprehension, both of which are complex tasks consisting of many cognitive units. Further exploration for other language-related networks related to different operations and how these networks could interact were explored as follows.

Syntax

One key set of functions that has not been well localized in language has been syntactic operations. In particular, localization of syntactic operations to one brain region has typically not resulted in consistent deficits. The one region of the language network whose role has shown some promise to be involved with syntactic operations has been the left inferior frontal gyrus. One study explored its role by combining fMRI and lesion analysis in patients with left hemisphere damage and healthy controls to assess syntactic processing (Tyler et al., 2011). In the fMRI study, control subjects made syntactic judgments and were found to co-activate the left hemisphere BA 45/47 and posterior middle temporal gyrus during these judgments. In addition, voxel-based correlational analyses of patients showed that preserved syntactic functions were correlated with intact left BA 45 and posterior middle temporal gyrus. The findings suggest that the left BA 45 may not be dedicated and essential to syntactic processing but contributes to the network supporting syntactic operations (Tyler et al., 2011).

Further studies delineating syntax-associated networks extended from a study of normal subjects and 21 patients with left frontal gliomas who received preoperative fMRI studies assessing picture–sentence matching syntactic judgments. Three networks related to syntactic processing were detected in the normal subjects using functional connectivity and diffusion tensor imaging (DTI). The first network included the left inferior frontal gyrus, left intraparietal sulcus, right frontal regions, presupplementary motor area, and right temporal regions. These regions were overactivated during the fMRI task in patients with gliomas in the left lateral premotor cortex. The second network consisted of the left lateral premotor cortex, left angular gyrus, lingual gyrus, and cerebellar nuclei. These regions were found to be overactivated during fMRI task performance in patients with gliomas in the left inferior frontal gyrus. The third network consisted of the left ventral frontal and posterior temporal regions. These regions were underactivated during fMRI in patients with gliomas in the left inferior frontal gyrus. The findings provide insight into how networks associated with syntactic processing reorganize after lesions disrupt two of the key nodes in normal syntactic networks—the left posterior inferior frontal gyrus and the left lateral premotor cortex—resulting in differential activation of the remaining nodes in the networks (Kinno et al., 2014).

Comprehension

Language comprehension involves a network of regions including cortical, subcortical, and white matter structures. Comprehension is not a cognitive unit, but it consists of multiple cognitive units linked together and thus is a clear example—as mentioned previously—of when the term network of anatomic regions is used but refers not to a network supporting a single cognitive unit but to multiple cognitive units working together supported by multiple regions, which may include CAUs. The term "comprehension" and investigations into it continue to be performed instead of more finer specified cognitive units because of comprehension's use in descriptions of classical aphasic syndromes (see Chapter 3).

VBLSM analysis of aphasic patients showed multiple left hemisphere brain regions engaged in comprehension: left posterior middle temporal gyrus, anterior BA 22 in the superior temporal gyrus, posterior superior temporal sulcus into BA 39, the orbital part of the inferior frontal gyrus, and the middle frontal gyrus (Dronkers et al., 2004). The white matter pathways engaged in this network were assessed with DTI tractography and functional connectivity assessed with fcMRI at rest. Fiber tractography and functional connectivity analyses indicated that left temporal regions including the left MTG, anterior STG, STS, and BA 47 represent an interconnected network that extends out to bilateral frontal and parietal regions involved in comprehension. The inferior occipitofrontal fasciculus, the arcuate fasciculus, the middle and inferior longitudinal fasciculi, and transcallosal projections were identified as key pathways connecting the temporal regions to other brain areas engaged in this comprehension network (Turken & Dronkers, 2011).

Another study examined how the language comprehension network realigns after an essential, central node (left posterior superior temporal gyrus) is temporarily disrupted. rTMS was applied to the left STG during performance of a language comprehension task while assessing whole brain function by performing concurrent fMRI. This resulted in decreased connectivity in language-related cortices and increased connectivity in regions of the brain known to engage in functional compensation after lesions occur in language areas (perilesional left STG, right STG, MFG, and posterior right hemisphere). Particularly with rTMS temporary lesioning of the lateral left STG, the contralesional right posterior STG and the perilesional left medial STG appeared to take over the function of the left STG. The MFG region is known to monitor discourse processing and could be recruited to adapt for lower-level (literal) comprehension processing when the left STG is lesioned. Overall, these findings show that for immediate reorganization after lesioning a key hub in the comprehension network (left STG), a nonlanguage network of regions is engaged to compensate (Mason et al., 2013).

Semantics

Some comprehension tasks engage semantic knowledge of items, semantic processing operations, and cognitive control circuits. To gain access to this knowledge, cognitive control units have been proposed to manipulate the semantic knowledge. Whereas some have proposed semantic-specific cognitive control circuits, others have suggested that these circuits are domain-general and engaged by the semantic system as needed. The left IFG has been implicated as a key node in a network that is either semantic-specific or domain-general for cognitive control when selecting a target item among multiple choices. Whitney et al. (2012) used rTMS in healthy controls to disrupt structures possibly part of a semantic control network: left IFG, left posterior middle temporal gyrus, and intraparietal sulcus. The impact of rTMS on tasks varying in semantic and nonsemantic control demands was examined for each region. The results suggested that the left IFG and pMTG jointly support both controlled retrieval and selection of semantic knowledge. The IPS participates in semantic selection and also responds to manipulations of nonsemantic control demands. These results suggest components of both a semantic cognitive control network and additional engagement of a domain-general region (IPS) are necessary to retrieve semantic knowledge (Whitney et al., 2012). Further studies are needed to confirm these findings and determine how cognitive control circuits aid in other semantic processing tasks.

Analogy reasoning is a form of semantic processing that includes analyzing conceptual relations. However, it is unknown if different types of analogies would engage different semantic processes. Schmidt et al. (2012) tested patients with left and right hemisphere lesions on two types of analogies: The analogical relationships were either an associative one (e.g., steeple–church) or a categorical one (e.g., appliance–toaster). VBLSM and behavioral performance demonstrated that the specific regions linked to associative analogies are a network including the left MTG, IFG, and frontal white matter, whereas categorical analogies engage the right MTG. When scores of the two analogy types were compared with VBLSM analysis, no regions were detected that were engaged at a general analogy level for both associative and categorical analogies. These findings support the claim that different types of analogical relations rely on different neural networks (Schmidt et al., 2012).

Effective use of semantic memory involves accessing and processing the representational meaning of words, pictures, objects, facts, actions, etc. At some point in the semantic processing stream, multimodality semantic processing occurs with integration of information from multiple semantic modalities (Hart & Gordon, 1990). Studies have delineated multiple cortical regions engaged in a semantic network (Binder et al., 2009) as well as subcortical regions (Hart et al., 2013) that may be engaged in multimodal semantic processing. The exact role of every region in these networks and the connections between nodes have not been fully delineated. One study investigating a specific white matter connection between nodes in the semantic system used intraoperative direct electrical stimulation in eight patients being operated on for gliomas. While performing a picture naming or a nonverbal semantic association task, direct electrical stimulation of the inferior fronto-occipital fascicle resulted in semantic disruption in each of the eight patients. This pathway is ideally situated to link multiple semantic brain regions, including those encoding for auditory and visual semantics (Figure 13.8) (Moritz-Gasser et al., 2013). Similar investigations for other white matter pathways show promise to further delineate the connections between nodes in the semantic and other networks.

Speech Perception

Left hemisphere temporal and frontal areas are connected via the temporal–parietal junction

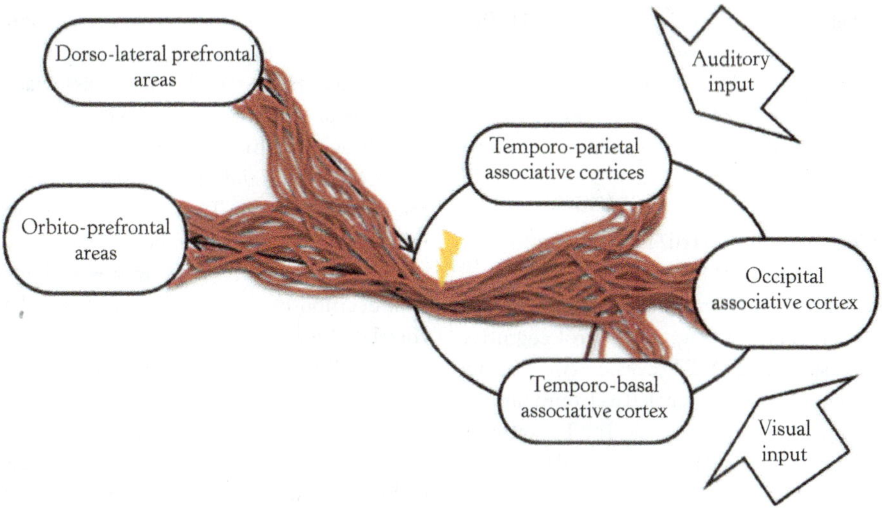

FIGURE 13.8: A proposed model of a network for semantic processing. Cortical regions are described in the ovals, with the inferior fronto-occipital fascicle (IFOF) white matter pathway depicted as red cables showing the connections between regions. The yellow lightning bolt shows where direct electrical stimulation was applied in a study by Moritz-Gasser et al. (2013) that was used to delineate aspects of the network connected by the IFOF. The arrows designate where different modalities of stimulus input come into the semantic network.

Source: Moritz-Gasser et al. (2013).

(Sylvian–parietal–temporal region referred to as area Spt), forming an auditory dorsal stream to map speech perception onto speech production processes. This network of regions is proposed to be able to direct articulatory motor function (Hickok & Poeppel, 2007). How this network links to the mouth motor area during speech perception, a proposed function of this network, has not been established. A study used rTMS in healthy subjects over the speech perception circuitry including the left TPJ and pIFG while assessing their connectivity to the mouth motor area. The findings demonstrated that the effective connectivity of the TPJ → M1 connection and the pIFG → M1 connections increased when listening to speech compared to white noise, supporting the claim that both regions contribute to sensorimotor integration in speech perception. rTMS over the pIFG reduced the connectivity between pIFG → M1 during speech perception, but it did not affect TPJ → M1. However, rTMS over TPJ reduced the task-dependent increased connectivity of both connections to M1. Thus, the network connectivity as demonstrated by lesioning shows that the TPJ node is hierarchically placed in the network controlling the connectivity of its own and the pIFG to the mouth motor region (Murakami et al., 2012). This use of transient lesioning with rTMS to determine the dynamics and organization of nodes in a network demonstrates optimal application of the rTMS technique in network analysis. As more studies similar to this application are conducted to elucidate network systems, a greater understanding of the role they play in cognition and behavior will emerge.

Prosody Network

The network of regions underlying emotional prosody perception has been reported to be lateralized to the right hemisphere, as was reported for individual CAUs in lesion studies. A quantitative meta-analysis of the neuroimaging literature was performed to investigate which brain areas were part of this network. A bilateral temporofrontal network was found to be implicated in emotional prosody perception, generally supporting previously proposed models of prosody perception, except that these were more lateralized to the right hemisphere (Ross & Monnot, 2008). A second analysis of the lesion literature found greater impairment in prosody performance following right rather than left hemisphere damage (Witteman et al., 2011). Overall, a right-sided "predominance" appears to be more consistent and can be accounted for by the right hemisphere's specialization for nonspeech acoustic sound analysis in the right posterior aspect of the superior temporal gyrus

(Witteman et al., 2012; Zatorre & Belin, 2001). This raises the point that without corresponding lesion studies to fcMRI and/or fMRI activation studies, these activation studies may overestimate the number of anatomic regions engaged in cognitive operations.

Cognitive Control/Executive Function Networks

Cognitive control functions refer to operations that coordinate, manage, regulate, or control cognitive processes. Task-related fMRI revealed two distinct cognitive control networks labeled as frontoparietal (FP) and cingulo-opercular (CO). The FP network consists of nodes proposed to act on a rapid timescale to initiate and adjust control of cognitive operations or tasks, whereas the CO network nodes act to provide signals that allow set maintenance over a longer time in a task (Dosenbach et al., 2006, 2007). In a study of 21 patients with heterogeneous, focal brain lesions, rest fcMRI imaging was collected and analyzed for connectivity. With heterogeneous damage to the two (FP and CO) functional networks, the analysis showed that the two networks appear to be independent of each other. This was determined by the finding that the degree of network damage after a lesion to one network correlated with a decrease in functional connectivity only within that network, while not affecting connectivity in the undamaged network. Overall, the study showed that cognitive control networks that were defined by their engagement in cognitive control processes during task performance demonstrated independence during resting state fcMRI (Nomura et al., 2010). This study provided another unique approach of applying multiple imaging studies to provide for converging evidence that the localization of cognitive operations to a region or set of regions can be more clearly established as a consistent correlation.

Another executive function/cognitive control operation, of a more complex nature, is decision-making. Decision-making functions have typically been probed using choice paradigms, which contain an element of risk to the choices presented in the task. Optimal choices typically require acquiring and integrating information about outcomes, calculating probabilities, and choices are then made. Previous studies have implicated a brain network including the ventromedial prefrontal cortex (vmPFC) and posterior parietal cortex (pPAR), with damage to the vmPFC previously shown to be associated with poor decision-making and increased risk-taking, whereas neuroimaging studies have implicated the pPAR in processing reward probability. However, this latter association with the parietal region has not been clearly established. In a study in which patients with lesions to the pPAR or vmPFC and healthy volunteers performed the Roulette Betting Task, both lesion groups were impaired in adjusting their bets to the probability of winning, and the pPAR group was also notable for slow decision-making. The "adjustment" deficit was correlated with the extent of pPAR lesion but not vmPFC. The findings demonstrated the roles and interactive relationship of both pPAR and vmPFC in a risk-sensitive choice network (Studer et al., 2015), suggesting that pPAR is also associated with making risk-sensitive choices, particularly contributing to the speed at which those choices are made.

NETWORKS IN RECOVERY

The recovery processes that occur after a lesion to a network can reveal a great deal about the organization of the network and its nodes. Groups have studied fMRI BOLD signal with tasks to determine if these studies can predict recovery from a lesion in patients with neglect, for example. Corbetta et al. (2005) and He et al. (2007) reported that in a group of neglect patients, task-evoked BOLD responses (Corbetta et al., 2005) and functional connectivity between regions within attention networks (He et al., 2007) showed systematic abnormalities within surviving intact brain regions, even those remote from the lesion. These remote anatomic abnormalities were related to increased activity within left parietal and frontal cortex, contralateral to the damaged hemisphere. Such contralesional hyperactivity in neglect had long been hypothesized on clinical and theoretical grounds (e.g., Kinsbourne, 1977) to be contributing to the inattention to half of a patient's personal space, but it had rarely, if ever, been demonstrated directly up until this time (although see Koch et al., 2008).

Recovery from neglect was also examined by measuring functional connectivity in two proposed separate attentional networks located in dorsal and ventral frontoparietal regions. Comparing the acute and chronic state of these networks revealed several prognostic markers. Most neglect patients had lesions involving brain regions that were part of the ventral network, and it was found that if connectivity was disrupted in this network, patients showed little or no recovery. In addition, if the interhemispheric connectivity in posterior parietal cortex in this network was found to be disrupted in the acute phase of neglect, it eventually recovered in terms of connectivity that was paralleled with improved performance. Notably in this study, disconnection of the white matter tracts connecting frontal and parietal cortices resulted in the most severe neglect symptoms and most disrupted connectivity (He et al., 2007). The point of the inclusion of this example is not validation of any model of attention or neglect but, rather, that in the process of assessing networks, the varying functions that a region can assume in the recovery process are factors to include in the assignment of roles in a network model.

There are two distinctions that have been made in terms of processing and their anatomic correlates, irrespective of whether the processing is supported by individual regions or networks. The two key types of processes are referred to as domain-general and domain-specific. Domain-general processes can perform the operations in multiple cognitive domains. For example, attention processes (also cognitive control, executive functions, etc.) are necessary for the successful performance of a variety of tasks from a variety of cognitive domains (e.g., language, episodic memory, and visuospatial tasks.).

Domain-General and Domain-Specific Processing in Network Recovery

One manner to view how domain-general functions have an impact in a network is the way in which these domain-general functions affect recovery when a network is damaged. One specific cognitive control network that is domain-general is the salience network that consists of regions including the dorsal anterior cingulate cortex and the superior frontal gyrus (midline frontal cortex). In a study of recovery from aphasic deficits in 16 stroke patients, the integrity of the domain-general activity in the midline frontal cortex (not involved in the stroke) was assessed using task-related fMRI before and after a rehabilitation program. The aphasics listened to simple sentences and then repeated them back during the fMRI scans. This task was targeted to engage both domain-general (attention to utterances, overcoming pre-response conflict, and decision uncertainty) and domain-specific (language—speech perception, comprehension, and verbal working memory) processes. For the aphasic patients, there was the expected activity in the superior temporal gyri for speech perception, and because subjects knew that they would have to repeat back the sentence, there was activation in speech production regions including the premotor (medial and lateral) and primary sensorimotor cortices, basal ganglia, thalami, and cerebellum. The study also assessed normal subjects on this task when speech was presented either in a normal or in a distorted manner to tax speech perception and engage domain-general systems. When comparison was made between the difficult and normal perception tasks, there was increased fMRI activity in the midline frontal cortical area. This same region was activated in aphasic patients for the normal-sounding sentence, suggesting these patients have difficulty perceiving the normal sentences. Following this region's activation over the recovery time of the aphasic patients receiving rehabilitation, it was found that midline frontal activity during fMRI tasks correlated with improvement in the patients' language abilities. The study showed that the response of a non-language region in the domain-general salience network (a cognitive control-related network) may play a key factor in recovery from what appears to be a language-specific deficit from strokes (Brownsett et al., 2014).

Another study of a group of aphasic patients assessed the results of functional activation detected by PET during a lexical decision task. This was performed in aphasic patients after middle cerebral artery stroke, with the findings demonstrating a network of regions showing compensatory increases in brain activity within the bilateral anterior inferior temporal areas and in the right posterior superior temporal gyrus. In addition, left perisylvian lesions were associated with decreased activation of left posterior inferior frontal cortex and extralesional remote decreases of activity within polar parts of the inferior temporal gyrus (Specht et al., 2009). A clearly useful application of network modeling is assessing brain reorganization in the recovery process after an acute injury.

As noted previously, aphasic patients can exhibit increased right hemisphere activity during language recovery. It is unclear whether this right hemisphere involvement is a recruitment of homologous brain regions, interference to recovery, or adaptation of alternate strategies to recover lost functions. To assess the role of the right hemisphere in aphasia recovery, syntactic comprehension was tested in 25 aphasic patients while performing a sentence–picture matching paradigm while concurrently recording electromagnetic measures off of patients scalps using magnetoencephalography (MEG). The sentences varied between being semantically reversible and semantically irreversible. In a semantically reversible sentence ("The snake is watching the monkey"), the sentence is still plausibly correct whether the subject and object are reversed ("The monkey is watching the snake"). Thus, even if a patient is confused or passive voice is being used ("The monkey was watched by the snake"), the patient cannot guess the correct answer simply from the order of which noun is first and which is second. In a semantically irreversible sentence ("The boy is eating the apple"), reversing the subject and object leads to a semantically implausible sentence ("The apple is eating the boy"). It is typically easier for patients to do sentence–picture matching with these sentences, even for patients with a syntactic comprehension problem, because they can use the order of the nouns in the sentence to guess the correctly matching picture. Each of these sentence types (reversible and irreversible) included sentences that varied at three levels of syntactic complexity. Patients performed best on irreversible sentences, and they performed at chance on reversible sentences of high syntactic complexity. Lesion analysis revealed that comprehension deficits for reversible sentences were predicted by damage to the left temporal lobe. Right temporal lobe regions were also activated on MEG but did not correlate with performance. Performance did correlate with increased activity in dorsal frontoparietal regions, regions previously shown to be associated with working memory. The findings were interpreted to show that strategic recruitment of alternative networks may account for some of the right hemisphere language activation in aphasia recovery (Meltzer et al., 2013).

OTHER NETWORK APPROACHES

Intermittently throughout this chapter, additional techniques have been discussed that allow for a network-based approach to be explored and assessed using techniques other than fcMRI (e.g., MEG and PET). It appears that the optimal approach to defining the regions involved in performing a specific task or function, and how lesions affect it, is to use multiple imaging modalities. An example of this approach is the investigation of elderly controls, mild cognitive impairment (MCI), and AD patients (Carter et al., 2014). The investigators studied both white matter and gray matter integrity in regional networks involving the Papez circuit and extending to neocortical association areas. This was accomplished by using the combined techniques of cortical volumetric measures and diffusion tensor imaging (3T MR imaging), PET with ^{18}F fluorodeoxyglucose, and comprehensive neuropsychological assessments. The results showed that atrophy of the medial temporal lobes was the strongest and most consistent abnormality in patients with MCI and AD, with atrophy in the temporal, frontal, and parietal regions being most strongly related to episodic memory deficits. Impairments in semantic processing in these patients were correlated with reductions of glucose metabolism in the posterior cingulate cortex and temporoparietal regions. The white matter tract maps demonstrated widespread decreases of fractional anisotropy (a measure of white matter integrity; for more details, see Chapter 12) in the major association tracts in MCI and even more significantly in AD; these included the cingulum, uncinate, and superior longitudinal fasciculus white matter pathways. PET studies showed that metabolic deficits in the posterior cingulate and orbitofrontal cortex were correlated with damage in projecting white matter tracts. In summary, multiple lesioned network components within the Papez circuit and its extended neocortical association areas were significantly associated with cognitive dysfunction in both MCI and AD. Although hippocampal atrophy was the most prominent lesion, other disruptions in the network are closely associated with these disease states (Carter et al., 2014).

CONCLUSIONS

The network approach to cognition has generated numerous accounts in which collection of gray matter nodes connected by white matter pathways support either one or multiple cognitive units. Many networks have been mentioned in this chapter without always a conclusion as to whether the network account provided a consensus account or competing accounts for the cognitive domains, tasks, or units being investigated. At times, these can appear as a list of anatomic regions attached to a function or task that became associated with the cognitive elements typically by an fMRI task-related study or an fcMRI resting state network study. In the case of an fMRI-generated network, the regions identified are linked to the experiments performed. Without corresponding lesion data, it is unclear what role the regions play in the network.

This chapter discussed the reported networks as this field is a new and evolving one. It is clear that CAUs provide a basis of cognitive–anatomic associations on which somenetworks build. Network accounts of cognition are also clearly able to account for numerous aspects of cognition, but will require delineation of the cognitive correlates and processing characteristics of nodes and connections within a network.

Many of the references in this chapter are recently published because this approach is a newly growing one. The test of time will determine the success and prevalence of the network approach to cognition. As the field matures, there will also be an increase in studies using multiple neuroinvestigative techniques to provide converging evidence of network–cognitive correlations and lesion studies of networks.

REFERENCES

Adriani, M., Maeder, P., Meuli, R., Thiran, A., Frischknecht, R., Villemure, J.-G., et al. (2003). Sound recognition and localization in man: Specialized cortical networks and effects of acute circumscribed lesions. *Experimental Brain Research, 153*, 591–604.

Amorapanth, P., Widick, P., & Chatterjee, A. (201). The neural basis for spatial relations. *Journal of Cognitive Neuroscience, 22*(8), 1739–1753.

Anderson, A., Douglas, P., Kerr, W., Haynes, V., Yuille, A., Xie, J., et al. (2014). Non-negative matrix factorization of multimodal MRI, fMRI and phenotypic data reveals differential changes in default mode subnetworks in ADHD. *Neuroimage, 102*, 207–219.

Anticevic, A., Repovs, G., & Barch, D. M. (2011). Working memory encoding and maintenance deficits in schizophrenia: Neural evidence for activation and deactivation abnormalities. *Schizophrenia Bulletin*, 10.1093/schbul/sbr107.

Anticevic, A., Cole, M., Murray, J., Corlett, P., Wang, X.-J., & Krystal, J. (2012). The role of default network deactivation in cognition and disease. *Trends in Cognitive Sciences, 16*(12), 584–592.

Beauchamp, M., Lee, K., Haxby, J., & Martin, A. (2002). Parallel visual motion processing streams for manipulable objects and human movements. *Neuron, 34*, 149–159.

Binder, J., Desai, R., Graves, W., & Conant, L. (2009). Where is the semantic system? A critical review and meta-analysis of 120 functional neuroimaging studies. *Cerebral Cortex, 19*, 2767–2796.

Brass, M., & von Cramon, D. (2004). Selection for cognitive control: A functional magnetic resonance imaging study on the selection of task-relevant information. *Journal of Neuroscience, 24*, 8847–8852.

Brownsett, S., Warren, J., Geranmayeh, F., Woodhead, Z., Leech, R., & Wise, R. (2014). Cognitive control and its impact on recovery from aphasic stroke. *Brain, 137*, 242–254.

Buckner, R., Snyder, A., Shannon, B., LaRossa, G., Sachs, R., Fotenos, A., et al. (2005). Molecular, structural, and functional characterization of Alzheimer's disease: Evidence for a relationship between default activity, amyloid, and memory. *Journal of Neuroscience, 25*, 7709–7717.

Capotosto, P., Tosoni, A., Spadone, S., Sestieri, C., Perrucci, M. G., Romani, G. L., . . . & Corbetta, M. (2013). Anatomical segregation of visual selection mechanisms in human parietal cortex. *The Journal of Neuroscience, 33*(14), 6225–6229.

Carhart-Harris, R., Erritzoe, D., Williams, T., Stone, J. M., Reed, L. J., Colasanti, A., et al. (2012). Neural correlates of the psychedelic state as determined by fMRI studies with psilocybin. *Proceedings of the National Academy of Sciences of the USA, 109*, 2138–2143.

Carter, A., Astafiev, S., Lang, C., Connor, L., Rengachary, J., Strube, M., et al. (2010). Resting inter-hemispheric fMRI connectivity predicts performance after stroke. *Annals of Neurology, 67*(3), 365–375.

Carter, S., Embleton, K., Anton-Rodriguez, J., Burns, A., Ralph, M., & Herholz, K. (2014). *American Journal of Neuroradiology, 35*(6 Suppl.), S18–S30.

Cataldi, M., Avoli, M., & de Villers-Sidani, E. (2013). Resting state networks in temporal lobe epilepsy. *Epilepsia, 54*(12), 2048–2059.

Catani, M., Dell'Acqua, F., Bizzi, A., Forkel, S., Williams, S., Simmons, A., et al. (2012). Beyond cortical localization in clinico-anatomical correlation. *Cortex, 48*, 1262–1287.

Chechlacz, M., Rotshtein, P., Hansen, P., Riddoch, J., Deb, S., & Humphreys, G. (2012). The neural underpinnings of simultanagnosia: Disconnecting the visuospatial attention network. *Journal of Cognitive Neuroscience, 24*(3), 718–735.

Corbetta, M. (2012). Functional connectivity and neurological recovery. *Developmental Psychobiology, 54*, 239–253.

Corbetta, M., Kincade, M., Lewis, C., Snyder, A., & Sapir, A. (2005). Neural basis and recovery of spatial attention deficits in spatial neglect. *Nature Neuroscience, 8*(11), 1603–1610.

Corbetta, M., & Shulman, G. (2002). Control of goal-directed and stimulus-driven attention in the brain. *Nature Reviews Neuroscience, 3*, 201–215.

Coull, J., & Nobre, A. (1998). Where and when to pay attention: The neural systems for directing attention to spatial locations and to time intervals as revealed by both PET and fMRI. *Journal of Neuroscience, 18*, 7426–7435.

Demeter, E., Hernandez-Garcia, L., Sarter, M., & Lustig, C. (2010). Challenges to attention: A continuous arterial spin labeling (ASL) study of the effects of distraction on sustained attention. *Neuroimage, 54*, 1518.

Dosenbach, N., Visscher, K. M., Palmer, E. D., Miezin, F. M., Wenger, K. K., Kang, H. C., et al. (2006). A core system for the implementation of task sets. *Neuron, 50,* 799–812.

Dosenbach, N., Fair, D. A., Miezin, F. M., Cohen, A. L., Wenger, K. K., Dosenbach, R. A. T., et al. (2007). Distinct brain networks for adaptive and stable task control in humans. *Proceedings of the National Academy of Sciences of the USA, 104,* 11073–11078.

Dronkers, N., Wilkins, D., Van Valin, R., Redfern, B., & Jaeger, J. (2004). Lesion analysis of the brain areas involved in language comprehension. *Cognition, 92,* 145–177.

Fodor, J. (1983). *The modularity of the mind.* Cambridge, MA: MIT Press.

Gallo, A., Esposito, F., Sacco, R., et al. (2012). Visual resting-state network in relapsing–remitting MS with and without previous optic neuritis. *Neurology, 79,* 1458–1465.

Gardner, R., Boxer, A., Trujillo, A., Mirsky, J., Guo, C., Gennatas, E., et al. (2013). Intrinsic connectivity network disruption in progressive supranuclear palsy. *Annals of Neurology, 73,* 603–616.

Grefkes, C., Ritzl, A., Zilles, K., & Fink, G. (2004). Human medial intraparietal cortex subserves visuomotor coordinate transformation. *Neuroimage, 23,* 1494–1506.

Greicius, M., Krasnow, B., Reiss, A., & Menon, V. (2003). Functional connectivity in the resting brain: A network analysis of the default mode hypothesis. *Proceedings of the National Academy of Sciences of the USA, 100,* 253–258.

Greicius, M., Srivastava, G., Reiss, A., & Menon, V. (2004). Default-mode network activity distinguishes Alzheimer's disease from healthy aging: Evidence from functional MRI. *Proceedings of the National Academy of Sciences of the USA, 101*(13), 4637–4642.

Gusnard, D., Akbudak, E., Shulman, G., & Raichle, M. (2001). Medial prefrontal cortex and self-referential mental activity: Relation to a default mode of brain function. *Proceedings of the National Academy of Sciences of the USA, 98,* 4259–4264.

Gusnard, D., & Raichle, M. (2001). Searching for a baseline: Functional imaging and the resting human brain. *Nature Reviews Neuroscience, 2,* 685–694.

Haneef, Z., Lenartowicz, A., Yeh, H., Engel, J., & Stern, J. (2012). Effect of lateralized temporal lobe epilepsy on the default mode network. *Epilepsy & Behavior, 25,* 350–357.

Hart, J., & Gordon, B. (1990). Delineation of single-word semantic comprehension deficits in aphasia, with anatomical correlation. *Annals of Neurology, 27,* 226–231.

Hart, J., Maguire, M., Motes, M. Mudar, R., Chiang, H-S., Womack, K., & Kraut, M. (2013). Semantic memory retrieval circuit: Role of BA6 and thalamus. *Brain and Language, 126*(1), 89–98.

He, B., Snyder, A., Vincent, J., Epstein, A., Shulman, G., & Corbetta, M. (2007). Breakdown of functional connectivity in frontoparietal networks underlies behavioral deficits in spatial neglect. *Neuron, 53,* 905–918.

Henson, R., Rugg, M., Shallice, T., Josephs, O., & Dolan, R. (1999). Recollection and familiarity in recognition memory: An event-related functional magnetic resonance imaging study. *Journal of Neuroscience, 19,* 3962–3972.

Hickok, G., & Poeppel, D. (2007). The cortical organization of speech processing. *Nature Reviews Neuroscience, 8*(5), 393–402.

Jacobs, H. I., Radua, J., Lückmann, H. C., & Sack, A. T. (2013). Meta-analysis of functional network alterations in Alzheimer's disease: toward a network biomarker. *Neuroscience & Biobehavioral Reviews, 37*(5), 753–765.

Kinno, R., Ohta, S., Muragaki, Y., Maruyama, T., & Sakai, K. (2014). Differential reorganization of three syntax-related networks induced by a left frontal glioma. *Brain, 137,* 1193–1212.

Kinsbourne, M. (1977). Hemi-neglect and hemisphere rivalry. *Advances in Neurology, 18,* 41–49.

Kircher, T., Senior, C., Phillips, M., Benson, P., Bullmore, E., Brammer, M., et al. (2000). Towards a functional neuroanatomy of self-processing: Effects of faces and words. *Cognitive Brain Research, 10,* 133–144.

Knauff, M., Fangmeier, T., Ruff, C., & Johnson-Laird, P. (2003). Reasoning, models, and images: Behavioral measures and cortical activity. *Journal of Cognitive Neuroscience, 15,* 559–573.

Koch, G., Oliveri, M., Cheeran, B., Ruge, D., Lo Gerfo, E., Salerno, S., Torriero, S., Marconi, B., Mori, F., Driver, J., Rothwell, J., & Caltagirone, C. (2008). Hyperexcitability of parietal-motor functional connections in the intact left-hemisphere of patients with neglect. *Brain, 131*(Pt. 12), 3147–3155.

Kummerer, D., Hartwigsen, G., Kellmeyer, P., Glauche, V., Mader, I., Kloppel, S., et al. (2013). Damage to ventral and dorsal language pathways in acute aphasia. *Brain, 136,* 619–629.

Le, T., Pardo, J., & Hu, X. (1998). 4T-fMRI study of nonspatial shifting of selective attention: Cerebellar and parietal contributions. *Journal of Neurophysiology, 79,* 1535–1548.

Leavitt, V., Wylie, G., Girgis, P., Deluca, J., & Chiaravalloti, N. (2014). Increased functional connectivity within memory networks following memory rehabilitation in multiple sclerosis. *Brain Imaging and Behavior, 8,* 394–402.

Lee, J., Ku, J., Han, K., Park, J., Lee, H., Kim, K., et al. (2013). rTMS over bilateral inferior parietal cortex induces decrement of spatial sustained attention. *Frontiers in Human Neuroscience, 11,* 26.

Liao, W., Zhang, Z., Pan, Z., Mantini, D., Ding, J., Duan, X., et al. (2011). Default mode network abnormalities in mesial temporal lobe epilepsy: A study combining fMRI and DTI. *Human Brain Mapping, 32,* 883–895.

Malhotra, P., Coulthard, E., & Husain, M. (2009). Role of right posterior parietal cortex in maintaining attention to spatial locations over time. *Brain, 132*, 645–660.

Mason, R., Prat, C., & Just, M. (2013). Neurocognitive brain response to transient impairment of Wernicke's area. *Cerebral Cortex*, doi: 10.1093/cercor/bhs423.

Mayer, A., Mannell, M., Ling, J., Gasparovic, C., & Yeo, R. (2011). Functional connectivity in mild traumatic brain injury. *Human Brain Mapping, 32*, 1825–1835.

Meltzer, J., Wagage, S., Ryder, J., Solomon, B., & Braun, A. (2013). Adaptive significance of right hemisphere activation in aphasic language comprehension. *Neuropsychologia, 51*, 1248–1259.

Mesulam, M. (1981). A cortical network for directed attention and unilateral neglect. *Annals of Neurology, 10*, 309–325.

Minzenberg, M., Yoon, J. H., & Carter, C. S. (2011). Modafinil modulation of the default mode network. *Psychopharmacology, 215*, 23–31.

Moritz-Gasser, S., Herbet, G., & Duffau, H. (2013). Mapping the connectivity underlying multimodal (verbal and non-verbal) semantic processing: A brain electrostimulation study. *Neuropsychologia, 51*, 1814–1822.

Mormino, E., Smiljic, A., Hayenga, A., Onami, S., Greicius, M. Rabinovici, G., et al. (2011). Relationships between beta-amyloid and functional connectivity in different components of the default mode network in aging. *Cerebral Cortex, 21*, 2399–2407.

Murakami, T., Hama, S., Yamashita, H., Onoda, K., Hibino, S., Sato, H., et al. (2014). Neuroanatomic pathway associated with attentional deficits after stroke. *Brain Research, 1544*, 25–32.

Murakami, T., Restle, J., & Ziemann, U. (2012). Effective connectivity hierarchically links temporoparietal and frontal areas of the auditory dorsal stream with the motor cortex lip area during speech perception. *Brain & Language, 122*, 135–141.

Nejad, A., Fossati, P., & Lemogne, C. (2013). Self-referential processing, rumination, and cortical midline structures in major depression. *Frontiers in Human Neuroscience, 7*, 666.

Nomura, E., Gratton, C., Visser, R., Kayser, A., Perez, F., & D'Esposito, M. (2010). Double dissociation of two cognitive control networks in patients with focal brain lesions. *Proceedings of the National Academy of Sciences of the USA, 107*, 12017–12022.

Perrin, J., Merz, S., Bennett, D. M., Currie, J., Steele, D. J., Reid, I. C., et al. (2012). Electroconvulsive therapy reduces frontal cortical connectivity in severe depressive disorder. *Proceedings of the National Academy of Sciences of the USA, 109*, 5464–5468.

Petersen, S., & Posner, M. (). The attention system of the human brain: 20 years after. *Annual Review of Neuroscience, 35*, 73–89.

Pievani, M., de Haan, W., Wu, T., Seeley, W., & Frisoni, G. (2011). Functional network disruption in the degenerative dementias. *Lancet Neurology, 10*(9), 829–843.

Pisella, L., Binkofski, F., Lasek, K., Tonid, I., & Rossetti, Y. (2006). No double-dissociation between optic ataxia and visual agnosia: Multiple sub-streams for multiple visuo-manual integrations. *Neuropsychologia, 44*, 2734–2748.

Price, C., Crinion, J., Leff, A., Richardson, F., Schofield, T., Prejawa, S., et al. (2010). Lesion sites that predict the ability to gesture how an object is used. *Archives Italiennes de Biologie, 148*, 243–258.

Ptak, R., & Schnidera, A. (2011). The attention network of the human brain: Relating structural damage associated with spatial neglect to functional imaging correlates of spatial attention. *Neuropsychologia, 49*, 3063–3070.

Rinne, P., Hassan, M., Goniotakis, D., et al. (2013). Triple dissociation of attention networks in stroke according to lesion location. *Neurology, 81*, 812–820.

Rocca, M., Valsasina, P., Absinta, M., et al. (2010). Default-mode network dysfunction and cognitive impairment in progressive MS. *Neurology, 74*, 1252–1259.

Rosen, H., Gorno-Tempini, M., Goldman, W., Perry, R., Schuff, N., Weiner, M., et al. (2002). Patterns of brain atrophy in frontotemporal dementia and semantic dementia. *Neurology, 58*, 198–208.

Ross, E., & Monnot, M. (2008). Neurology of affective prosody and its functional–anatomic organization in right hemisphere. *Brain and Language, 104*, 51–74.

Rounis, E., Yarrow, K., & Rothwell, J. (2007). Effects of rTMS conditioning over the fronto-parietal network on motor versus visual attention. *Journal of Cognitive Neuroscience, 19*(3), 513–524.

Rushworth, M., Krams, M., & Passingham, R. (2001). The attentional role of the left parietal cortex: The distinct lateralization and localization of motor attention in the human brain. *Journal of Cognitive Neuroscience, 13*, 698–710.

Sacco, R., Bonavita, S., Esposito, F., Tedeschi, G., & Gallo, A. (2013). The contribution of resting state networks to the study of cortical reorganization in MS. *Multiple Sclerosis International, 2013*, Article ID 857807.

Samuelsson, H., Hjelmquist, E., Jensen, C., Ekholm, S., & Blomstrand, C. (1998). Nonlateralized attentional deficits: An important component behind persisting visuospatial neglect? *Journal of Clinical and Experimental Neuropsychology, 20*, 73–88.

Saygin, A. (2007). Superior temporal and premotor brain areas necessary for biological motion perception. *Brain, 130*, 2452–2461.

Saygin, A., Wilson, S., Hagler, D., Bates, E., & Sereno, M. (2004). Point-light biological motion perception activates human premotor cortex. *Journal of Neuroscience, 24*, 6181–6188.

Schmidt, G., Cardillo, E., Kranjec, A., Lehet, M., Widick, P., & Chatterjee, A. (2012). Not all analogies are created equal: Associative and categorical analogy processing following brain damage. *Neuropsychologia, 50*(7), 1372–1379.

Seeley, W., Crawford, R., Zhou, J., Miller, B., & Greicius, M. (2009). Neurodegenerative diseases target large-scale human brain networks. *Neuron, 62*(1), 42–52.

Sheline, Y., Barch, D. M., Price, J. L., Rundle, M. M., Vaishnavi, S. N., Snyder, A. Z., et al. (2009). The default mode network and self-referential processes in depression. *Proceedings of the National Academy of Sciences of the USA, 106*, 1942–1947.

Singh-Curry, V., & Husain, M. (2009). The functional role of the inferior parietal lobe in the dorsal and ventral stream dichotomy. *Neuropsychologia, 47*(6), 1434–1448.

Smith, S., Miller, K. L., Moeller, S., Xu, J., Auerbach, E. J., Woolrich, M. W., et al. (2012). Temporally-independent functional modes of spontaneous brain activity. *Proceedings of the National Academy of Sciences of the USA, 109*, 3131–3136.

Specht, K., Zahn, R., Willmes, K., Weis, S., Holtel, C., Krause, B., et al. (2009). Joint independent component analysis of structural and functional images reveals complex patterns of functional reorganization in stroke aphasia. *NeuroImage, 47*, 2057–2063.

Spreng, R. (2012). The fallacy of a "task-negative" network. *Frontiers in Psychology, 3*, 145.

Steinmetz, M., & Constantinidis, C. (1995). Neurophysiological evidence for a role of posterior parietal cortex in redirecting visual attention. *Cerebral Cortex, 5*, 448–456.

Stevens, M., Lovejoy, D., Kim, J., Oakes, H., Kureshi, I., & Witt, S. T. (2012). Multiple resting state network functional connectivity abnormalities in mild traumatic brain injury. *Brain Imaging and Behavior, 6*, 293–318.

Studer, B., Manes, F., Humphreys, G., Robbins, T., & Clark, L. (2015). Risk-sensitive decision-making in patients with posterior parietal and ventromedial prefrontal cortex injury. *Cerebral Cortex, 25*, 1–9.

Tana, M., Montin, E., Cerutti, S., & Bianchi, A. (2010). Exploring cortical attentional system by using fMRI during a continuous performance test. *Computational Intelligence and Neuroscience, 2010*, 329213.

Tomasi, D., & Volkow, N. (2012). Resting functional connectivity of language networks: Characterization and reproducibility. *Molecular Psychiatry, 17*(8), 841–854.

Turken, A., & Dronkers, N. (2011). The neural architecture of the language comprehension network: converging evidence from lesion and connectivity analyses. *Frontiers in Systems Neuroscience, 5*, 1.

Tyler, L., Marslen-Wilson, W., Randall, B., Wright, P., Devereux, B., & Zhuang, J., et al. (2011). Left inferior frontal cortex and syntax: Function, structure and behavior in patients with left hemisphere damage. *Brain, 134*, 415–431.

Vaina, L., Solomon, J., Chowdhury, S., Sinha, P., & Belliveau, J. (2001). Functional neuroanatomy of biological motion perception in humans. *Proceedings of the National Academy of Sciences of the USA, 98*, 11656–11661.

Vuilleumier, P. (2013). Mapping the functional neuroanatomy of spatial neglect and human parietal lobe functions: progress and challenges. *Annals of the New York Academy of Sciences, 1296*, 50–74.

Westlye, L., Grydeland, H., Walhovd, K., & Fjell, A. (2011). Associations between regional cortical thickness and attentional networks as measured by the attention network test. *Cerebral Cortex, 21*, 345–356.

Whitney, C., Kirk, M., O'Sullivan, J., Lambon Ralph, M., Jefferies, E. (2012). Executive semantic processing is underpinned by a large-scale neural network: Revealing the contribution of left prefrontal, posterior temporal, and parietal cortex to controlled retrieval and selection using TMS. *Journal of Cognitive Neuroscience, 24*(1), 133–147.

Witteman, J., Van Heuven, V., & Schiller, N. (2012). Hearing feelings: A quantitative meta-analysis on the neuroimaging literature of emotional prosody perception. *Neuropsychologia, 50*, 2752–2763.

Witteman, J., van Ijzendoorn, M., van de Velde, D., van Heuven, V., & Schiller, N. (2011). The nature of hemispheric specialization for linguistic and emotional prosodic perception: A meta-analysis of the lesion literature. *Neuropsychologia, 49*, 3722–3738.

Zatorre, R., & Belin, P. (2001). Spectral and temporal processing in human auditory cortex. *Cerebral Cortex, 11*, 946–953.

Zhang, Z., Lu, G., Zhong, Y., Tan, Q., Liao, W., Wang, Z., et al. (2010). Altered spontaneous neuronal activity of the default mode network in mesial temporal lobe epilepsy. *Brain Research, 1323*, 152–160.

Zhou, J., Gennatas, E., Kramer, J., Miller, B., & Seeley, W. (2012). Predicting regional neurodegeneration from the healthy brain functional connectome. *Neuron, 73*, 1216–1227.

Zhou, J., & Seeley, W. (2014). Network dysfunction in Alzheimer's disease and frontotemporal dementia: Implications for psychiatry. *Biological Psychiatry, 75*, 565–573.

14

Caveats and Conclusions

Dating back to the pioneering work of Broca, Wernicke, Dejerine, Marie, Lichtheim, and Geschwind, localization of cognitive operations has been sought after and refined. At the Montreal Neurological Institute, Penfield and Jasper performed the ultimate test of cognitive–brain modular localization by inducing deficits with direct cortical electrical stimulation of the brain in the operating room while patients were awake and functioning to identify "eloquent" cortical regions to avoid during surgical resections. Geschwind, Goodglass, and Kaplan refined the localization of language functions in stroke patients at the Boston VA. Corkin and colleagues' extensive case studies of the amnestic patient H. M., who had received bilateral temporal lobectomies, have provided the groundwork of our understanding of episodic memory and human amnesia. Kwong's development of functional magnetic resonance imaging (fMRI) and Biswal's development of functional connectivity MRI (fcMRI) have led to major advances in the noninvasive localization of cognitive operations in normal humans and elucidated the role that resting networks play in cognition.

SOME CAVEATS

All of these advances and changes have led to the present dynamic state of discovery in cognitive neuroscience. There are clear caveats that need be considered with this large volume of information. The first is that we must consider the assumptions underlying the techniques being used to make these cognitive–anatomic associations. These assumptions have been described in detail throughout this book as the techniques were discussed. The second caveat is that we should carefully assess the conclusions made from the analyses performed. For example, the regions that we assume are engaged with a cognitive task or operation that subjects are performing in an fMRI study may overstate the number of regions essential to the task. One manner by which this could occur is by assuming that at times there are several cognitive operations performed by brain regions that the investigators think are just one cognitive operation. This will lead to false localizations of many brain regions associated with what is thought to be one operation. A more likely error in localization is that one assumes all of the regions involved are essential for the operation being studied. In reality, these regions may be only involved with, but not essential to, the cognitive operation. Another assumption that needs to be considered carefully is whether a brain region shown to be associated with cognitive function in a study is truly the only region engaged in that function or is instead part of a network of regions that support that operation. This is one of the reasons why, in confirming the designation that a cognitive unit is associated with a brain region such that a lesion to that region produces a consistent impairment in the performance related to that unit (e.g., a cognitive–anatomic unit (CAU)), lesion studies are useful by producing cognitive unit disruption. Lesion studies are also critical at times in delineating the roles of nodes in a network-supporting cognitive unit(s). A key example of how this combination works is reported in Chapter 13 with the study by Murakami et al. (2012). To recount, speech perception was studied at two left hemisphere sites identified as part of a network supporting speech perception—the temporoparietal junction (TPJ) and the posterior inferior frontal gyrus (pIFG). Repetitive transcranial magnetic stimulation (rTMS) of these two regions confirmed the connectivity between the regions, and transient lesioning of these two regions identified that the TPJ node is hierarchically placed in the network, controlling the pIFG connectivity (Murakami et al., 2012). This clarified the roles of the nodes in the network and established that both regions are involved in the operation of speech perception. This use of combining the results of several neuroinvestigative techniques to obtain confirmatory evidence that a given cognitive operation is correlated with a specific anatomic region provides converging evidence for identifying a cognition–brain association.

For any of these neuroinvestigative techniques, there is variability in anatomic localizations that needs to be considered. Whenever group studies of the anatomic localizations across individuals are conducted, there may be a warping process to place all of the brains in the same template. When a template-fitting approach is used, there will be an inherent variability in the anatomic localizations. In addition, there is notable variability in the size of individuals' brains, gyral sizes, and gyral patterns. As a result, one cannot expect localizations to be exact. Also, one cannot expect that there will be 100% concordance that the occurrence of a specific lesion in every individual will yield the same results. Localizations must be viewed as generalized regularities of correlation of a cognitive operation to an anatomic region. Furthermore, we must consider the effects of warping brains to a template with regard to localizing lesions with possible white matter involvement and how well the co-registration of tracts across individuals was performed. Finally, from an anatomic perspective, the precision of anatomic localization for each individual study is limited by the thickness of the imaging slices that are acquired. The precision of the localization of a cognitive function to a brain region cannot have a finer resolution (in millimeters) than the resolution of acquisition of the imaging that produced the data.

Since Fodor's (1983) *The Modularity of the Mind*, there has been considerable debate as to what is a "module." A cognitive module was the focus of that monograph, and debate circled around the definition of such a unit. In essence, the definition of a cognitive unit is variable across the cognitive domains under study. Once a unit is delineated, it will likely change over time as further experimental procedures refine the cognitive unit into further subunits. Because the cognitive constructs are abstractions (e.g., search, inhibit, switch, match, phonological matching, etc.) that do not relate directly to neural function or even neurotransmitter actions, there will continually be reducibility to cognitive units until there exists a close to direct match of the description of a cognitive function to the physiology of a neural circuit. Thus, it must be accepted that the delineation of cognitive units will be a dynamic process.

Another clear factor that has not been addressed concerns interpretation of cognitive performance after a lesion occurs. For example, how little of a cognitive deficit has to be present to state that a region is involved in the cognitive operation? How much of a deficit is needed to assume that the anatomic region is the sole region that supports that cognitive operation? It is difficult to make these judgments based solely on the errors that a subject produces after a lesion. The following is an example of how false conclusions can occur after a lesion: A task that requires four CAUs to be performed is disrupted by a lesion removing the third CAU. One might assume that the output performance would be errors that resemble the output from the second CAU. This would assume serial processing and that the output from the second CAU allows for interpreting that behavioral errors observed originated from the second CAU. These assumptions may not be met, and false conclusions can be formed. Even if all of these assumptions are met, this does not take into consideration that the brain might adapt and reorganize, leading to some unknown error, or detour to other unspecified cognitive operations, leading to a variety of error patterns. Thus, when considering such a dynamic system, it is extremely difficult to infer from the performance of the individual how much a lesion has damaged a cognitive operation.

The technique of resting state fcMRI has shown promise in being be useful in distinguishing between disease states. For this to be applied to clinical decision-making, it must be tested and verified in single subjects. The most important issue to discuss with regard to fcMRI at this point is how hypotheses can be generated and tested and how fcMRI can mechanistically account for cognitive states. Much of what has been generated from fcMRI is correlated fluctuations at frequencies of 0.1 Hz or below that are recorded during a "rest state." First, it is unclear how frequencies 0.1 Hz or below physiologically contribute to cognition. Because information about these frequencies and the networks derived from them are obtained from the brain at "rest," it is unclear what these networks' relationship is to cognition. This leads to the difficulty that we cannot generate a great deal of hypotheses or testing of these networks because this may require applying experiments; subsequently, this would nullify the brain being in a rest state. This "catch-22" of it being difficult to experiment on the rest state because subjects are no longer in a rest state during an experiment lessens some applications of this technique. This limits to a degree how rest state fcMRI can be used to account for cognitive mechanisms. Studies of task-related functional connectivity has promise of providing further insights into cognitive mechanisms. Thus far, however, the rest state fcMRI appears to offer the most promise as a marker of disease states or cognitive function because one can compare these networks in dysfunctional individuals to those in control groups. An excellent opportunity for application of the technique is in the use of seed regions to assess connectivity between regions. This type of approach of hypothesis-driven assessment of disrupted connectivity, again typically in a rest state scanning acquisition, can provide a great deal of insight into explaining dysfunctional cognitive performance if there is a decrease in the connectivity between the regions proposed to account for that performance. It would be ideal, however, if this measure of connectivity was obtained during task performance, which is possible. This can also be obtained with electrophysiological measures (e.g., electroencephalography and magnetoencephalography) but without the spatial resolution of MRI, whereas MRI can provide the spatial resolution (including subcortical extent) but without the range of frequency and time resolution measures of electrophysiology.

Another issue with fcMRI is the use of the term "rest state" and determining what rest state means in terms of what is going on in the brain cognitively. The attributions applied to this condition have been many, none of which of course can be verified as a "rest state." Further investigations addressing these issues will likely lead to even more widespread use of the technique.

One case in which lesions to networks can provide important explanatory insights is in the study of aspects of cognitive control. Nomura et al. (2010) reported a study that was able to demonstrate two independent cognitive control networks. Studies in patients with damage to these networks' nodes showed that they support different cognitive operations such that altered connectivity within one damaged network resulted in no changes detected in the undamaged network. This was also true when the lesions were to the other network. What was of special interest is that damage to nodes in the network resulted in dysfunction in the performance related to regions that were remote from but interconnected to the damaged nodes. This finding has been reported for years in clinical neurology and has been referred to as diaschisis. Diaschisis refers to temporary clinical deficits related to areas remote from an area of brain damage. The previous major explanation for diaschisis was that the lesion resulted in withdrawal of excitatory influences to these brain regions that are remotely located but nonetheless connected to the lesioned area. Evidence for this hypothesis has never been convincing. Nomura et al. now have an account for diaschisis, which allows for testable hypotheses that predict diaschisis-related effects because these should occur only in regions that are connected functionally to the lesioned region.

There are multiple advances in analytic tools available for assessing networks, which show promise in being able to measure the magnitude of correlations between single nodes. For example, graph theory allows for quantifying the organization of network nodes at both the whole brain and local levels. With the addition of lesioning techniques (e.g., rTMS) and following lesion patients, knowledge of the roles of nodes in a network will also increase our knowledge about how these brain regions support cognitive processes.

CONCLUSIONS

The localizations presented here have a pattern of occurrence that may not necessarily appear obvious in the current organizational structure of the chapters in this book. The organization of the chapters was believed to be optimal to present cognitive–anatomic correlations, but this may have obscured patterns present in localizations across cognitive domains.

Viewing across the cognitive–anatomic correlations described, it appears *first that the strongest evidence of localization of functions to anatomic regions are those that are related in some manner to speech and language*. Irrespective of the type of study, most agree that the *speech* mechanism is strongly lateralized to the left hemisphere in greater than 90% of individuals (Drane et al., 2012). This laterality to the left hemisphere and specific localization of key speech and language functions to perisylvian regions such as the posterior inferior frontal gyrus and posterior superior temporal gyrus provide key anchors to cognition that are both lateralized to the left hemisphere and localized to focal, circumscribed regions.

This localization of speech to the left hemisphere, and to a lesser degree language localization to the left hemisphere, provides an anchor, via extramodality connections, to a variety of other cognitive domains that are intimately connected to the language system. For example, praxis, which in part includes the connection of the language system to the motor system, is by definition attached to the language architecture and thus will be lateralized and localized to an extensive degree by its anatomic connections to specific language processing regions. Similarly, verbal episodic memory has a degree of lateralization to the left hemisphere due to its direct connections to the verbal language system.

Other localizations that follow different patterns are discernible based on separate sets of neurobiological principles. *Agnosias, disorders of recognizing items within a given modality, are tightly linked anatomically to the sensorimotor cortices of the modality affected and are localized to some degree in focal circumscribed regions.* For example, agnosias associated with specific sensory modalities (e.g., visual, auditory, and tactile agnosias) are typically tightly localized to regions neighboring the primary sensory cortices where the primary perceptual input from the peripheral nervous system first is encoded in the cerebral cortices for that specific modality. Memory systems that are also tightly linked to specific modalities and are essential to the item recognition process are localized in some cases near the primary sensory cortices. For example, the visual memory system (the "what" system) that contributes to processes of recognition is localized bilaterally in areas neighboring the primary visual cortices.

These localizations of dysfunction with agnosias to include higher-order sensory association cortices engaged in cognition and sensory-linked memory systems are different from the pattern of localizations associated with the speech/language system. One clear difference is that the higher-order sensorimotor cognitive localizations are often bilateral, whereas the localizations associated with speech/language functions are predominantly left-hemisphere. This is believed to be secondary to the bilateral localization of the anchors which are sensorimotor systems.

Another set of functions that localize to specific regions are those that have long been associated with dedicated brain regions. In the case of cognition, episodic memory and amnesia are strongly associated with limbic system structures—the Papez circuit. Although there is still a continuing discovery as to the cognitive operations that the medial temporal lobe and frontal lobe play in episodic memory, there is a localization of episodic memory functions, in general, to the structures in these regions. The unique aspect of this cognitive system and its localization consistency is that this dedicated anatomic system for predominantly this cognitive domain emanates from primitive brain structures. The limbic system Papez circuit is evolutionarily a primitive brain structure, which is unique for cognitive functions. MacLean (1949) noted that the limbic system developed to aid in the fight-or-flight circuitry and is referred to as the "old mammalian brain" in that only the primitive structure of the "reptilian brain" is evolutionarily more remote in development.

The patterns of focal localizations being related to the laterality of language, agnosias associated with sensorimotor systems, and episodic memory with the Papez circuit form a set of biological principles in the human brain. Because language is a basic *human* function, compared to other species, the left hemisphere lateralized and localized functions demonstrate a unique occurrence in nature for brain organization.

The left hemisphere anatomic framework for language organization has its roots in the prenatal stages of development. The genetic instructions for cell migration to specific anatomic regions in the developing brain in utero lead to the general anatomic framework for developing language once the human is born and has interactions with the environment, showing that laterality and localization has its origin in the embryological development stages. This is most clearly evident in those cases in which cell migration abnormalities have led to specific deficits and localizations. Examples that typify this most clearly are the cases of developmental dyslexia, in which neuronal migration deficits were detected postmortem in dyslexics compared to controls (Chang et al., 2005; Galaburda & Kemper, 1979; Galaburda et al., 1985, 1994, 2006). In one case of developmental dyslexia that went to autopsy, abnormal cortical folding was detected in the parietal lobes and neurons were detected that migrated only into the subcortical white matter rather than to the language-related cortices that were their targets (Drake, 1968). The most consistent pathologic finding in these developmental dyslexia cases is nests of neurons, termed ectopias or heterotopias, in language-related regions (Galaburda et al., 1985). Technology has progressed so that dyslexic individuals can receive an MRI with the resolution to detect hetertopias indicative of neuronal migration dysfunction (Chang et al., 2005).

Impaired cell migration in embryological development is not the only factor in the early disruption of functional localization in the brain. It has also been shown in the newborn cat brain's visual system. If there is a lack of environmental interaction with light within a critical period of time after birth, there is inadequate development of the visual cortices that cannot be overcome (Friauf et al., 1990; Garraghty et al., 1988; Shatz, 1985; Shatz & Kliot, 1982). Thus, although early neonatal changes to neural architecture can affect functional–anatomic correlations, later changes that occur after birth, such as interaction with environmental stimuli, also alter brain structures and affect these correlations.

In addition to this environmental interaction role that shapes functional–anatomic organization, developmental neurobiological functions also affect this organization after birth. For example, synaptic pruning, the active reduction of synapses in the brain, shapes anatomical regions from near birth to puberty (Paolicelli et al., 2011). This sculpting of the synaptic connections throughout the brain frames the cognitive architecture of an individual, and although the biological mechanism underlying pruning remains unclear, it is likely influenced greatly by genetic factors and the individual's experiences with the environment. To what degree this affects processing nodes (or representational nodes) or representational-based distributed networks is unknown, although one would speculate that it is more likely that the networks (e.g., pruning connections), as opposed to processing nodes, are most affected.

It is proposed that there is a general framework of cell migration that produces a framework for brain functions including cognition. This framework results in a lateralized organization for the development of speech and language and higher cognitive sensorimotor systems. Interaction with the environment leads to development of these systems and further drives the lateralization and localization of these functions. Developmental mechanisms, such as pruning, solidify the localization of these functions, as white matter development continues to develop connections between regions into young adulthood (Reiss et al., 1996).

Another emerging principle of cognitive neural organization is that although a cortical lesion may lead to a consistent deficit in a cognitive operation, that deficit may recover notably over time. When a cognitive deficit persists after a lesion occurs in a cortical region associated with a cognitive unit, the white matter underlying that cortical region is typically involved in the lesion. It appears that after a lesion involves a cortical region, cortical neurons neighboring the lesion can adapt and assume the cognitive operation previously performed by that damaged region. However, for effective recovery of cognitive operations to occur, the white matter pathways that connect the lesioned and surrounding area to its target cortical and subcortical regions involved in cognition need to be intact. One of the key reasons this is the case is white matter's lack of plasticity, regeneration, or reassignment of connections; thus, cortical regions cannot newly attach or reconnect to other brain regions by the mechanism of white matter adaptive processes. Typically, then, the involvement of the cortex *and* its underlying white matter in a lesion leads to a long-lasting deficit of the cognitive function associated with that cortical region. In addition, Chapter 12 on white matter and connections showed that with the ability to better image white matter, there is more consistency in detecting cognitive deficits that are associated with white matter lesions. These CAUs, in which white matter is the anatomic correlate, represent true "disconnection" syndromes and are an emerging field of brain–behavior correlations.

Thus, four factors that appear to strongly influence if a cognitive function has a consistent localization are the following:

1. If that function is associated with speech/language as aspects of speech/language are in general lateralized and localized in a consistent manner.
2. Higher-order cognitive sensory functions as these are generally localized near that modalities primary sensory cortex.
3. Functions that are subserved by evolutionarily consistent dedicated brain regions (e.g., episodic memory functions and the Papez circuit).
4. For a cognitive deficit to be persistently present, the lesion typically is in the cortical region associated with that cognitive function AND the white matter underlying that cortical region (that connects it to its target cortical and subcortical regions).

The localizations in this book were also made in relation to the processing schema described in Chapter 1. Some of the localizations described perform specific functions independent of other regions and functions. Other localizations may well exist within a network of regions to perform a specific operation or a task. When a region is located within a network, then that region's function can and should be investigated for its contribution to that function and its relationship to the other anatomic units in that network vis-à-vis that function. There are multiple ways that the nodes in a network can interact with each other to perform a complex function (e.g., serial, cascade, parallel). New or modified approaches and models will have to be elaborated to provide functional–anatomic correlations for these types of neural systems.

It is also clear that specific regions can be involved in several networks, serving varying functions. A brain region can also be involved with other regions in one network performing a specific operation and yet may combine with other regions forming a network subserving an entirely different function. In fact, a specific region in isolation, without being involved in any networks, can be linked with two distinct discrete functions. It appears that there are numerous regions in the brain, particularly those associated with cognition, that do not necessarily serve just one specific function but, rather, can be selectively engaged in several different functions. There are multiple plausible mechanisms explaining how the same brain region can be engaged in multiple functions. One well-described example is that by neurons in a region firing in different frequencies (e.g., time-frequency or power analyses) or at different times in the course of a task or operation, the same region can be engaged in multiple functions.

An example of a region that appears to assume multiple functions is the lingual and fusiform gyri, with roles in semantic object operations, face processing, and color processing. That a specific region can assume different functions in the human brain is an important principle to recognize and understand in the mapping of cognition and behavior. A better understanding of different firing patterns of groups of neurons, which lead to distinct brain rhythm frequencies (e.g., beta, theta, delta, and gamma) to which other groups of neurons selectively respond, has led to a better understanding of how one region can perform multiple functions. In addition, further delineating a brain region into subpopulations of neurons that contribute to different operations will also provide greater insight about regions that appear to be involved in multiple cognitive functions.

As the field of the application of cognitive neuroscience principles to treatments emerges, it may be essential to understand these brain rhythm frequencies. Groups of neurons performing cognitive operations and communicating with other brain regions can accomplish this via trains of action potentials that occur rhythmically and are measured by the frequency of these trains (called time-frequency brain rhythms—theta, alpha, gamma frequency, etc.). Treating disease states may benefit by modulating disrupted frequencies that are negatively affecting cognitive operations. However, clinicians currently consider the application of a variety of treatment options after an injury, including cognitive rehabilitation training, electromagnetic stimulation (e.g., rTMS, transcranial direct current stimulation (tDCS), and "cognitive pacemakers" using depth electrodes), and neurotransmitter modulation (e.g., medications adjusting dopamine, acetylcholine, etc.). Because neurotransmitters are the chemical substrates involved in triggering neuronal firings, modulation of neurotransmitters has been the hallmark of treatment of behavioral symptoms in mental illnesses (e.g., schizophrenia and affective disorders). Neurotransmitter systems have been more approachable to modulation for behavioral–emotional symptoms because these systems are organized in such a way that a type of neurotransmitter is more likely to be dedicated to a behavioral symptom and not as likely involved in other functions (sensorimotor, cognitive, autonomic body regulation, etc.) that the brain performs. Thus, medications modulating neurotransmitters associated with emotion have been selective enough to change only behavioral symptoms without adversely disrupting multiple other brain functions. Unfortunately, neurotransmitters engaged in cognition are not as selective as those involved with behavioral symptoms but are ubiquitous throughout the brain, involved not only with cognition but also with other brain functions. Currently, modulating neurotransmitters of cognition may affect multiple brain systems, positively and negatively, in addition to affecting the targeted cognitive process. Future designs for modulating neurotransmitters of cognition should target specific neuronal populations engaged in cognition. Modification of cognition via stabilizing brain rhythm frequencies offers promise, particularly with the development of electromagnetic interventions (e.g., rTMS and tDCS). Also, intuitively, continuing to seek a better understanding of cognition and behavior will lead to more effective cognitive training programs.

Overall, this book is used as a best approximation of reliable cognitive–anatomic correlates given the technological advances at the present time. Future developments in technology, network model analyses, white matter functional correlations, and finer-level cognitive dissociations will further advance these findings and lead to better refinement of the architecture of cognition and behavior in the brain. These advances will also assuredly lead to more effective means of treating cognitive and behavioral dysfunction.

REFERENCES

Chang, B., Ly, J., Appignani, B., Bodell, A., Apse, K. A., Ravenscroft, R. S., et al. (2005). Reading impairment in the neuronal migration disorder of periventricular nodular heterotopia. *Neurology, 64,* 799–803.

Drake, W. (1968). Clinical and pathological finding in a child with a developmental learning disability. *Journal of Learning Disabilities, 1,* 486–502.

Drane, D., Roraback-Carson, J., Hebb, A., et al. (2012). Cortical stimulation mapping and Wada results demonstrate a normal variant of right hemisphere language organization. *Epilepsia, 53*(10), 1790–1798.

Fodor, J. (1983). *The modularity of the mind.* Cambridge, MA: MIT Press.

Friauf, E., McConnell, S., & Shatz, C. (1990). Functional synaptic circuits in the subplate during fetal and early postnatal development of cat visual cortex. *Journal of Neuroscience, 10*(8), 2601–2613.

Galaburda, A., & Kemper, T. (1979). Cytoarchitectonic abnormalities in developmental dyslexia: A case study. *Annals of Neurology, 6*(2), 94–100.

Galaburda, A., LoTurco, J., Ramus, F., Fitch, R., & Rosen, G. (2006). From genes to behavior in developmental dyslexia. *Nature Neuroscience, 9*(10), 1213–1217.

Galaburda, A., Menard, M., & Rosen, G. (1994). Evidence for aberrant auditory anatomy in developmental dyslexia. *Proceedings of the National Academy of Sciences of the USA, 91,* 8010–8013.

Galaburda, A., Sherman, G., Rosen, G., Aboitiz, F., & Geschwind, N. (1985). Developmental dyslexia: Four consecutive cases with cortical anomalies. *Annals of Neurology, 18,* 222–233.

Garraghty, P., Shatz, C., Sretavan, D., & Sur, M. (1988). Axon arbors of X and Y retinal ganglion cells are differentially affected by prenatal disruption of binocular inputs. *Proceedings of the National Academy of Sciences of the USA, 85*(19), 7361–7365.

MacLean, P. (1949). Psychosomatic disease and the visceral brain; Recent developments bearing on the Papez theory of emotion. *Psychosomatic Medicine, 11*(6), 338–353.

Murakami, T., Restle, J., & Ziemann, U. (2012). Effective connectivity hierarchically links temporoparietal and frontal areas of the auditory dorsal stream with the motor cortex lip area during speech perception. *Brain & Language, 122,* 135–141.

Nomura, E., Gratton, C., Visser, R., Kayser, A., Perez, F., & D'Esposito, M. (2010). Double dissociation of two cognitive control networks in patients with focal brain lesions. *Proceedings of the National Academy of Sciences of the USA, 107*(26), 12017–12022.

Paolicelli, R., Bolasco, G., Pagani, F., et al. (2011). Synaptic pruning by microglia is necessary for normal brain development. *Science, 333*(6048), 1456–1458.

Reiss, A., Abrams, M., Singer, H., Ross, J., & Denckla, M. (1996). Brain development, gender and IQ in children: A volumetric imaging study. *Brain, 119,* 1763–1774.

Shatz, C. (1985). Visual neurobiology: Development of visual pathways in mammals. *Science, 228*(4695), 67–68.

Shatz, C., & Kliot, M. (1982). Prenatal misrouting of the retinogeniculate pathway in Siamese cats. *Nature, 300*(5892), 525–529.

INDEX

Page numbers followed by *f* and *t* indicate figures and tables, respectively.